2019

ADVANCES IN MOLECULAR PATHOLOGY

EDITOR-IN-CHIEF

Gregory J. Tsongalis, PhD, HCLD, CC

SECTION EDITORS

Ahmad N. Abou Tayoun, PhD, FACMG

Kevin Alby, PhD, D(ABMM)

Guru Ananda, PhD

Andrea Ferreira-Gonzalez, PhD, HCLD(ABB), CC(ABB), FACB

Christopher Korch, PhD

Eric Y. Loo, MD

Ann M. Moyer, MD, PhD

ELSEVIER

Director, Continuity Publishing: Taylor Ball
Editor: Lauren Boyle
Developmental Editor: Laura Fisher

Editorial Office:
Elsevier, Inc.
1600 John F. Kennedy Blvd,
Suite 1800
Philadelphia, PA 19103-2899

International Standard Serial Number: 2589-515X
International Standard Book Number: 13: 978-0-323-70950-7

ADVANCES IN MOLECULAR PATHOLOGY

CONTRIBUTORS

MICHELLE AFKHAMI, MD
Medical Director of Clinical Molecular Diagnostic Laboratory, City of Hope National Cancer Center, Duarte, California, USA

MIR B. ALIKHAN, MD
Molecular Hematopathologist, Department of Pathology, Division of Molecular Diagnostics, North Shore University Health System, Clinical Assistant Professor of Pathology, The University of Chicago Pritzker School of Medicine, Evanston, Illinois, USA

MUSTAFA AL-KAWAAZ, MD
Fellow, Molecular Genetic Pathology, Department of Pathology, The University of Chicago/NorthShore University HealthSystem, Evanston, Illinois, USA

MARIA E. ARCILA, MD
Director, Diagnostic Molecular Pathology Laboratory, Department of Pathology, Memorial Sloan Kettering Cancer Center, New York, New York, USA

ARJUN P. ATHREYA, MS, PhD
Assistant Professor, Department of Molecular Pharmacology and Experimental Therapeutics, Mayo Clinic, Rochester, Minnesota, USA

DANIEL BABU, MD
Assistant Professor, Department of Pathology, University of New Mexico, Albuquerque, New Mexico, USA

TEJUS A. BALE, MD, PhD
Assistant Attending Pathologist, Department of Pathology, Memorial Sloan Kettering Cancer Center, New York, New York, USA

LINNEA M. BAUDHUIN, PhD
Associate Professor of Laboratory Medicine and Pathology, Mayo Clinic, Rochester, Minnesota, USA

SEBASTIAN BOEGEL, PhD
Johannes Gutenberg University, Mainz, Germany

JOHN C. CASTLE, PhD
Agenus Inc, Lexington, Massachusetts, USA

SRIKAR CHAMALA, PhD
Assistant Professor, Department of Pathology, Immunology and Laboratory Medicine, University of Florida, Gainesville, Florida, USA

HARSHPREET CHANDOK, MS
Bioinformatician, Computational Sciences, The Jackson Laboratory for Genomic Medicine, Farmington, Connecticut, USA

SOK CHING CHEONG, PhD
Senior Group Leader, Head and Neck Cancer Research Team, Cancer Research Malaysia, Subang Jaya Medical Centre, Subang Jaya, Selangor, Malaysia; Department of Oral and Maxillofacial Clinical Sciences, Faculty of Dentistry, University of Malaya, Kuala Lumpur, Malaysia

MACKENZIE E. COLLINS, BS
Medical Laboratory Scientist, Clinical Microbiology Laboratory, University of North Carolina Health Care, Chapel Hill, North Carolina, USA

DANIEL L. DUNCAN, MD
Senior Pathologist and Associate Medical Director, Foundation Medicine, Morrisville, North Carolina, USA

ANDREA FERREIRA-GONZALEZ, PhD, HCLD(ABB), CC(ABB), FACB
Professor and Chair Molecular Diagnostics Division, Department of Pathology, Virginia Commonwealth University, Richmond, Virginia, USA

JOSHY GEORGE, PhD
Associate Director, Computational Sciences, The Jackson Laboratory for Genomic Medicine, Farmington, Connecticut, USA

RAVISHANKAR K. IYER, PhD
Professor, Department of Electrical and Computer Engineering, University of Illinois at Urbana-Champaign, Urbana, Illinois, USA

DARREN K. JOHNSON, MS
Geisinger Genomic Medicine Institute, Forty Fort, Pennsylvania, USA

SHEILA M. JOHNSON, PhD
Medical Microbiology and Public Health Fellow, Clinical Microbiology Laboratory, University of North Carolina Health Care, Chapel Hill, North Carolina, USA

R. KRISHNA MURTHY KARUTURI, PhD
Senior Director, Computational Sciences, The Jackson Laboratory for Genomic Medicine, Farmington, Connecticut, USA

KAREN KAUL, MD, PhD
Chair, Department of Pathology and Laboratory Medicine, Duckworth Family Chair, NorthShore University HealthSystem, Clinical Professor of Pathology, The University of Chicago Pritzker School of Medicine, Evanston, Illinois, USA

BERNARD KOK BANG LEE, PhD
Research Associate, Division of Medical Oncology, Department of Medicine, University of Colorado Anschutz Medical Campus, Aurora, Colorado, USA; Head and Neck Cancer Research Team, Cancer Research Malaysia, Subang Jaya Medical Centre, Subang Jaya, Selangor, Malaysia; Department of Oral and Maxillofacial Clinical Sciences, Faculty of Dentistry, University of Malaya, Kuala Lumpur, Malaysia

ERIC Y. LOO, MD
Assistant Professor of Pathology & Laboratory Medicine, Department of Pathology and Laboratory Medicine, Dartmouth-Hitchcock Medical Center, Lebanon, New Hampshire, USA

JESSICA MESTER, MS
Senior Genetic Counselor, GeneDx Inherited Cancer Program, Gaithersburg, Maryland, USA

MELISSA B. MILLER, PhD
Director, Clinical Microbiology Laboratory, University of North Carolina Health Care, Professor, Department of Pathology and Laboratory Medicine, University of North Carolina School of Medicine, Chapel Hill, North Carolina, USA

NATHAN D. MONTGOMERY, MD, PhD
Assistant Professor, Department of Pathology and Laboratory Medicine, The University of North Carolina at Chapel Hill, Chapel Hill, North Carolina, USA

ANN M. MOYER, MD, PhD
Assistant Professor of Laboratory Medicine and Pathology, Department of Laboratory Medicine and Pathology, Mayo Clinic, Rochester, MN, USA

JAVAD NOORBAKHSH, PhD
Associate Research Scientist, The Jackson Laboratory for Genomic Medicine, Farmington, Connecticut, USA

RINI PAULY, MS
Greenwood Genetic Center, Greenwood, South Carolina, USA

THOMAS N. PERSON, MS
Geisinger Genomic Medicine Institute, Forty Fort, Pennsylvania, USA

TINA PESARAN, MS, MA
Director, Variant Assessment Program, Ambry Genetics, Aliso Viejo, California, USA

LUCAS H. RIFKIN, MD
Department of Pathology and Laboratory Medicine, Dartmouth-Hitchcock Medical Center, Lebanon, New Hampshire, USA

MARIE-CLAIRE ROWLINSON, PhD, D(ABMM)
Florida Department of Health, Bureau of Public Health Laboratories, Jacksonville, Florida, USA; Emerging Pathogens Institute, Department of Medicine, University of Florida, Gainesville, Florida, USA

LINDA SABATINI, PhD
Director, Department of Pathology, Division of Molecular Diagnostics, Department of Pathology and Laboratory Medicine, North Shore University Health System, Evanston, Illinois, USA

STEVEN E. SCHERER, PhD
Professor, Department of Molecular and Human Genetics, Baylor College of Medicine, Human Genome Sequencing Center, Houston, Texas, USA

CHARLES E. SCHWARTZ, PhD
Greenwood Genetic Center, Greenwood, South Carolina, USA

PATRICIA J. SIMNER, PhD, D(ABMM)
Associate Professor of Pathology, Director of Bacteriology and Parasitology, Division of Medical Microbiology, Department of Pathology, Johns Hopkins School of Medicine, Baltimore, Maryland, USA

AIK CHOON TAN, PhD
Professor of Bioinformatics, Division of Medical Oncology, Department of Medicine, University of Colorado Anschutz Medical Campus, Aurora, Colorado, USA; Vice Chair and Senior Member, Department of Biostatistics and Bioinformatics, Moffitt Cancer Center, Tampa, Florida, USA

LAURA N. TOTH, DO, MPH
Fellow, Department of Pathology, University of New Mexico, Albuquerque, New Mexico, USA

ANTHONY TRAN, DrPH, MPH, D(ABMM)
District of Columbia Department of Forensic Sciences, Public Health Laboratory Division, Washington, DC, USA

NEPHI A. WALTON, MD, MS, FACMG
Assistant Professor, Geisinger Genomic Medicine Institute, Forty Fort, Pennsylvania, USA

LIEWEI WANG, MD, PhD
Professor, Department of Molecular Pharmacology and Experimental Therapeutics, Mayo Clinic, Rochester, Minnesota, USA

RICHARD M. WEINSHILBOUM, MD
Professor, Department of Molecular Pharmacology and Experimental Therapeutics, Mayo Clinic, Rochester, Minnesota, USA

REBECCA YEE, PhD
Division of Medical Microbiology, Department of Pathology, Johns Hopkins School of Medicine, Baltimore, Maryland, USA

JOSHUA F. ZEIDNER, MD
Assistant Professor of Medicine, Division of Hematology/Oncology, The University of North Carolina at Chapel Hill, Chapel Hill, North Carolina, USA

CONTENTS

VOLUME 2 • 2019

Advances in Molecular Pathology 2 (2019) xv
ADVANCES IN MOLECULAR PATHOLOGY

Erratum

Errors were made in Volume 1 of *Advances in Molecular Pathology* on page 196 in "Therapy Implications of DNA Mismatch Repair Deficiency, Microsatellite Instability, and Tumor Mutation Burden" by Maryam Shirazi and Antonia R. Sepulveda. The last sentence in the "Assessment of Tumor Mutation Burden Using Next-Generation Sequencing Platforms" section should be as follows:

To determine TMB, the number of detected somatic mutations in the fraction of genome sequenced by NGS was quantified and this value was extrapolated to the whole exome using a validated algorithm in which all short variant alterations, base substitutions, indels, and coding variants (including the silent alterations) were counted; whereas, noncoding variants, alterations with known or likely pathogenic (known somatic alterations in the COSMIC database and truncations in tumor suppressor genes, respectively), and predicted germline mutations were excluded. TMB was measured as the number of eligible alterations per Mb of genome and was divided into 3 groups: low (1–5 mutations/Mb), intermediate (6–19 mutations/Mb), and high (≥20 mutations/Mb) [39,40].

https://doi.org/10.1016/j.yamp.2019.08.005
2589-4080/19/

Advances in Molecular Pathology 2 (2019) xvii–xviii
ADVANCES IN MOLECULAR PATHOLOGY

Preface

Molecular Pathology: Unraveling the Underlying Complexities of Human Disease

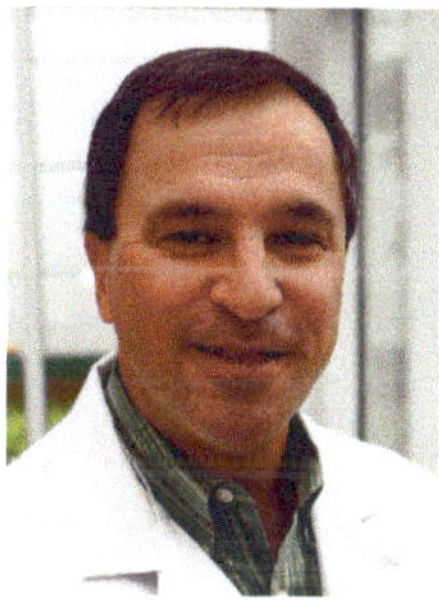

Gregory J. Tsongalis, PhD, HCLD
Editor

Molecular pathology, the use of nucleic acid interrogation to better diagnose, prognosticate, and treat human diseases, continues to advance at a pace that is unprecedented in medicine. With a focus on precision medicine initiatives, molecular pathology is the hub from which these initiatives radiate and are driven by new technologies and therapeutic drugs. While much of the precision medicine promises have focused on oncology, the scope of such an approach passes well beyond cancer and has significant impact on genetic diseases, infectious diseases, and population health.

Implementation of massively parallel sequencing in many laboratories across the globe for somatic and constitutional testing has brought the advantages and disadvantages of this powerful technology to the forefront. The wet bench nuances of technical expertise, how to interpret the many variants identified, and the growing shortfall of trained professionals for data analytics/informatics and genetic counseling must be addressed. Sequencing has not been the only technology to emerge in the era of precision medicine. Microarray, nanostring, and mass spectroscopy technologies have given laboratories a means to provide higher-throughput, multiplexed analyses of the human genome, while cartridge-based assays, such as the Biocartis Idylla system, have made it possible for smaller laboratories to engage in molecular pathology testing.

In this second issue of *Advances in Molecular Pathology*, we highlight some of the latest developments in the field of molecular pathology as testing for genetic diseases, hematologic diseases, infectious diseases, pharmacogenomics, solid tumors, and for identity testingcontinues to impact routine clinical practice. We have included articles that touch upon variant interpretation and inclusion of this information into electronic health records, new applications for hematologic malignancy, novel applications for antimicrobial stewardship, a resurgence of pharmacogenomics, further characterization of solid tumors, machine learning,

https://doi.org/10.1016/j.yamp.2019.08.004
2589-4080/19/

and identity testing. Molecular pathology and clinical genomics promise to continue to revolutionize our approaches to diagnosing disease, to establishing more accurate prognoses, and to developing more robust and effective treatment strategies.

It is very clear that one application or one technology does not define our field with respect to human disease, but they all represent individual pieces of the puzzle needed in order to better understand human disease and wellness. We continue to strive for more successful outcomes, improved quality of life, and maintenance of wellness through all of our efforts. I am grateful to those friends and colleagues who once again agreed to becoming section editors and to all of the authors who contributed articles for this issue.

Happy reading!

Gregory J. Tsongalis, PhD, HCLD
Department of Pathology and
Laboratory Medicine
The Audrey and Theodore Geisel
School of Medicine at Dartmouth
Hanover 03755, NH, USA

Laboratory for Clinical Genomics and
Advanced Technology
Department of Pathology and
Laboratory Medicine
Dartmouth Hitchcock Medical Center
1 Medical Center Drive
Lebanon, NH 03756, USA

E-mail address: Gregory.j.tsongalis@hitchcock.org

Genetics

Advances in Molecular Pathology 2 (2019) 1–11
ADVANCES IN MOLECULAR PATHOLOGY

The Evolution of Constitutional Sequence Variant Interpretation

Jessica Mester, MS[a,*], Tina Pesaran, MS, MA[b]
[a]GeneDx Inherited Cancer Program, Gaithersburg, MD, USA; [b]Variant Assessment Program, Ambry Genetics, 15 Argonaut, Aliso Viejo, CA 92656, USA

KEYWORDS
• Variant classification • Genetic testing • Population data • Functional studies • In silico • de novo • Quantitative • ACMG-AMP

KEY POINTS

- A combination of different types of evidence incorporating population data, functional studies, clinical data, and predictive tools is necessary for thorough, thoughtful variant classification.
- Variant classification criteria may be optimized in a quantitative, gene-specific manner using validated predictors of pathogenicity for genes or conditions with sufficient information.
- Large-scale data (genome sequencing of healthy and affected cohorts, high-throughput functional studies, and in silico metapredictors) increase the robustness of evidence used for variant classification and lend themselves to incorporation in quantitative frameworks.
- Collaborative efforts by laboratories and disease-specific expert groups reduce variant classification discrepancies and improve the quality of variant interpretation information available to patients and researchers.

INTRODUCTION

Sequence variants may be detected in an individual's germline DNA by molecular genetic testing performed in diagnostic, predictive, or preventive clinical settings. Interpretation of variants detected via this testing is complex and requires gathering multiple pieces of information to be analyzed in the context of the clinical presentation and the gene or disorder under consideration. This article reviews the history of germline sequence variant interpretation, highlighting the lines of evidence used in current variant interpretation practices. It also considers how developments in sequencing and other technologies have provided data that have enhanced the ability to interpret genetic variants.

SIGNIFICANCE

Molecular germline genetic testing has evolved from a niche service consisting of single-gene testing for affected individuals exclusively by genetics providers, to multigene panels or exome testing for either affected or unaffected individuals offered by any clinician, and will one day involve routine genome sequencing of healthy individuals as a part of primary care preventive medical practice. Expanding the scope of genetic testing as well as the population undergoing analysis brings new challenges to analyzing results. Inaccurate variant interpretation can have dire consequences for patients. For genes associated with high cancer risks, detection of a variant deemed pathogenic can lead patients to make surgical decisions that are irreversible should

Disclosure: J. Mester is an employee of GeneDx, Inc., a wholly owned subsidiary of OPKO Health, Inc. T. Pesaran is an employee of Ambry Genetics, a wholly owned subsidiary of Konica-Minolta.

*Corresponding author. 1425 Grace Ave, Lakewood, OH 44107. *E-mail address:* jmester@genedx.com

https://doi.org/10.1016/j.yamp.2019.06.001
2589-4080/19/

the variant classification subsequently change based on new information. Specific medications or therapies to treat seizure disorders or metabolic conditions may be offered to or contraindicated for patients with pathogenic variants in specific genes. These factors drive the need for a careful, evidence-based approach to variant interpretation for individuals pursuing molecular genetic testing regardless of the clinical indication.

A BRIEF HISTORY OF SEQUENCE VARIANT INTERPRETATION

Clinical testing for sequence variants and copy number changes may be performed on an individual's germline DNA to diagnose a hereditary disorder based on clinical phenotype or family history, or may also be undertaken to screen healthy individuals for disease risk. This testing seeks to identify changes, or variants, in the patient's DNA that differ from a "healthy" reference sequence. Inevitably, the more genes that are analyzed, the more variants are bound to be detected. The challenge then becomes interpretation of these variants: gathering evidence to determine whether they should be considered pathogenic (disease causing) or benign (not associated with disease risk).

Although it may seem logical to assume that a truncating variant (one that disrupts the protein's reading frame, leading to its decay or removal of an essential functional domain) in a gene for which loss of function is the mechanism of disease would be pathogenic, this does not always hold true. For example, exons 26 and 32 of *TSC2* (GenBank NM000548.3), also described as exons 25 and 31 using alternate exon numbering, are subject to alternative splicing, and truncating or frameshift variants in these regions have been identified in adults lacking features consistent with tuberous sclerosis complex [1]. Likewise, it can be tempting to consider a missense variant as pathogenic if it occurs in a functionally important protein domain, but subsequent functional studies may reveal no impact, or the variant may be present at high population frequency. It is therefore necessary to have gene-specific rules to guide the process of variant classification that take into account multiple lines of evidence and combine them to determine variant pathogenicity.

More than 20 years ago, Cotton and Scriver [2] suggested criteria for determining whether a DNA variant was phenotype-modifying or neutral, specifying type of variant, segregation studies, population frequency, and functional studies, along with the extent of DNA analysis performed, as helpful pieces of information for variant classification. These lines of evidence continued to serve as core criteria for other qualitative and quantitative gene-specific variant classification models [3–7]. However, one laboratory or expert group might place a higher or lower level of importance on the same piece of evidence, leading to discrepant classifications for the same variant, and to confusion for patients and providers [8].

Major steps forward in harmonizing the approach to variant classification occurred with publications from the American College of Medical Genetics and Genomics (ACMG) in 2000 [9] and 2008 [10] and coauthored with the Association for Molecular Pathology (AMP) in 2015 [11]. The 2015 ACMG/AMP guidelines outline a qualitative approach to variant classification incorporating data from several lines of evidence: population data, computational and predictive data, functional data, segregation data, de novo data, allelic data, phenotype specificity, co-occurrence data, and expert opinion. These guidelines have also been adopted by the UK-based Association for Clinical Genomic Science. Variant curation expert panels developed under the auspices of ClinGen (www.clinicalgenome.org) are using the ACMG/AMP guidelines as a framework, publishing modified versions of the guidelines tailored for gene-specific use. Of note, these guidelines were crafted for use in the classification of mendelian disorders, as opposed to more common and complex polygenic conditions or somatic cancer, and are relevant to sequence variants detected by Sanger, next-generation, or other sequencing methodologies as opposed to copy number variants. In addition, the ACMG/AMP guidelines provide guidance regarding the nomenclature used to define pathogenicity and likelihood for each category [12] (Fig. 1).

This article focuses on each line of evidence specified in the ACMG/AMP guidelines (Fig. 2), providing background regarding the utility of each criterion for sequence variant classification purposes. Readers are referred to the ACMG/AMP guidelines [11] for definitions regarding the proposed evidence codes (eg, PVS1, PM5, PP4) that are referred to in this article.

LINES OF EVIDENCE USED IN SEQUENCE VARIANT INTERPRETATION

Predicted Effect on Protein and Disease Mechanism

The first step in variant interpretation is to understand the nature of the gene-disease mechanism. Does the

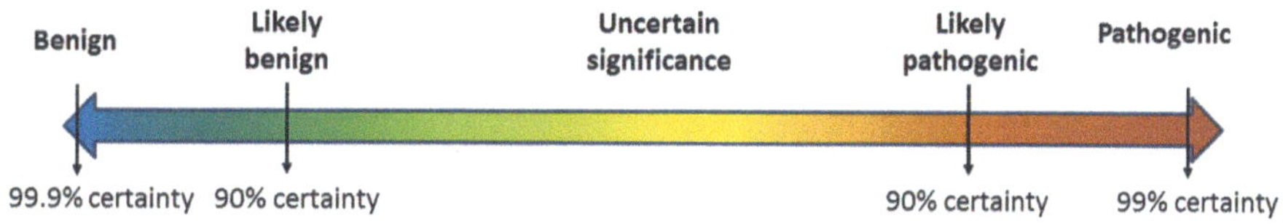

FIG. 1 Thresholds used for variant classification in the ACMG/AMP framework.

gene act via a loss-of-function (LoF) mechanism or a gain-of-function/dominant-negative effect? Protein-truncating variants, most of which lead to nonsense-mediated decay and haploinsufficiency, in genes with an LoF mechanism have a high prior probability of being pathogenic. This probability is captured in the ACMG/AMP rule code PVS1, which is considered to be very strong evidence supporting pathogenicity. PVS1 also encompasses other types of alterations that have a high probability of leading to haploinsufficiency, such those that affect the initiation site, canonical plus or minus 1 or 2 splice sites, certain intragenic tandem duplications, and single-exon or multiexon deletions. It may be inappropriate to apply a very strong evidence level toward pathogenicity for LoF variants in the following situations:

- The gene's mechanism of disease is not LoF
- The variant causes protein truncation but does not result in NMD
- The variant results in an in-frame deletion
- The variant occurs in a region that is subject to alternative splicing

However, the ACMG/AMP guidelines do not expand on how these caveats would affect use of the PVS1 code. Abou Tayoun and colleagues [13] provide a decision tree for modifying the strength of PVS1 that takes into account the type of variant, location within the protein, and other evidence.

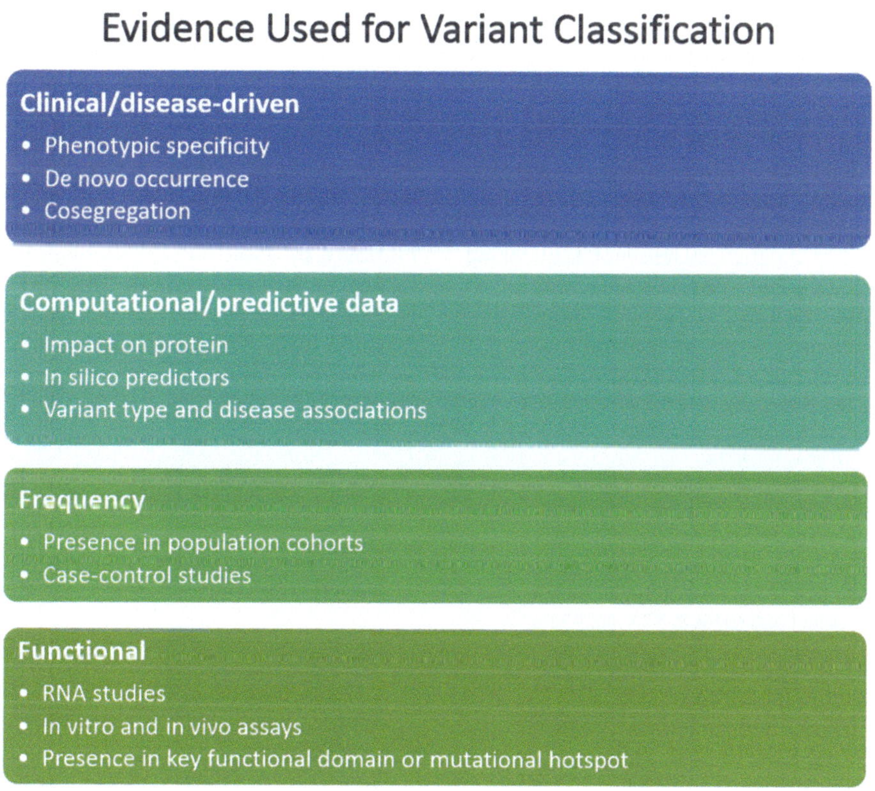

FIG. 2 Evidence incorporated into variant classification.

Other ACMG/AMP criteria based on protein impact and knowledge regarding variant spectrum include:

- PP2: used to support a possible role in disease causation for a missense variant in a gene in which (1) missense variants are a common disease mechanism, and (2) benign missense variants are uncommon. BP1: used to support a benign role for a missense variant in a gene in which only truncating variants are known to cause disease.
- PM4: moderate pathogenic evidence for variants that change the length of the protein; this may include inframe deletions or duplications or variants that extend protein length.
- BP3: supports a benign role for an in-frame deletion of a repetitive sequence in a region with no known function.
- BP7: supports a benign role for a synonymous (silent) variants not proved or predicted to affect splicing.

Population Data

Historically, a polymorphism was defined as an allele present in at least 1% of the general population [14]. Given their high frequency and the rare nature of most genetic disorders, it follows that variants present at high enough population frequency, to be defined as polymorphisms, would be considered harmless, with several notable exceptions (Table 1).

Early work to understand the diversity of alleles in global populations was limited by high sequencing cost, quality control limitations, and lack of sufficiently powered sequencing studies in diverse ancestral groups [15,16]. As the efficiency of sequencing technology has increased, genome-wide studies of larger, apparently healthy, or general population cohorts have allowed better understanding of the global allele diversity. In particular, gnomAD [17] (https://gnomad.broadinstitute.org/) includes exome sequencing data from more than 125,000 unrelated individuals and whole-genome sequencing for an additional 15,000 persons, with specific allele frequencies available for several subpopulations. Other databases focusing on specific subpopulations are listed in Table 2.

Population data may provide evidence leading to either a benign or pathogenic classification. A variant with population frequency greater than 5% can take a variant directly to benign through application of the ACMG/AMP stand-alone benign criterion BA1. Strong evidence toward a benign classification may also be achieved when a variant is present at a high enough allele frequency to be inconsistent with disease causation. No allele frequency threshold for BS1 (strong benign evidence) application was purposefully set so that cutoffs could be established in a disease-specific or gene-specific manner. Whiffin and colleagues [18] published a strategy to set disease-specific population frequency cutoffs taking into consideration condition prevalence, allelic and genetic heterogeneity, and disease penetrance, and created a freely available online calculator for maximum credible allele frequency calculation (https://cardiodb.org/allelefrequencyapp/). Absence of a variant within a large unaffected population cohort may hint at disease association, and is designated as moderate evidence toward pathogenicity by ACMG/AMP (PM2), although caution must be taken regarding this. Although the emergence of population-specific allele frequency data is vastly improved by resources such as gnomAD, not all populations are well represented. Thus, if the particular patient is from a population that may not have been captured in existing population resources, it remains

TABLE 1
Examples of Pathogenic Sequence Variants at 1% or Higher Allele Frequency in Specific Populations

Gene and Variant	Disorder	Approximate Population Frequencies
CFTR c.1521_1523delCTT (p.Phe508del), commonly referred to as delta F508 (ΔF508) (NM_000492.3)	Cystic fibrosis	1 in 25 white people
HBB c.20A>T (p.Glu7Val) (NM_000518.5)	Sickle cell disease	1 in 10 African Americans
BRCA1 c.68_69delAG (p.Glu23Valfs) (NM_007294.3) *BRCA2* c.5946delT (p.Ser1982Argfs) (NM_000059.3)	Hereditary breast and ovarian cancer, Fanconi anemia	1 in 100 Ashkenazi Jews 1 in 62 Ashkenazi Jews
GJB2 c.109G>A (p.Val37Ile) (NM_004004.5)	Deafness	1 in 10 east Asians

TABLE 2
Ancestry-Specific Population Allele Frequency Databases

Database	Description	URL
The Greater Middle East Variome	Genome sequencing of 2497 Middle Eastern individuals	http://igm.ucsd.edu/gme/
Al Mena	Genomes and exome sequencing from 2115 Arab, Middle Eastern, and North African individuals	http://clingen.igib.res.in/almena/
Institute of Precision Medicine	Genome sequencing from 100 healthy volunteers and exome sequencing from 648 normal individuals; most persons of Singaporean Chinese ancestry	http://beacon.prism-genomics.org/
Korean Variant Archive	Exome sequencing of 1055 healthy Korean individuals	https://www.kobic.re.kr/kova/
Integrative Japanese Genome Variation	Genome sequencing of >3500 Japanese individuals	https://ijgvd.megabank.tohoku.ac.jp/

possible that the variant in question is a benign finding endemic to the patient's ancestral group. In addition, rarity in and of itself may not be a specific predictor of pathogenicity [19].

For highly penetrant conditions for which onset is expected before adulthood, identifying a variant in multiple unaffected individuals suggests a benign classification (ACMG/AMP BS2). However, the natural history of the disorder as well as the demographic features of the unaffected control population being studied are important considerations.

Functional Studies

Studying organisms and genes that have acquired changes in their nucleotide sequences is a fundamental practice in biology. In vivo or in vitro functional studies, assessing germline variant impact, is often an important aspect of making gene-disease associations and, once established, can be used in the classification of that alteration. For rare variants, robust, clinically validated functional studies are often the key to classification, especially when other lines of evidence, such as cosegregation or case-control data, are scarce [20].

A well-established, statistically validated functional study can be weighted as a strong line of evidence for or against pathogenicity (PS3 and BS3, respectively). The ACMG/AMP guidelines recommend that, for a well-established study, the following be considered:

- The biological environment
- Whether the assay reflects the full spectrum of functions of the protein
- The validation, reproducibility, and robustness of the assay

Assays with high positive and negative predictive values that are reproducible and functionally appropriate can be weighted as strong evidence. However, it can be challenging to find studies that meet these criteria, and the ACMG/AMP guidelines do not provide guidance on what data are needed to deem an assay well established. After evaluating the evidence at hand, expert groups may decide to consider the body of functional evidence as strong if multiple studies replicate the same result. Alternatively, the weight of functional evidence could be decreased if appropriate functional studies are available but have not been statistically validated or replicated [21].

To keep up with the increasing rates of variants identified by multigene panel testing, functional studies that are both high throughput and clinically validated will be of critical importance. An early example of large-scale functional analysis was published in 2003 by Kato and colleagues [22], who used comprehensive site-directed mutagenesis in a yeast-based assay to evaluate all possible missense substitutions caused by single nucleotide variants throughout the p53 protein. As new technologies such as saturation mutagenesis are more widely used, multiplexed functional assays for large numbers of variants in single experiments will become more readily available [23]. Depending on the sensitivity and specificity of the assays, these could have a significant impact for variant classification, particularly for rare variants that lack other helpful evidence.

In Silico Predictors

In the absence of functional studies, computational in silico tools may provide a lower-confidence prediction as a proxy. These tools can be grouped into those that examine potential splicing defects and those that predict whether an amino acid change, mostly missense, is likely to damage the protein. Under the ACMG/AMP framework, in silico predictors are given the lowest level of evidence (supporting) when multiple predictors are in complete concordance. However, these guidelines do not specify how many predictors should be explored or which should be used, which can lead to variant classification discrepancies between clinical laboratories because using different predictors may increase the rates of variants classified as being of uncertain significance if 1 discordant prediction prevents application of the PP3 (pathogenic evidence) or BP4 (benign evidence) criteria [24,25]. Sun and Yu [26] found that the predictive accuracy increases until an optimal performance is reached using 2 or 3 tools, but that sensitivity began to decrease when additional models were incorporated.

Variants that cause splicing defects can occur in introns or exons, and they may disrupt the consensus splice site, alter splicing regulatory sequences such as exonic and intronic splice enhancers and silencers, activate a cryptic splice site, or create an entirely new alternate splice site. Computational splicing predictors based on a variety of algorithms, including position weighted matrix, neural network analysis, maximum entropy distributions, and other machine learning methods, have been developed to predict potential splice defects [27]. Most of the models are designed to predict changes in the strength of the splice sites for U2-type introns (GT-AG), which account for 99% of introns [28]. Although U12-type introns (AT-AC) are rare, clinicians should be careful not to use models designed for U2-type introns to predict U12-type splice sites.

Predicting the pathogenicity of missense variants relies on a combination of features including evolutionary conservation and structural and/or functional features of the amino acid change [26,29]. Each computational tool is based on different principles and has its own strengths and weaknesses [30,31], but improved performance may be seen when complementary models are combined to create a metapredictor [32,33]. Given that different metapredictors may include some of the same individual predictors in their algorithms, selecting one that performs the best after testing on a set of validated pathogenic and benign variants is the preferred strategy compared with using results from several different metapredictors to avoid circularity. However, complete avoidance of circularity may be impossible, because predictors might have been trained on the variants or proteins currently under analysis, leading to overfitting [34].

Phenotypic Specificity and Case-Control Studies

Identifying a rare variant in an individual with a phenotype highly specific to a rare disorder may provide evidence supporting pathogenicity, in line with the ACMG/AMP PP4 criteria. For disorders with genetic heterogeneity, it may be wise to ensure that, to the extent possible, other candidate genes have also been analyzed with no pathogenic variants identified. Targeted exome studies may be particularly helpful toward this goal [35–37]. The rarity of the variant is also an important consideration. If a variant is present at significant allele frequency in the general population, 1 (or more) affected individuals with the relevant phenotype will be found to harbor the variant based on chance alone.

Case-control evidence may apply when multiple affected individuals share the same variant. In order to warrant evidence toward pathogenicity, particularly for strong evidence as awarded by the ACMG/AMP PS4 criteria, cases and controls must include well-phenotyped populations; be well-matched with respect to age, gender, ancestry, and other potential confounding factors; and should include enough individuals (be sufficiently powered) to detect statistically significant odds ratios [38]. However, given the rare nature and allelic heterogeneity observed in most mendelian diseases, it is uncommon that a case-control study for a rare mendelian disorder is sufficiently powered. For this reason, the ACMG/AMP criteria allow for a relaxed use of the PS4 case-control criteria to count multiple unrelated probands showing phenotypic specificity with the same variant.

Cosegregation with Disease

Cosegregation of a variant with disease is a valuable quantitative data point used in assessing the pathogenicity of germline variants, particularly for rare mendelian disorders. This concept is similar to genetic linkage analysis in that likelihood ratios are derived similarly to logarithm of the odds scores in linkage, but specifically concerning the segregation of the variant and not a linked marker [39]. The seminal linkage models, developed from the 1950s through the 1980s [40,41], are based on the degree of relationship of the probands and the genotype and disease status of the tested relatives. The derived likelihood ratio is also a function of an assumed penetrance that includes the risk of disease and can be stratified by age and/or sex as well as the frequency of the disease allele. Jarvik and Browning [42] proposed a simpler approach for use with qualitative frameworks such as the ACMG/AMP guidelines. Given that segregation supports linkage to the allele as opposed to a specific variant, the strength of evidence assigned for segregation data may be adjusted based on the number of genes associated with the disease and degree of certainty that all potential disease-causing variants were identified during the testing process.

De Novo Occurrence

Identification of de novo variants has been greatly accelerated by the emergence of exome and genome trio sequencing, in which concordant analysis of the affected proband along with both parents can identify genetic variants unique to the proband while concordantly excluding nonpaternity and/or nonmaternity, providing evidence supporting a strong pathogenic criterion (PS2) per ACMG/AMP [43]. Before the advent of trio testing as a means to confirm parentage, separate analyses, such as microsatellite marker studies, could prove parentage but may not have been pursued. A nonpaternity rate of 1.9% has been identified among men with high paternity confidence, and higher rates (some greater than 10%) have been reported in other studies [39]. Thus, the ACMG/AMP guidelines give a lower, moderate evidence strength (PM6) for an assumed de novo variant in the absence of studies confirming parentage.

Although de novo occurrence can be helpful evidence supporting pathogenicity, any newborns may have up to 100 de novo variants within their genomes, with 1 or 2 predicted to alter the coding sequence [43,44]. For genes with expansive coding sequences, de novo variation has a higher a priori risk of occurring by chance [45]. Thus, the requirement that the patient's phenotype be consistent with the disease caused by the gene in question is key to the appropriate application of de novo criteria. The ClinGen Sequence Variant Interpretation Working Group has crafted guidelines for tempering the strength of evidence applied for de novo occurrence when phenotype specificity is lacking or the disorder has high heterogeneity, or for increasing strength when multiple probands with de novo occurrence are identified (https://clinicalgenome.org/site/assets/files/3461/svi_proposal_for_de_novo_criteria_v1_0.pdf).

Additional Evidence

Other types of evidence that may play a role in variant classification include:

- Presence in a mutational hotspot functional domain: moderate pathogenic evidence may be considered if a variant occurs in a critical functional domain or region known to harbor multiple pathogenic missense variants without any benign variation, indicating functional importance (ACMG/AMP PM1).
- Allelic data: whether a second known pathogenic variant occurs on the same (in cis) or opposite (in trans) allele as the variant of interest. Use of this criterion depends on the inheritance and mechanism of disease.
  - For autosomal recessive disorders, a variant of interest appearing in trans with a known pathogenic variant supports pathogenicity (ACMG/AMP PM3).
  - For dominant conditions for which biallelic pathogenic variants are incompatible with life or cause a severe phenotype, finding a variant in trans with a known pathogenic variant supports a benign classification (ACMG/AMP BP2).
  - Variants in cis or with unknown phase require a thoughtful approach. A variant occurring in cis with a variant predicted to result in nonsense-mediated decay would not be expressed, or 2 missense variants occurring on the same allele may work synergistically. If phase is unknown, other observations of the same 2 rare variants together in multiple individuals suggests they are in cis; likewise, observations of each variant independent of the other, or co-occurring with other variants, suggest they are in trans.
- Co-occurrence with other pathogenic variants: observation of a variant in an individual harboring other pathogenic variants explaining the patient's phenotype is an evidence against pathogenicity (ACMG/AMP BP5). Caution should be exercised for phenotypes with significant heterogeneity (eg, breast cancer) because there are multiple reports of individuals with rare pathogenic variants in more than 1 breast cancer predisposition gene [46,47].

TABLE 3
Odds of Pathogenicity for American College of Medical Genetics and Genomics/Association for Molecular Pathology Criteria

ACMG/AMP Criterion	Tavtigian et al [51], Odds of Pathogenicity
Pathogenic: very strong	350.0
Pathogenic: strong	18.7
Pathogenic: moderate	4.33
Pathogenic: supporting	2.08
Benign: strong	0.05
Benign: supporting	0.48

Data from Tavtigian SV, Greenblatt MS, Harrison SM, et al. Modeling the ACMG/AMP variant classification guidelines as a Bayesian classification framework. Genet Med.2018;20(9):1054-60.

PRESENT RELEVANCE AND FUTURE AVENUES TO CONSIDER OR TO INVESTIGATE

The Shift to Quantitative and Bayesian Approaches

This article outlines a primarily qualitative, categorical approach to variant assessment. This approach is purposefully general so that the ACMG/AMP criteria can be used for classification of variants in any mendelian disorder. For well-studied genes with validated functional studies, in silico models, and clinical correlates, it is possible to make gene-specific variant classification criteria using a quantitative approach. Calls for variant interpretation to be driven by a quantitative, bayesian approach have echoed in the literature for more than a decade, when bayesian approaches began to be used to classify variants in cancer predisposition genes [48–50]. More recently, Tavtigian and colleagues [51] developed a bayesian framework that takes the current ACMG/AMP categories and shifts them from a qualitative to a quantitative structure (Table 3). Among the benefits of this system are the opportunity to combine pathogenic and benign criteria when determining classification, as well as permitting clinicians to more clearly recognize where on the spectrum of benign to pathogenic a variant of uncertain significance may be.

VARIANT CURATION OUTCOMES USING QUALITATIVE AND QUANTITATIVE APPROACHES

Variant 1: PTEN c.392C>T (p.Thr131Ile)

Germline pathogenic *PTEN* variants are causative for PTEN Hamartoma Tumor syndrome (PHTS), an autosomal dominant disorder causing increased risk for benign and malignant tumors as well as neurodevelopmental phenotypes. This missense variant was curated by the ClinGen PTEN Variant Curation Expert Panel [21] and classified as pathogenic based on the following data:

- Functional data: strong impact on phosphatase activity (PS3)
- Clinical data: multiple probands with presumed de novo occurrence (PM6_Strong) and phenotypes highly specific for PHTS (PS4_Moderate)
- Population data: variant absent or very rare in large population cohorts (PM2)
- Computational/predictive: *PTEN* shows missense constraint, and missense variants are a common mechanism of disease in PHTS (PP2)

Under the qualitative ACMG/AMP framework, this variant has 2 strong, 2 moderate, and 1 supporting pathogenic criteria, leading to a final classification of pathogenic. Using the bayesian framework proposed by Tavtigian and colleagues [51], even starting with a low prior probability of 0.10 (generic prior proposed by investigators and reasonable for a missense variant), a combined odds of pathogenicity of 13,617.91 is achieved, leading to a posterior probability of 0.999, consistent with the pathogenic classification achieved by the qualitative method.

Variant 2: MYH7 c.5588G>A (p.Arg1863Gln)

Germline pathogenic variants in *MYH7* are associated with risk for cardiomyopathy. This missense variant was curated by the ClinGen Inherited Cardiomyopathy Variant Curation Expert Panel [52] and classified as being of uncertain significance based on the following data:

- Clinical data: variant identified in 2 individuals with cardiomyopathy (PS4_Supporting).
- Population data: variant absent or very rare in large population cohorts (PM2).
- Computational/predictive: in silico tools predict damaging effect (PP3).

Under the ACMG/AMP framework, this evidence results in classification of uncertain significance. However, under the bayesian framework, again using a prior probability of 0.10, the combined odds of pathogenicity equals 38.91, leading to a posterior probability of pathogenicity of 0.812. Although this still results in a final classification of uncertain significance, the quantitative method shows that the variant is approaching the threshold to be classified as likely pathogenic and has potential to be reclassified in that direction with minimal additional evidence.

ClinGen and Data Sharing

The Clinical Genome Resource (ClinGen, www.clinicalgenome.org), funded by the United States National Institutes of Health, is dedicated to improving the understanding of genomic variation for use in clinical care and research [53]. Under the auspices of ClinGen, expert panels including clinicians, researchers, and diagnostic laboratory representatives are being organized to tailor the ACMG/AMP criteria for gene-specific variant curation [54]. Collaborative efforts such as those driven by ClinGen will enhance data sharing efforts and increase the quality and consistency of variant classification efforts among participating groups [55].

SUMMARY

As the improvements in technologies used for variant detection have increased rapidly, so have the quality and quantity of data points available for use during the variant classification process. The numbers and diversity of individuals in the general population exome and genome sequencing cohorts have expanded; high-throughput techniques have functionally interrogated variants before their observation in a single patient; trio-based and other familial testing strategies have enabled detection of de novo variants and provided segregation data helpful to the variant classification process. At the same time, relationships among disease-specific experts and clinical laboratories will continue to grow through involvement in efforts such as the ClinGen project, providing opportunities to share expertise and data with the ultimate goal to benefit patients.

REFERENCES

[1] Ekong R, Nellist M, Hoogeveen-Westerveld M, et al. Variants within TSC2 Exons 25 and 31 are very unlikely to cause clinically diagnosable tuberous sclerosis. Hum Mutat 2016;37(4):364–70.

[2] Cotton RG, Scriver CR. Proof of "disease causing" mutation. Hum Mutat 1998;12(1):1–3.

[3] Easton DF, Deffenbaugh AM, Pruss D, et al. A systematic genetic assessment of 1,433 sequence variants of unknown clinical significance in the BRCA1 and BRCA2 breast cancer-predisposition genes. Am J Hum Genet 2007;81(5):873–83.

[4] Miller PJ, Duraisamy S, Newell JA, et al. Classifying variants of CDKN2A using computational and laboratory studies. Hum Mutat 2011;32(8):900–11.

[5] Sosnay PR, Siklosi KR, Van Goor F, et al. Defining the disease liability of variants in the cystic fibrosis transmembrane conductance regulator gene. Nat Genet 2013;45(10):1160–7.

[6] Thompson BA, Spurdle AB, Plazzer J-P, et al. Application of a 5-tiered scheme for standardized classification of 2,360 unique mismatch repair gene variants in the InSiGHT locus-specific database. Nat Genet 2014;46(2):107–15.

[7] Walsh R, Mazzarotto F, Whiffin N, et al. Quantitative approaches to variant classification increase the yield and precision of genetic testing in Mendelian diseases: the case of hypertrophic cardiomyopathy. Genome Med 2019;11(1):5.

[8] Harrison SM, Dolinsky JS, Knight Johnson AE, et al. Clinical laboratories collaborate to resolve differences in variant interpretations submitted to ClinVar. Genet Med 2017;19(10):1096–104.

[9] ACMG recommendations for standards for interpretation of sequence variations. Genet Med 2000;2:302.

[10] Richards CS, Bale S, Bellissimo DB, et al. ACMG recommendations for standards for interpretation and reporting of sequence variations: Revisions 2007. Genet Med 2008;10(4):294–300.

[11] Richards S, Aziz N, Bale S, et al. Standards and guidelines for the interpretation of sequence variants: a joint consensus recommendation of the American College of Medical Genetics and Genomics and the Association for Molecular Pathology. Genet Med 2015;17(5):405–24.

[12] Plon SE, Eccles DM, Easton D, et al. Sequence variant classification and reporting: recommendations for improving the interpretation of cancer susceptibility genetic test results. Hum Mutat 2008;29(11):1282–91.

[13] Abou Tayoun AN, Pesaran T, DiStefano MT, et al. Recommendations for interpreting the loss of function PVS1 ACMG/AMP variant criterion. Hum Mutat 2018;39(11):1517–24.

[14] Brookes AJ. The essence of SNPs. Gene 1999;234(2):177–86.

[15] International HapMap 3 Consortium, Altshuler DM, Gibbs RA, et al. Integrating common and rare genetic variation in diverse human populations. Nature 2010;467(7311):52–8.

[16] 1000 Genomes Project Consortium, Auton A, Brooks LD, Durbin RM, et al. A global reference for human genetic variation. Nature 2015;526(7571):68–74.

[17] Lek M, Karczewski KJ, Minikel EV, et al. Analysis of protein-coding genetic variation in 60,706 humans. Nature 2016;536(7616):285–91.

[18] Whiffin N, Minikel E, Walsh R, et al. Using high-resolution variant frequencies to empower clinical genome interpretation. Genet Med 2017;19(10):1151–8.

[19] Young EL, Feng BJ, Stark AW, et al. Multigene testing of moderate-risk genes: be mindful of the missense. J Med Genet 2016;53(6):366–76.

[20] Brnich SE, Rivera-Muñoz EA, Berg JS. Quantifying the potential of functional evidence to reclassify variants of uncertain significance in the categorical and Bayesian

interpretation frameworks. Hum Mutat 2018;39(11):1531–41.
[21] Mester JL, Ghosh R, Pesaran T, et al. Gene-specific criteria for PTEN variant curation: recommendations from the ClinGen PTEN expert panel. Hum Mutat 2018;39(11):1581–92.
[22] Kato S, Han S-Y, Liu W, et al. Understanding the function-structure and function-mutation relationships of p53 tumor suppressor protein by high-resolution missense mutation analysis. Proc Natl Acad Sci U S A 2003;100(14):8424–9.
[23] Gasperini M, Starita L, Shendure J. The power of multiplexed functional analysis of genetic variants. Nat Protoc 2016;11(10):1782–7.
[24] Maxwell KN, Hart SN, Vijai J, et al. Evaluation of ACMG-guideline-based variant classification of cancer susceptibility and non-cancer-associated genes in families affected by breast cancer. Am J Hum Genet 2016;98(5):801–17.
[25] Ghosh R, Oak N, Plon SE. Evaluation of in silico algorithms for use with ACMG/AMP clinical variant interpretation guidelines. Genome Biol 2017;18(1):225.
[26] Sun H, Yu G. New insights into the pathogenicity of non-synonymous variants through multi-level analysis. Sci Rep 2019;9(1):1667.
[27] Moles-Fernández A, Duran-Lozano L, Montalban G, et al. Computational tools for splicing defect prediction in breast/ovarian cancer genes: how efficient are they at predicting RNA alterations? Front Genet 2018;9:366.
[28] Sibley CR, Blazquez L, Ule J. Lessons from non-canonical splicing. Nat Rev Genet 2016;17(7):407–21.
[29] Katsonis P, Koire A, Wilson SJ, et al. Single nucleotide variations: biological impact and theoretical interpretation. Protein Sci 2014;23(12):1650–66.
[30] Tavtigian SV, Greenblatt MS, Lesueur F, et al, IARC Unclassified Genetic Variants Working Group. In silico analysis of missense substitutions using sequence-alignment based methods. Hum Mutat 2008;29(11):1327–36.
[31] Jordan DM, Ramensky VE, Sunyaev SR. Human allelic variation: perspective from protein function, structure, and evolution. Curr Opin Struct Biol 2010;20(3):342–50.
[32] Ioannidis NM, Rothstein JH, Pejaver V, et al. REVEL: an ensemble method for predicting the pathogenicity of rare missense variants. Am J Hum Genet 2016;99(4):877–85.
[33] Hart SN, Hoskin T, Shimelis H, et al. Comprehensive annotation of BRCA1 and BRCA2 missense variants by functionally validated sequence-based computational prediction models. Genet Med 2019;21(1):71–80.
[34] Grimm DG, Azencott C-A, Aicheler F, et al. The evaluation of tools used to predict the impact of missense variants is hindered by two types of circularity. Hum Mutat 2015;36(5):513–23.
[35] Polla DL, Cardoso MTO, Silva MCB, et al. Use of targeted exome sequencing for molecular diagnosis of skeletal disorders. PLoS One 2015;10(9):e0138314.
[36] Weinberg CR, Umbach DM. Choosing a retrospective design to assess joint genetic and environmental contributions to risk. Am J Epidemiol 2000;152(3):197–203.
[37] Campbell H, Rudan I. Interpretation of genetic association studies in complex disease. Pharmacogenomics J 2002;2(6):349–60.
[38] Anderson KG. How well does paternity confidence match actual paternity?: Evidence from worldwide nonpaternity rates. Curr Anthropol 2006;47(3):513–20.
[39] Goldgar DE. Collection and analysis of pedigree data. Birth Defects Orig Artic Ser 1984;20(6):61–76.
[40] Morton NE. Sequential tests for the detection of linkage. Am J Hum Genet 1955;7(3):277–318.
[41] Lalouel JM, Morton NE. Complex segregation analysis with pointers. Hum Hered 1981;31(5):312–21.
[42] Jarvik GP, Browning BL. Consideration of cosegregation in the pathogenicity classification of genomic variants. Am J Hum Genet 2016;98(6):1077–81.
[43] Ku CS, Polychronakos C, Tan EK, et al. A new paradigm emerges from the study of de novo mutations in the context of neurodevelopmental disease. Mol Psychiatry 2013;18(2):141–53.
[44] Acuna-Hidalgo R, Veltman JA, Hoischen A. New insights into the generation and role of de novo mutations in health and disease. Genome Biol 2016;17(1):241.
[45] MacArthur DG, Manolio TA, Dimmock DP, et al. Guidelines for investigating causality of sequence variants in human disease. Nature 2014;508(7497):469–76.
[46] Couch FJ, Shimelis H, Hu C, et al. Associations between cancer predisposition testing panel genes and breast cancer. JAMA Oncol 2017;3(9):1190–6.
[47] Frey MK, Sandler G, Sobolev R, et al. Multigene panels in Ashkenazi Jewish patients yield high rates of actionable mutations in multiple non-BRCA cancer-associated genes. Gynecol Oncol 2017;146(1):123–8.
[48] Goldgar DE, Easton DF, Byrnes GB, et al. Genetic evidence and integration of various data sources for classifying uncertain variants into a single model. Hum Mutat 2008;29(11):1265–72.
[49] Tavtigian SV, Greenblatt MS, Goldgar DE, et al, IARC Unclassified Genetic Variants Working Group. Assessing pathogenicity: overview of results from the IARC Unclassified Genetic Variants Working Group. Hum Mutat 2008;29(11):1261–4.
[50] Goldgar DE, Easton DF, Deffenbaugh AM, et al. Integrated evaluation of DNA sequence variants of unknown clinical significance: application to BRCA1 and BRCA2. Am J Hum Genet 2004;75(4):535–44.
[51] Tavtigian SV, Greenblatt MS, Harrison SM, et al. Modeling the ACMG/AMP variant classification guidelines as a Bayesian classification framework. Genet Med 2018;20(9):1054–60.
[52] Kelly MA, Caleshu C, Morales A, et al. Adaptation and validation of the ACMG/AMP variant classification framework for MYH7-associated inherited cardiomyopathies: recommendations by ClinGen's Inherited

Cardiomyopathy Expert Panel. Genet Med 2018. https://doi.org/10.1038/gim.2017.218.

[53] Rehm HL, Berg JS, Brooks LD, et al. ClinGen–the clinical genome resource. N Engl J Med 2015;372(23):2235–42.

[54] Rivera-Muñoz EA, Milko LV, Harrison SM, et al. ClinGen Variant Curation Expert Panel experiences and standardized processes for disease and gene-level specification of the ACMG/AMP guidelines for sequence variant interpretation. Hum Mutat 2018; 39(11):1614–22.

[55] Harrison SM, Dolinksy JS, Chen W, et al. Scaling resolution of variant classification differences in ClinVar between 41 clinical laboratories through an outlier approach. Hum Mutat 2018;39(11):1641–9.

Advances in Molecular Pathology 2 (2019) 13–19
ADVANCES IN MOLECULAR PATHOLOGY

The Future of Clinical Diagnosis

Moving Functional Genomics Approaches to the Bedside

Rini Pauly, MS*, Charles E. Schwartz, PhD
Greenwood Genetic Center, JC Self Research Institute, 113 Gregor Mendel Circle, Greenwood, SC 29646, USA

KEYWORDS

- Whole-genome sequencing (WGS) • RNA sequencing • Genome wide methylation/Epi-signatures
- Functional assay • Metabolomics • Proteomics • Multi-omic analysis

KEY POINTS

- Whole-genome sequencing (WGS) identifies critical alterations in the genome that are not present in the coding genes.
- Genome-wide methylation studies identify epi-signatures that allow clarification and proper classification of variants of uncertain significance.
- RNA-seq, both targeted and untargeted, allows diagnosis of human disorders, particularly those in patients with a suspicious phenotype and no obvious genomic alteration.
- Bioinformatics tools, and neural networks, allow for the association of apparently unrelated events.
- Multi-omic analysis—the integrated analysis of data from various omic studies (WGS, methylation, RNAseq)—identifies coordinated interaction of variants leading to a phenotype.

INTRODUCTION

Sequencing techniques are limited by the interpretation of a large number of coding and noncoding, sequence and structural, variants. In-silico tools for predicting the impact of coding variants and regulatory elements have become increasingly advanced. However, the evidence from these tools is generally not sufficient for accurate variant classification. In this article, the authors discuss a multi-omic approach that they foresee will enable genome-wide characterization and classification of variants by integrating several omics data, assisted by bioinformatics tools and deep learning algorithms for variant prioritization. These prioritizations can then be quantified using advanced high-throughput functional assays.

SIGNIFICANCE

Interpreting the clinical impact of variants of uncertain significance (VUSs) and eventually the joint effect of having multiple variants in the same or different genes is complex. A multi-omic approach promises to address this compound issue of variant assessment by combining genomic, transcriptomic, epigenomic, and functional proteomic data using novel computational tools. Accumulation and accessibility of these data will eventually lead to a comprehensive variant effect map, a significant step toward accurate clinical interpretation of genetic variants.

CURRENT CLINICAL VARIANT INTERPRETATION APPROACHES

Rapid advances in genomic technologies is changing the traditional practice of medicine to primarily include predictive, preventive, and personalized medicine approaches [1,2]. However, the central

*Corresponding author, *E-mail address:* rpauly@ggc.org

https://doi.org/10.1016/j.yamp.2019.08.001
2589-4080/19/

challenge for clinical genomics remains in conclusive interpretation of the numerous novel variants found through DNA sequencing. Increasingly, sequencing-based technologies in research and clinical laboratories are detecting large number of variants for which the clinical significance is unknown. Such variants are also called variants of uncertain significance (VUSs). In 2015, the American College of Medical Genetics and Genomics and the Association for Molecular Pathology [3] published standards and guidelines for sequence variant interpretation and to ensure accurate and consistent variant classification. This guideline outlines the evidence used in variant classification including population, computational, functional, segregation and allelic data, and conservation analyses among other variant evidence. Different pieces of evidence are weighed differently (supporting, moderate, strong, very strong) and then combined to reach a final classification (pathogenic, likely pathogenic, VUSs, likely benign, benign) for any given variant.

Often times, there is not enough clinical or functional evidence to support variant classification leading to an assimilation of a large number of VUSs. Therefore, there is a need for additional testing modalities across laboratories to improve the reproducibility and objectivity of variant interpretation. These might include primarily genomic, epigenetic, transcriptomic, proteomic, and metabolomic modalities. Data from all such modalities may then be combined and analyzed, using high-throughput computational systems, to determine the clinical significance of the relevant genetic variant (Fig. 1).

WHOLE-GENOME SEQUENCING

The implementation of genomic medicine in the clinic has long being recognized as an essential component in providing good clinical care. Although exome

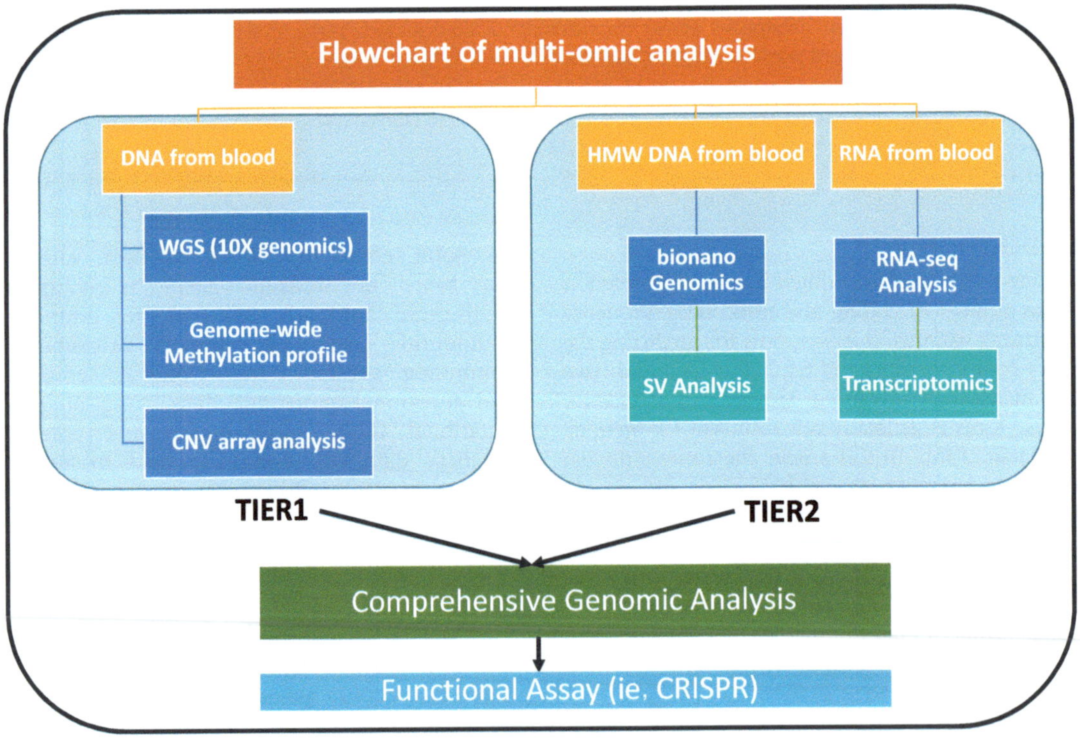

FIG. 1 Steps for human multi-omic analysis that combines multiple technologies to identify and characterize non-linear relationships between variants and genes in a single disorder or several related disorders. WGS; Whole-genome sequencing, CNV; Copy number variants, HMV; High Molecular Weight, bionano genomics; non-sequencing-based genome mapping technology to identify structural variants and create de *novo* genome assemblies, SV; Structural Variant, CRISPR; Clustered Regularly Interspaced Short Palindromic Repeats.

sequencing is cost and time efficient, it focuses on only ~1% to 2% of the genome, unlike whole-genome sequencing (WGS) that covers 95% to 98% of the genome. WGS has several advantages when compared with exome and targeted panels including uniform coverage in coding and noncoding regions, which allows detection of copy number variants (CNVs) and structural variants. Specifically, WGS has demonstrated the use of paired-end sequencing to obtain breakpoint resolution of CNVs, rearrangements, and other structural variations [4–7]. Several medical centers and commercial laboratories across the United States have now implemented genome sequencing programs with "in-house" sequencing and analysis of variants with review and sign-out by a board-certified clinical molecular geneticist. However, the pace of the clinical application of WGS has been limited due to various factors including cost, insurance coverage, and data storage limitations.

EPIGENOMICS AND PREDICTION OF VARIANTS IMPACT

Epigenetic changes, through DNA methylation and histone modifications, can modulate gene expression and the overall cellular and/or systems phenotype [8–10]. There are several ways to obtain enriched methylated sequences, for example, methylated DNA immunoprecipitation-sequencing, methylated CpG island recovery assay, or whole-genome shotgun bisulfite sequencing (WGBS) [11,12]. WGBS, considered the "gold standard", enables the detection of DNA methylation at single base-pair resolution. The treatment of DNA with sodium bisulfite allows the discrimination of methylated and unmethylated cytosines. However, this technology is limited by the DNA quantity and quality that can be compromised by the desulfonation process.

Furthermore, the epigenetic modifications can be used as markers for molecular diagnostics and disease screening. For example, there are 3 commercially available DNA methylation-based diagnostic tests for colorectal cancer: EpiproColon, ColoVantage, and Real-Time mS9 that are designed to detect hypermethylated *SEPT9* in a blood sample. EpiproColon is the most clinically validated diagnostic epigenetic biomarker for colon cancer. Noninvasive tests such as these are preferred over colonoscopy by patients, thereby serving as an efficient tool for molecular screening and diagnosis [13].

Schenkel and colleagues [14] developed specific DNA methylation signature assays for Fragile X syndrome by identifying differential methylation levels at the *FMR1* gene promoter. Separately, Choufani and colleagues [15] used the same approach to identify additional aberrant methylation loci across the genome for Sotos syndrome. Recently, syndrome-specific epi-signatures were characterized and used to support the classification of VUSs and the unambiguous identification of affected individuals. In 2018, Aref-Eshghiand colleagues [16] used genomic DNA methylation signatures to support the classification of variants in neurodevelopmental syndromes, including 14 Mendelian disorders. This novel approach was further developed to characterize overlapping peripheral blood DNA methylation epi-signatures in individuals with Coffin-Siris and Nicolaides Baraitser syndromes [17]. More recently, this application was expanded to include 19 conditions [18] and became the first epigenetic signature test (EpiSign) for inherited disorders in the United States and Europe [19].

RNA-SEQ ANALYSIS AND PREDICTION OF VARIANTS IMPACT

RNA-seq is increasingly being seen as a powerful clinical tool to improve diagnostic yield in genetically unresolved and complex cases [20,21]. In 2017, Kremer and colleagues [22] investigated the utility of RNA-seq in diagnosing patients with mitochondrial disorders. The study identified several genes with aberrant expression, abnormal splicing events, and/or allele-specific expression (mono-allelic expression), whereby one allele is silenced, leaving only the other allele expressed. These findings lead to the molecular diagnosis of 5 out of 48 undiagnosed patients with mitochondriopathies along with and identification of candidate genes to establish novel disease-gene association in other cases. In another publication, Cummings and colleagues [23] explored RNA-seq as a complementary diagnostic tool to genomic sequencing by systematically detecting transcript level changes, mainly aberrant splicing events. The added diagnostic yield of RNA-seq in this study was 35%. Using this approach, a highly recurrent, disruptive intronic variant was identified in the *COL6A1* gene in a total of 27 genetically unsolved collagen VI-like dystrophy patients. Overall, both these studies demonstrated the power of RNA-seq for detection and classification of variants missed by standard genomic diagnostic approaches.

Gonorazky and colleagues [24] developed PAGE (Panel Analysis of Gene Expression), a web-based tool to promote RNA sequencing-based diagnostics for rare Mendelian diseases. PAGE supports the comparison of gene expression across multiple tissues and identification of variants and splicing changes through this analysis. This study focused on monogenetic neuromuscular disorders as proof of principle to provide genetic resolution in 36% (9/25) of cases. Their diagnostic algorithm compared 70 undiagnosed individuals with an in-house database and with control transcriptome data obtained from the Genotype-Tissue Expression (GTEx) project. GTEx is a database of 53 nondisease tissue sites across nearly 1000 individuals. It includes tissue-specific gene expression data (RNA-seq) combined with WGS or WES data [25]. This transcriptome database catalogs many naturally occurring genetic variants that modulate alternative splicing and consequently influence phenotypic variability and disease susceptibility in human populations.

APPLICATION OF VARIANT FUNCTIONAL ASSAYS IN METABOLOMICS

Metabolomics is the comprehensive analysis of metabolites within a biological system and can be a valuable tool in deciphering the clinical significance of VUSs. Chong and colleagues [26] developed an open source tool, MetaboAnalyst, which facilitates integrative analysis to identify biologically meaningful patterns in quantitative metabolomic data. Such tools are valuable in rapidly classifying multiple patterns in complex datasets. In 2013, Boccuto and colleagues [27] used phenotype microarrays for metabolic profiling of lymphoblastoid cells from 137 patients with neurodevelopmental disorders with or without autism spectrum disorders (ASDs) and 78 normal individuals. Phenotype MicroArray assays are mammalian cell-based assays used to investigate up to 1400 metabolites in mammalian cells in a high-throughput manner. Using this system, the investigators identified decreased tryptophan metabolism as a potential unifying biochemical basis for patients with ASDs, which could be pursued further as a first diagnostic assay for ASDs. This platform also allows the characterization of the metabolic profile of ASD cells, which will then help in understanding the impact of rare novel variants on ASD genes. Another neurologic disorder, Snyder-Robinson syndrome, was first reported in 1969 [28] as an X-linked intellectual disability syndrome and until very recently was the only known genetic disorder associated with the polyamine metabolic pathway. Li and colleagues [29] successfully uncovered some of the mechanisms underlying the pathologic consequences of abnormal polyamine metabolism in the nervous system by identifying a distinctive shift in the metabolism of carbon energy sources that further indicates a compromised mitochondrial function. This is another example where such a specific metabolic signature can be used to characterize VUSs associated with this disease.

HIGH-THROUGHPUT FUNCTIONAL ASSAYS AND DEEP LEARNING MODELS

In 2018, Findlay and colleagues [30] developed a saturation genome editing assay to characterize 96.5% of all possible single-nucleotide variants (SNVs) in 13 (out of 24) exons of the *BRCA1* gene. This region is known to play a key role in the tumor suppressor function. This assay was designed using the CRISPR/Cas9 approach to alter each nucleotide for a total of about 4000 possible individual mutations. The frequency of the induced variant was used to score its effect on *BRCA1* function. It was found that the functional effects were concordant with assessments of pathogenicity from ClinVar. This included more than 400 missense SNVs, as well as around 300 SNVs that disrupt expression. This approach can be extended to overcome the challenge of VUSs in additional clinically actionable genes.

Separately, Starita and colleagues [31] also developed and published a multiplex Homology-directed DNA Repair Assay to measure the effects of more than 1000 *BRCA1* missense substitutions on DNA repair in breast and ovarian cancer. They were able to demonstrate an accurate discrimination of loss-of-function versus benign missense variants with 87.5% sensitivity and 100% specificity.

Taking a different approach, Drost and colleagues [32], in 2018, developed a Cell-free *In vitro* Mismatch Repair Activity (CIMRA) assay to enhance the classification of VUSs in the DNA mismatch repair genes in Lynch syndrome. Their CIMRA assay allows generation and functional analysis of several variants of the MLH1 protein in vitro at the same time. The investigators tested 26 *MLH1* variants and of these, 15 had lost activity. Further, these results match up with the in silico and pathology data. High-throughput functional assays such as this will enable fast and accurate classification of VUSs; however, their clinical implementation still requires more work to address feasibility, clinical validity, and infrastructure requirements.

A well-validated functional assay could ultimately be used as a clinical annotation tool to study the impact of the variant on a protein's function, its effect on cellular function, and its ability to be used as a drug target [33]. The major bottleneck for functional studies is that most VUSs are rare (ie, seen in one or very few patients) but are collectively numerous. Therefore, fast, cost-effective and high-throughput functional assays are needed to assess the effect of a large number of possible variants in any given gene or molecular pathway. Three benchmark studies in 2010 to 2011 by Fowler and colleagues [34], Ernst and colleagues [35], and Hietpas and colleagues [36] led to the development of deep mutational scanning. These studies initiated the use of multiplexed assays for variant effect (MAVEs) that could create comprehensive atlas of functional data for 10^4–10^6 variants in a single experiment. The multiplexed assays accomplished this by linking the genotype of each variant to its effect in a functional assay [37]. Different MAVE approaches have been established, but they share a common process. Variants are synthesized, introduced into a model system, and carefully chosen for a phenotype of interest.

Massively parallel reporter assays use a library of mutagenized promoter sequences, to calculate the effect of a promoter variant on expression by using the read ratio of RNA-seq to DNA-seq data [38,39]. Researchers at the University of Alabama at Birmingham (UAB) developed a blood-based functional RNA assay for the *NF1* (*neurofibromin 1*) gene, which enabled identification of 2.5% (>65 different locations harboring deep intronic splice variants) of all known pathogenic deep intronic splice variants in the *NF1*UAB cohort [40–42].

Recently, Evans and colleagues [43] used clinical sequencing data from more than 17,000 patients to train a disease-specific variant pathogenicity predictor that approached 100% accuracy for several epilepsy, cardiomyopathy, and RASopathies genes. Another deep neural network application predicts the clinical impact of a human mutation using primate species. Unlike previous efforts that lacked adequately sized datasets containing confidently labeled benign and pathogenic variants for training, Sundaram and colleagues [44] demonstrated that common missense variants in other primate species are largely clinically benign in human, enabling pathogenic mutations to be systematically identified by the process of elimination. Using thousands of common variants from population sequencing of 6 nonhuman primate species, they trained a deep neural network that identifies pathogenic mutations in patients with rare disease with 88% accuracy and enabled the discovery of 14 new candidate genes in intellectual disability genome wide. This kind of comprehensive cataloging of common variation from additional primate species would advance genome variant interpretation and further improve the clinical utility of human genome sequencing.

MULTI-OMIC ANALYSIS

The technologies mentioned in this article have the potential to improve the characterization of molecular phenotypes in normal and disease tissues by capturing of genomic, epigenomic, and transcriptomic profiles. However, an integrated analysis of these heterogeneous data sets to diagnose diseases is not straight forward and is still not within the capacity of most clinical laboratories. Argelaguet and colleagues [45] introduced MOFA, a framework for unsupervised integration of multi-omics data sets in chronic lymphocytic leukemia (CLL) and mouse embryonic stem cells. MOFA was done in 2 steps. In step 1, data were collected from 200 patients to assess single-cell RNA expression and DNA methylation and their response to drugs. In step 2, the single-cell expression and methylation data were used to identify coordinated transcriptional and epigenetic changes along cell differentiation. This application accurately detected mislabeled samples and imputed missing values but most importantly was able to identify major sources of disease heterogeneity in CLL, that is, somatic mutation status of the immunoglobulin heavy-chain variable region gene and chromosome 12 trisomy status. Another study by Singh and colleagues [46–48], used a factor model integrative approach for identifying key molecular drivers from multi-omic assays. Data Integration Analysis for Biomarker discovery using Latent Components identifies both known and novel multi-omics biomarkers consisting of mRNAs, miRNAs, CpGs, proteins, and metabolites. Although most studies integrate omics data for testing marginal associations between different data types, they still lack an overall interpretability. A major limitation of this approach is relying on a linear model, which means that it would not detect nonlinear relationships between the input features. The authors propose a multi-omics strategy that aims to go from genotype to phenotype.

However, in order for this approach to attain its full potential, one needs an interactive omics platform to fully understand the choreography of genes, cells, tissues, organs, and environment [1]. The platform should enable building and implementation of computational analytical tools to be able to identify nonlinear relationships between variants and genes and across different datasets.

Although a comprehensive omic analysis platform is set in place, advanced functional assays are still needed to quantify these findings. For instance, CRISPR could be applied to create multiple single edits in a control cell line to recapitulate the original patient profile

[48]. The advantages of this technique is that it allows in situ modification, which can be done at a genome-wide scale for specific sites of interest and it can be used in the proper cell type using iPS cell technology. This platform would certainly serve as an accomplished start for clinical reporting and personalized genomic medicine.

SUMMARY

Recent years have seen an exponential increase in VUS findings. A large number of missense variant entries in ClinVar are classified as VUSs [33]. Although there have been some commendable coordinated efforts to produce, analyze, and share these large complex datasets, we are long way from addressing the variant interpretation challenge. In order to progress, we need to recognize intermediate steps that lie between genomic discovery research and evidence-based clinical implementation.

Comprehensive variant assessment programs need to be implemented to assess a variant's impact on protein function and to integrate multiple lines of evidence to expedite efficient variant classification, providing improved benefit for patients [49,50]. In addition, it will become necessary to undertake what we term human multi-omic analysis to solve disorders resulting from a single variant or from the interaction of multiple variants. Finally, using high-throughput functional assays will be a powerful tool for VUS classification in Mendelian and complex disorders.

ACKNOWLEDGMENT

This work is supported in part by a grant from the South Carolina Department of Disabilities and Special Needs (SCDDSN).

REFERENCES

[1] Green ED, Guyer MS. Charting a course for genomic medicine from base pairs to bedside. Nature 2011; 470(7333):204–13.

[2] MuzafarBeigh M. Next-generation sequencing: the translational medicine approach from "bench to bedside to population" (vol. 3). Medicines 2016;3(2):14.

[3] Richards S, Aziz N, Bale S, et al. Standards and guidelines for the interpretation of sequence variants: a joint consensus recommendation of the American College of Medical Genetics and Genomics and the Association for Molecular Pathology. Genet Med 2015;17(5): 405–24.

[4] Stavropoulos DJ, Merico D, Jobling R, et al. Whole genome sequencing expands diagnostic utility and improves clinical management in pediatric medicine. NPJ Genom Med 2016;1:15012.

[5] Caspar SM, Dubacher N, Kopps AM, et al. Clinical sequencing: from raw data to diagnosis with lifetime value. Clin Genet 2018;93(3):508–19.

[6] Mostovoy Y, Levy-Sakin M, Lam J, et al. A hybrid approach for de novo human genome sequence assembly and phasing. Nat Methods 2016;13:587.

[7] Barseghyan H, Tang W, Wang RT, et al. Next-generation mapping: a novel approach for detection of pathogenic structural variants with a potential utility in clinical diagnosis. Genome Med 2017;9(1):90.

[8] Egger G, Liang G, Aparicio A, et al. Epigenetics in human disease and prospects for epigenetic therapy. Nature 2004;429(6990):457–63.

[9] Gibney ER, Nolan CM. Epigenetics and gene expression. Heredity 2010;105:4.

[10] Lim DH, Maher ER. DNA methylation: a form of epigenetic control of gene expression. Obstet Gynaecol 2010;12:37–42.

[11] Li D, Zhang B, Xing X, et al. Combining MeDIP-seq and MRE-seq to investigate genome-wide CpG methylation. Methods 2015;72:29–40.

[12] Li Y, Tollefsbol TO. DNA methylation detection: bisulfite genomic sequencing analysis. MethodsMol Biol 2011; 791:11–21.

[13] Issa IA, Noureddine M. Colorectal cancer screening: an updated review of the available options. World J Gastroenterol 2017;23(28):5086–96.

[14] Schenkel LC, Schwartz C, Skinner C, et al. Clinical validation of fragile X syndrome screening by DNA methylation array. J Mol Diagn 2016;18(6):834–41.

[15] Choufani S, Cytrynbaum C, Chung BHY, et al. NSD1 mutations generate a genome-wide DNA methylation signature. Nat Commun 2015;6:10207.

[16] Aref-Eshghi E, Rodenhiser DI, Schenkel LC, et al. Genomic DNA methylation signatures enable concurrent diagnosis and clinical genetic variant classification in neurodevelopmental syndromes. Am J Hum Genet 2018;102(1):156–74.

[17] Aref-Eshghi E, Bend EG, Hood RL, et al. BAFopathies' DNA methylation epi-signatures demonstrate diagnostic utility and functional continuum of Coffin–Siris and Nicolaides–Baraitser syndromes. Nat Commun 2018;9(1):4885.

[18] Aref-Eshghi E, Bend EG, Colaiacovo S, et al. Diagnostic utility of genome-wide DNA methylation testing in genetically unsolved individuals with suspected hereditary conditions. Am J Hum Genet 2019. https://doi.org/10.1016/j.ajhg.2019.03.008.

[19] Genome web, April 2019. Available at: https://www.genomeweb.com/molecular-diagnostics/first-epigenetic-signature-test-inherited-disorders-launch-us-europe. Accessed July 22, 2019.

[20] Li D, Tian L, Hakonarson H. Increasing diagnostic yield by RNA-Sequencing in rare disease-bypass hurdles of interpreting intronic or splice-altering variants. Ann Transl Med 2018;6(7):126.

[21] Byron SA, Van Keuren-Jensen KR, Engelthaler DM, et al. Translating RNA sequencing into clinical diagnostics: opportunities and challenges. Nat Rev Genet 2016;17:257.

[22] Kremer LS, Bader DM, Mertes C, et al. Genetic diagnosis of Mendelian disorders via RNA sequencing. Nat Commun 2017;8:15824.

[23] Cummings BB, Marshall JL, Tukiainen T, et al. Improving genetic diagnosis in Mendelian disease with transcriptome sequencing. Sci Transl Med 2017;9(386) [pii: eaal5209].

[24] Gonorazky HD, Naumenko S, Ramani AK, et al. Expanding the boundaries of RNA sequencing as a diagnostic tool for rare mendelian disease. Am J Hum Genet 2019;104(3):466–83.

[25] GTEx portal. Available at: https://gtexportal.org/home/. Accessed July 22, 2019.

[26] Chong J, Soufan O, Caraus I, et al. MetaboAnalyst 4.0: towards more transparent and integrative metabolomics analysis. Nucleic Acids Res 2018;46(W1):W486–94.

[27] Boccuto L, Chen C-F, Pittman AR, et al. Decreased tryptophan metabolism in patients with autism spectrum disorders. Mol Autism 2013;4(1):16.

[28] Lauren Cason A, Ikeguchi Y, Skinner C, et al. X-linked spermine synthase gene (SMS) defect: the first polyamine deficiency syndrome. Eur J Hum Genet 2003;11:937.

[29] Li C, Brazill JM, Liu S, et al. Spermine synthase deficiency causes lysosomal dysfunction and oxidative stress in models of Snyder-Robinson syndrome. Nat Commun 2017;8(1):1257.

[30] Findlay GM, Daza RM, Martin B, et al. Accurate classification of BRCA1 variants with saturation genome editing. Nature 2018;562(7726):217–22.

[31] Starita LM, Islam MM, Banerjee T, et al. A multiplex homology-directed DNA repair assay reveals the impact of more than 1,000 BRCA1missense substitution variants on protein function. Am J Hum Genet 2018;103(4): 498–508.

[32] Drost M, Tiersma Y, Thompson BA, et al. A functional assay–based procedure to classify mismatch repair gene variants in Lynch syndrome. Genet Med 2018. https://doi.org/10.1038/s41436-018-0372-2.

[33] Starita LM, Ahituv N, Dunham MJ, et al. Variant Interpretation: Functional Assays to the Rescue. Am J Hum Genet 2017;101(3):315–25.

[34] Fowler DM, Araya CL, Fleishman SJ, et al. High-resolution mapping of protein sequence-function relationships. Nat Methods 2010;7(9):741–6.

[35] Ernst A, Gfeller D, Kan Z, et al. Coevolution of PDZ domain-ligand interactions analyzed by high throughput phage display and deep sequencing. MolBiosyst 2010;6(10):1782–90.

[36] Hietpas RT, Jensen JD, Bolon DNA. Experimental illumination of a fitness landscape. Proc Natl Acad Sci U S A 2011;108(19):7896–901.

[37] Weile J, Roth FP. Multiplexed assays of variant effects contribute to a growing genotype-phenotype atlas. Hum Genet 2018;137(9):665–78.

[38] Movva R, Greenside P, Marinov GK, et al. Deciphering regulatory DNA sequences and noncoding genetic variants using neural network models of massively parallel reporter assays. PLoS One 2019;14(6):e0218073.

[39] Hoskinson DC, Dubuc AM, Mason-Suares H. The current state of clinical interpretation of sequence variants. CurrOpin Genet Dev 2017;42:33–9.

[40] Koczkowska M, Chen Y, Callens T, et al. Genotype-phenotype correlation in NF1: evidence for a more severe phenotype associated with missense mutations affecting <em>NF1</em>codons 844–848. Am J Hum Genet 2018;102(1):69–87.

[41] RNA-based NF1testing on blood: Available at: https://www.uab.edu/medicine/genetics/medical-genomics-laboratory/testing-services/nf1-legius-syndrome-and-rasopathies/nf1-via-rna. Accessed July 22, 2019.

[42] Zhou J, Theesfeld CL, Yao K, et al. Deep learning sequence-based ab initio prediction of variant effects on expression and disease risk. Nat Genet 2018;50(8): 1171–9.

[43] Evans P, Wu C, Lindy A, et al. Genetic variant pathogenicity prediction trained using disease-specific clinical sequencing data sets. Genome Res 2019 Jul;29(7): 1144–51.

[44] Sundaram L, Gao H, Padigepati SR, et al. Predicting the clinical impact of human mutation with deep neural networks. Nat Genet 2018;50(8):1161–70.

[45] Argelaguet R, Velten B, Arnol D, et al. Multi-omics factor analysis-a framework for unsupervised integration of multi-omics data sets. Mol Syst Biol 2018;14(6):e8124.

[46] Singh A, Shannon CP, Gautier B, et al. DIABLO: an integrative approach for identifying key molecular drivers from multi-omics assays. Bioinformatics 2019. https://doi.org/10.1093/bioinformatics/bty1054.

[47] Ipe J, Swart M, Burgess KS, et al. High-throughput assays to assess the functional impact of genetic variants: a road towards genomic-driven medicine. ClinTranslSci 2017; 10(2):67–77.

[48] Perrino C, Barabási AL, Condorelli G, et al. Epigenomic and transcriptomic approaches in the post-genomic era: path to novel targets for diagnosis and therapy of the ischaemic heart? Position Paper of the European Society of Cardiology Working Group on Cellular Biology of the Heart. Cardiovasc Res 2017;113(7):725–36.

[49] Zhu Y, Tazearslan C, Suh Y. Challenges and progress in interpretation of non-coding genetic variants associated with human disease. ExpBiol Med (Maywood) 2017; 242(13):1325–34.

[50] Woods NT, Baskin R, Golubeva V, et al. Functional assays provide a robust tool for the clinical annotation of genetic variants of uncertain significance. NPJ Genom Med 2016;1:16001.

Advances in Molecular Pathology 2 (2019) 21–33
ADVANCES IN MOLECULAR PATHOLOGY

Genomic Data in the Electronic Health Record

Nephi A. Walton, MD, MS[a,*], Darren K. Johnson, MS[a], Thomas N. Person, MS[a], Srikar Chamala, PhD[b]
[a]Geisinger Genomic Medicine Institute, 100 N Academy Ave, Danville, PA 17822, USA; [b]Department of Pathology, Immunology and Laboratory Medicine, University of Florida, 1600 Southwest Archer Road, Gainesville, FL 32610, USA

KEYWORDS

• EHR • Genomic data • HL7 • FHIR • Clinical decision support • GACS • Infobuttons • Precision medicine

KEY POINTS

- Integration of genomic data into the electronic health record (EHR) is in its infancy.
- Current genomic data standards Health Level Seven International/Fast Healthcare Interoperability Resource are not adequate to scale genomic data integration.
- Genetic phenotypes are poorly defined and need standard definition to facilitate delivery of phenotypic information from the laboratory to the EHR and vice versa.
- Clinical decision support (CDS) holds great promise for genomics but has had limited utility because executing CDS has required manual entry of genetic conditions into the problem list for decision support.
- To further enable progress in this field of research, EHR vendors should provide an infrastructure for structured genetic data with open application programming interfaces.

INTRODUCTION

Precision medicine holds significant promise to improve patient health. In order to achieve the goals of precision medicine, genomic information must be integrated into clinical care. This integration can be accomplished through the integration of genomic data into the electronic health record (EHR), thus enabling effective clinical use. Providing clinical decision support (CDS) tools and targeted information to both patients and providers based on genomic sequence information holds significant promise in improving health. This need has long been recognized and is being made a priority by several large research initiatives as more genetic data become available. The current landscape is in a primitive state that is ripe for research and innovation. This article compares and contrasts genomic data storage systems with PACS (Picture Archiving and Communication Systems) and devises several paths forward to accomplish a scalable integration of genomic data.

SIGNIFICANCE

This topic is of great importance to medicine because it has been a recent focus of several major research initiatives. Innovation, standards development, and external information resources are needed to enable a scalable integration of genomic data into the EHR. This article gives a thorough overview of the landscape and provides gaps and research needs for several key areas.

Disclosure: This article was Funded by NIH/NHGRI EMR Linked Biobank to Assess Outcomes in Participants and their Relatives Receiving Genomic Results U01HG8679 (eMERGE) and NIH/NHGRI A Unified Clinical Genomics Database U41HG009650 (ClinGen).

*Corresponding author, *E-mail address:* nawalton@geisinger.edu

https://doi.org/10.1016/j.yamp.2019.07.001
2589-4080/19/

PRESENT RELEVANCE AND FUTURE AVENUES TO CONSIDER OR TO INVESTIGATE

This article presents the current state and suggests several potential options for moving forward, along with many challenges that are currently being faced to integrate genomic data into the EHR. This article provides a clear landscape on which to build tools to enable precision medicine and improve patient care.

SUMMARY

EHRs are not well equipped for structured genetic data. Although several paths forward have been devised, there is still significant research needed to achieve a scalable integration of genomic data. Most integration has been performed at academic centers with ancillary systems. EHR vendors only recently offered the native ability to incorporate structured genetic data with limited clinical implementation. Health Level Seven International (HL7) and Fast Healthcare Interoperability Resource (FHIR) standards for genomics are evolving and need further development. There is a lack of available resources to deliver targeted information on genetic variants to patients and providers. Standards development is needed to enable delivery of genetic and phenotypic information from the laboratory into the EHR and vice versa.

Current State and Emerging Technology

Precision medicine has long been touted as a means to improve health through targeted clinical management based on genetic information. With this goal in mind, the integration of genetic information into health care is viewed as major priority around the world. These efforts hold such importance that several national and international initiatives have been launched with substantial funding to pursue this goal [1]. Although the idea holds promise, most genetic data currently exist in the EHR as a scanned document, usually from a fax, and are stored as portable document format (PDF) files [2,3]. The nature of this type of data storage limits extraction of discrete result elements, which prevents automated data extraction. This limitation hinders the ability to implement CDS and translational biomedical research [4] and requires that a human finds and reads the document to act on it, leaving the information subject to inaction, mixed interpretation, and variable courses of action. To bypass the lack of infrastructure to accommodate structured genomic data, several health care systems have manually entered these results into other structured data fields, such as listing pharmacogenomic variants as allergies or genetic findings as items on the problem list [5]. Although these solutions were not ideal, they did allow decision support to be executed around this information.

Even if the PDF were a computable format, it only reports the findings of interest for the testing indication. Whole-exome sequencing (WES) is becoming a more common form of genetic testing, and there is a considerable amount of potentially useful data that is available from this testing that is largely ignored and never enters the EHR in any form. Laboratories do report American College of Medical Genetics (ACMG) secondary findings [6] from WES, which appear in sequencing reports as part of the scanned PDF; however, a large portion of other, potentially valuable information is left locked in a laboratory, unable to be used in clinical care. This information has a value that is likely to increase over the patients' lifetimes as they age and succumb to more disease.

Because sequencing data are rapidly becoming more available, it is important that clinicians are able to harness the full potential of the information. It is also important to ensure these genomic data are integrated into the EHR in a way that allows them to be used to further direct patient care and provide optimal patient outcomes. This goal is currently far from the present situation. EHRs have only recently allowed storage of discrete genomic information. Of the top 3 EHR vendors, only 1 has implemented this in a clinical setting, although another has announced plans for that capability at the time of writing. These early implementations have considerable deficiencies and there is much work needed to facilitate the useful implementation of genomic data into the EHR [7]. Most of the work that has been done to this point has been through ancillary systems connected to the EHR. Pharmacogenomic variants are perhaps the most widely implemented form of genetic data that enters the EHR. Nearly all of these data are implemented and stored through third-party software or homegrown software developed at academic hospitals [8,9]. Despite the recent growth in availability of tools for pharmacogenomics, most health care systems have yet to implement these systems, partly because of poorly defined clinical workflows for these new data. This critical area of research needs attention [10]. Third-party, disease-focused systems (outside of the EHR) are beginning to emerge that can house large stores of genetic data and allow connections to the EHR, interpret variants, and provide decision support or other information [11,12]. This area of precision medicine is new and evolving, and will grow quickly over the next few years.

The scientific and academic health care community has recognized the need for integration of genomic data into the EHR, and several research collaborations have made this area of research a priority, including the Electronic Medical Records and Genomics (eMERGE) network [2,13], the Clinical Sequencing Exploratory Research (CSER) consortium [2,14], and the Implementing Genomics in Practice (IGNITE) network [7,15]. Significant progress has been made through these efforts; however, there is still substantial research needed to achieve true integration and realize the goals of precision medicine.

Types of Genomic Variants

DNA of any 2 unrelated individuals is about 99.5% identical [16], and the small fraction of differences are called genomic (or genetic) variations. The amount of genomic variation among close family or related members is even smaller, whereas, conversely, the variation increases between individuals from different populations or ethnic groups. These genomic variations are one of the main factors, along with lifestyle and environmental factors, that dictates people's physical phenotypes (eg, skin or eye color, height), disease susceptibility, medication response [17], and microbiota [18]. Identification of genomic variants among people has been standardized by comparing their DNA sequence with a reference human genome generated by the Human Genome Project. This genome is continuously being updated, and the improved versions have been numbered (eg, hg19, hg38). These genomic differences come in different sizes. Some are simple single base differences, and others involve several thousands of bases. Sometimes major portions of chromosomes or even whole chromosomes are involved in genomic variation [19].

Modern systems are not well suited to capture the breadth of this genomic variation. Although existing systems may do well with capturing single nucleotide changes, there are many diseases driven by multiple types of complex variation. For example, Beckwith-Wiedemann syndrome (BWS), one of the most common pediatric cancer predisposition syndromes, can be caused by single nucleotide variants, multiple nucleotide variants, microdeletions, microduplications, or methylation changes [20]. Therefore, to drive precision medicine around this disease, the EHR must be able to accurately and adequately accommodate all these types of variation. Descriptions of some of the most commonly reported genomic variant types used in clinical genomic testing are provided here.

Single nucleotide variants

These are the most common genetic variants, in which a single nucleotide at a specific position on the reference genome is substituted with a different nucleotide. On average they occur every 1000 nucleotides in an individual's genome [21]. Most of these substitutions are benign, but a few have severe impacts on human health. For example, substitution of the A nucleotide with T on chr11 position 5,248,232 causes sickle cell anemia [22].

Multiple nucleotide variants

This genomic variant category is similar to single nucleotide variants (SNVs), but, instead of single nucleotide base pair substitution, it involves the substitution of multiple base pairs with the same number but different sequence of base pairs [23].

Insertions, deletions, and indels

These genomic variants are the second most frequent. Additional nucleotide base pairs in these variants tend to be inserted, and/or existing base pairs are deleted from a DNA sequence. By definition, the insertions and deletions can be from 1 to 1000 base pairs (bp) in length [19,24]. The larger insertions and deletions (>1000 bp) are grouped into separate genomic variant categories called structural variants, which include translocations, inversions, and copy number variants [19,24].

Translocation and inversions

In the case of both translocations and inversions, segments of DNA sequences are rearranged. Translocations occur when a portion of a continuous nucleotide sequence is translocated to a new position within the genome, whereas inversions maintain genomic positions but are backward from their original orientation [23]. Examples of human diseases caused by inversions and translocations are hemophilia A [25–27] and Ewing sarcoma [28,29].

Copy number variations

Copy number variation (CNV) genomic variants are increases or decreases in the copy number of a given region in the genome [23]. These variations are also referred to as deletions, duplications, microdeletions, or microduplications. It is common to find CNVs in the human genome and most of the CNVs are not deleterious. Up to 100 genes could be completely deleted without having any phenotypic consequences [30]. However, CNVs are also known to be responsible for many genetic syndromes and other human diseases [31–35].

Short tandem repeats

Short tandem repeats (STRs) are short (1–6 bp) DNA nucleotide base pairs repeated consecutively [36]. STRs are also known as microsatellites and microsatellite instability (MSI) in the somatic/cancer world [37]. It is estimated that 3% of the human genome and 6% of human coding regions constitute STRs [38,39]. Numerous STRs have been shown to play crucial roles in several human diseases [40,41], such as Huntington disease [36,42] and fragile X [43]. In addition, MSIs may serve as biomarkers in certain cancers [37,44,45].

DNA methylation

DNA methylation is modification of DNA through the addition of methyl groups. These modifications are one of the most well-understood epigenetic mechanisms of gene regulation. Several diseases are diagnosed through assessment of DNA methylation, including Prader-Willi syndrome [46], and BWS [20]. These epigenetic markers also have an emerging role in cancer diagnosis and treatment [47,48].

Aneuploidy

Aneuploidy is having an abnormal number of 1 or more chromosomes [49]. This condition is typically diagnosed through a karyotype. Down syndrome is the result of having 3 copies of chromosome 21 [50]. Aneuploidies also play a significant role in cancer [51,52].

Primary Genetic Testing Methodologies and Trends

Karyotype

A karyotype is a visual depiction of an individual's chromosomes. Creating a karyotype requires that living cells are cultured and chemically arrested in metaphase. Cells are then fixed on a microscope slide and stained to allow the chromosomes to be visualized, digitally imaged, and then arranged in order on a computer. Karyotypes are used to determine large (>5 Mb) chromosomal abnormalities that can be seen visually, such as aneuploidy, translocations (balanced and unbalanced), insertions, or deletions [53].

Chromosome microarray

Chromosomal microarrays (CMAs) are a microchip testing platform that uses labels or probes that bind to specific regions of the DNA. The microarray is built like a grid, with thousands of probes that can span across all 46 chromosomes. A computer analyzes the microarray to detect differences between a control sample and the patient's DNA. CMAs can detect CNVs, most chromosomal abnormalities (trisomy, monosomy), and unbalanced translocations or rearrangements. CMAs do not detect point mutations or very small duplications or deletions. They are also unable to detect balanced chromosomal rearrangements, thus limiting their potential to replace the karyotype [54].

Single gene/variant testing

The goal of these tests is to confirm 1 or more suspected genetic variants in a single gene or locus. These tests are inexpensive and commonly ordered. For example, mutations in *F2* and *F5* genes are screened to assess increased risk for thrombosis [55]. A second example is detection of actionable genetic variants in specific cancers. Mutations in *BRAF* and *KRAS* genes are routinely tested for in colorectal cancer [56].

Gene panel

The goal of these tests is to identify several genomic variants across multiple genes corresponding with a single disease or group of similar diseases. This form of genetic testing is currently one of the most popular because it is a cost-effective way to screen for disease-relevant mutations across multiple genes. However, WES is gaining ground in replacing some of the large panels as the price comes down [57]. Gene panels are also offered for many inherited disease categories, including but not limited to autism, cardiomyopathy, hearing loss, drug metabolism (pharmacogenomics), and epilepsy [57–60].

Whole-genome and whole-exome sequencing

Whole-genome sequencing (WGS) has the potential to identify genomic variants across an entire genome. In contrast, whole-exome tests are limited to identifying variants within only the exonic regions of the genome, covering approximately 1.1% of the genome [61]. These testing methods tend to be more costly, although the cost of WES is nearing that of some panels [62]. Also, they generate several hundreds of thousands of genomic variants (with no known functional relevance), thus making clinical interpretation and reporting difficult [63]. These testing methods are typically used in clinical situations in which the disease or phenotype under study either does not have applicable gene panel tests or existing gene panel tests have failed [63]. Although WES theoretically covers all expressed genes, focused genetic panels still tend to have better coverage of genes for the targeted disorder [64]. WES platforms have increasingly been able to detect CNVs but have not achieved the level of accuracy of CMA for detecting large variants [65], partly because of the limited coverage in noncoding regions. WGS is better suited to detect CNV's because of the increased coverage [66].

There have been significant changes in approach to genetic diagnoses of patients over time. As technology progresses, clinicians have been able to look closer at the genome and look at more of it at once. They started with karyotyping using microscopic images to detect large structural variation and improved on the ability to detect smaller structural changes with microarrays. They began sequencing single genes or variants, then moved to gene panels, then to WES, and are embarking on an era of WGS. As they have progressed, each prior testing technology has a more limited role but has not lost its utility. At present, WGS is rarely ordered clinically. As WGS becomes cheaper it could replace single gene testing, gene panels, WES, and even CMA [66]. One of the continued challenges for adoption of WGS is that it generates a large number of variants with uncertain significance, which sometimes complicates clinical care [67]. As clinicians learn more about the genome, this limitation will get weaker and the case for more comprehensive sequencing will become stronger, which is likely to lead to an increased use of comprehensive testing and the large amount of sequencing data that come along with it.

Tissue-Specific Testing

To complicate things further, any given cell in the human body could have a different DNA sequence than other cells because of errors in replication or mosaicism. Genomic testing is typically classified as either germline or somatic testing. Germline testing is primarily used to identify inheritable genetic variants, whereas somatic testing is performed for detecting genetic variants that are present in certain types of tissue. Somatic testing is primarily used for testing tumor samples in oncology. However, many diseases are caused by somatic changes, such as vascular malformations [68] and overgrowth syndromes [69], which require testing of affected tissues beyond blood to capture genetic changes. Effective integration of genomic data into the EHR will need to support both somatic and germline testing. Current ancillary systems tend to be focused solely on either germline or somatic testing. Native EHR infrastructure is not currently well suited for somatic testing.

Which Data to Store

The storing of next-generation sequencing (NGS) genomic data for dynamic access through the EHR is a major challenge that has yet to be fully solved. There are 2 primary challenges to address: (1) determining how to store genetic information, and (2) determining which information to store. A standard NGS pipeline flows as follows: FASTQ data (the raw genomic sequencing reads) [70] are aligned against the human reference genome generating a BAM (binary alignment map) file [71]. This file is then used to identify genomic variants to create a VCF (variant call format) file [72]. These genomics variants are interpreted for their impact on patient health, whereas only clinically actionable variants are reported into the EHR. At each step in the process, several magnitudes of data are lost, giving rise to more meaningful data. For example, typically the FASTQ files range from several gigabytes to more than 100 GB, whereas the resulting VCF file measures only several megabytes and contains up to several thousands of genetic variants. Furthermore, the final genomic test reports that are imported into the EHR are only several kilobytes and contain only a handful of genetic variants. The size and complexity of raw and intermediate genomic data prohibit storing them in the EHR. This limitation is well recognized.

One trending solution involves storing raw and intermediate genomic data externally to the EHR in a genomic archiving and communication system (GACS) while housing only the variants or reported data that are actively being used in patient care in the native EHR (Fig. 1) [73,74]. These systems are analogous to existing PACS used in radiology. PACS can serve as a successful model on which to build a new genetic data storage and access system. There are several similarities between systems that store imaging and those that store genetic data:

1. Both involve large data sets that EHRs are not inherently built to store or manipulate.
2. Both data sets are analyzed by a specialist who provides an interpretative report that is transmitted to the EHR.
3. Both present the opportunity for reporting of incidental findings.

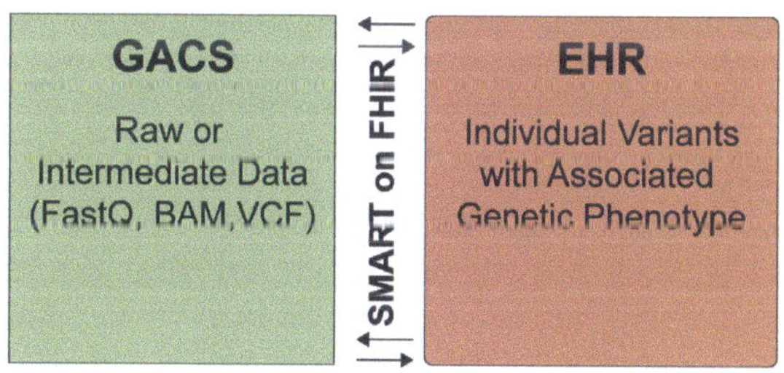

FIG. 1 GACS. FHIR, Fast Healthcare Interoperability Resource.

4. Both require a special viewer to view and interpret the larger data set.
5. Both can be reanalyzed by a clinician in the context of the current state of the patient to glean additional information not contained in the report.
6. Domain specialists often have expertise in certain areas of interpretation that may exceed those of the specialist writing the original report (eg, neurologists are good at looking at brain imaging). Many specialists are becoming experts in genetics related to their domain and should be enabled to view the pertinent genetic data in the context of the patient.

As genetic data systems are developed it is equally important to realize there are also several ways in which they are different from PACS:

1. Interpretation of genetic data may change over time with frequent reanalysis needed as more information becomes available, necessitating additional variants to be pushed into the EHR.
2. The relative value of genetic data does not degrade over time and may even become more valuable. For example, a chest radiograph at age 5 years is unlikely to be informative for a pneumonia at age 40 years, whereas a pathogenic variant in *BRCA1* discovered at birth becomes actionable at age 25 years.
3. Image interpretation is not highly dependent on outside knowledge databases. Genetic databases are updated constantly, and changes may dramatically alter interpretation.
4. Standard methods to view imaging data existed before the invention of PACS. Such standard viewers do not currently exist for genomics data.

Assuming that the GACS architecture is adopted, there is still considerable research that needs to be done surrounding the selection of variants that will be stored locally in the EHR. The local variants are to likely consist of those that may or may not be actionable but are known to cause a particular phenotype/disease in the patient, and those that are actionable in that they have clinical value even in the absence of the phenotype. Examples of such variants include pharmacogenomic variants and variants in cancer predisposition syndromes. Guidelines for actionability have been developed, but there is still considerable debate over which genes are actionable and even more so the variants that would be considered actionable [75,76]. To complicate matters further, as patients develop additional phenotypes over time, more variants in the ancillary system will become actionable and these systems must have ways to accommodate this.

Another challenge with the GACS-type system is that the use of genetic data outside of laboratory interpretation assumes the ancillary system can perform several functions of a clinical laboratory. Variant interpretation is a complex process that presents several challenges [77], foremost of which is that there is no comprehensive source of truth for variant interpretation. ClinVar is arguably the most robust knowledge base for clinical interpretation of pathogenicity of variants [78] but, as of the end of 2018, more than 75% of all ClinVar variants were represented by a single submitter providing little evidence for classification. The discordance in interpretations among laboratories shows the complexity of the interpretation process [79]. There is also concern regarding the clinical use of genetic data outside of that reported by a CLIA (Clinical Laboratory Improvement Amendments)-certified laboratory. Even if the exome data used were generated in a CLIA laboratory, there may be challenges using data for clinical decision making that is not on the laboratory report.

Dynamic Nature of Genetic Data

Systems developed to manage genomic data should be able to accommodate the dynamic nature of these data. Data that may not be actionable now could become actionable in the future, and variants considered pathogenic may change classification to benign. The actionability of some genetic changes depends on the presence of the corresponding phenotype. For example, variants in genes causing epilepsy may direct treatment in patients with a seizure disorder; however, not all patients with these pathogenic epilepsy variants have seizures, and therefore they do not need any treatment [80,81]. The interpretation of variants does change over time [82], which creates a situation in which the structured data in the EHR may become discordant with the scanned laboratory report, causing confusion and possibly inappropriate patient management. WES reanalysis over time has been shown to have significant diagnostic value, producing variants that had not been reported on the prior analysis [83,84]. This value underscores the importance of having a system that stores the structured data but also includes a tracking and maintenance system, which allows for updating and recording changes in patients' records over time.

The dynamic nature of genetic data raises the important question as to whether a physician or laboratory has a duty to reanalyze and return to the new clinically actionable information. The ACMG has released a statement regarding reanalysis of sequencing data that is focused on the laboratory performing the reanalysis

[85]. If these same data were housed as a native part of a patient's medical record or in an ancillary system, it raises the possibility that the health care system could be liable for its maintenance and interpretation over time.

Moving Genetic Data into the Electronic Health Record

To effectively enable integration of genetic data into the EHR in a scalable way requires standards for storing and transmitting genomic data, and standard application programming interfaces (APIs) that allow ancillary genomics systems to interface with the EHR, and these are both evolving areas in genomics. Epic Systems has built its native genetic data structure based on the HL7 Clinical Genomics Report standard. HL7 has been a leader in producing health care data standards for sharing and reusing information within many health care domains, including genomics. There is considerable push to adopt FHIR standards for genomics from research collaboratives [86]. FHIR is a standards framework for exchanging health care information developed by the HL7 community. FHIR has a strong foundation in Web standards, including XML, JSON, and HTTP, and incorporates support for RESTful architectures. The FHIR infrastructure is the basis of the Sync for Genes effort of the Precision Medicine Initiative to promote interoperability and data sharing for genomics [86]. The FHIR Molecular Sequence was designed for NGS data and holds promise as a standard for genomics. EHRs and laboratories have been hesitant to adopt FHIR for genomics in the early stages of maturity. Both the HL7 genetic data format and FHIR sequencing resource are evolving standards that have challenges that need to be addressed [73,87]. The eMERGE network is actively working with HL7 to improve the FHIR architecture for genomics. GACSs have been suggested to communicate with the EHR via a Smart-on-FHIR interface. However, most of the current EHRs do not support FHIR genomics standards [73,88].

At present, laboratories use HL7 messaging to pass laboratory results to a laboratory information system (LIS), where they are relayed to the EHR. Despite the use of HL7, laboratories are not using the HL7 Genomic Laboratory Report format to pass these data and are overwhelmingly not passing any structured genetic data at all. The LIS is designed to support laboratory operations and facilitate the ordering and return of laboratory tests; however, most of them have not been designed to facilitate the use of discrete genetic data in the EHR. For this reason, there is some question as to role of the LIS with regard to genetic data because it potentially adds another layer of complexity to the solution if an EHR is enabled to handle genetic data and the LIS is not. Discrete genomic data in the LIS cannot be used in clinical care and the easiest path to integration may be to maintain existing workflows for genetic data in the LIS and enable a separate data stream into the EHR from the laboratory, as shown in Fig. 2A. Fig. 2B shows the flow of data into an LIS that can manage and pass structured genetic data into the EHR. Fig. 2C shows a work flow with a GACS implemented. Some vendors are suggesting that a modified version of the LIS might function as a GACS, as shown in Fig. 2D.

Phenotype in Relation to Genetic Variants

With the millions of possible variants encompassing human differentiation, it is difficult to construct and maintain decision support and information delivery models at the variant level. An exception may be made for common highly penetrant variants; however, most diseases are driven by one of hundreds or thousands of different pathogenic variants in a gene. For example, as of May 2019, there were 2969 pathogenic variants documented in ClinVar for *BRCA1* alone, which underscores the importance of having a genetic phenotype as a point of decision making and decision support, as shown in Fig. 3. This phenotype can be a disease, a drug metabolizer status, or even a subphenotype in which a modifier variant changes disease risk and alters the recommended path of care. Even polygenic risk scores ultimately drive a phenotype on which to provide decision support. Some systems have been designed to require that variants drive these phenotypes with mappings from variant to phenotype performed within in the EHR. The problem with this approach is that it is recreating the work of the sequencing laboratory whose job is to assign a phenotype to a variant. The better solution may be to standardize genomic phenotypes so they can be passed uniformly from different laboratories into the EHR. For example, laboratories may report *BRCA1* variants under *BRCA1* and *BRCA2* Associated Hereditary Breast Cancer, whereas another may report them under the phenotype Breast-ovarian cancer, familial 1. Similarly, for pharmacogenomic variants one laboratory may report an extensive metabolizer, whereas another may report the phenotype as normal metabolizer. Assignment of these variants to the correct phenotype is critical because the phenotype is the data element on which all decision support is constructed and to which all information resources are mapped. Without standardization, the hospital system either has to result to manual assignment of the phenotype or mapping of phenotypes for each laboratory they use and for every condition the laboratory tests for. For exome sequencing mapping all these phenotypes becomes an impossible task because new genetic disorders are

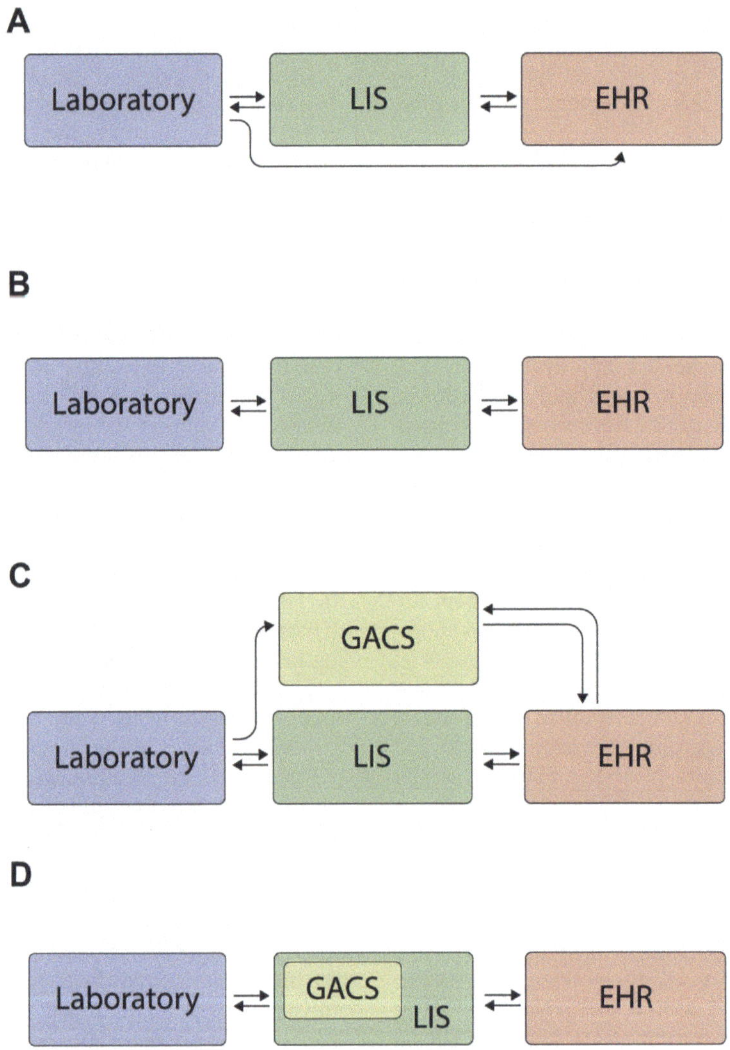

FIG. 2 Genetic data flows from the laboratory to the EHR. Data flow (**A**) demonstrates maintenance of current data flow while an separate data stream sends genetic information from the lab to the EHR. Data flow (**B**) illustrates the flow of data into an LIS that can manage and pass structured genetic data into the EHR. Data flow (**C**) demonstrates the incorporation of an ancillary GACS system that stores and provides access to genetic data. Data flow (**D**) demonstrates the integration of GACS capability within an LIS. (*Courtesy of* Nephi Walton, MD, MS, FACMG, Forty Fort, PA.)

discovered frequently. The granularity of phenotypes on which decision support is based also needs some standardization; for example, patients with *BRCA1* pathogenic variants have different surveillance guidelines than those with *BRCA2* pathogenic variants, so grouping them together under *BRCA1* and *BRCA2* Associated Hereditary Breast Cancer is probably not ideal. To further complicate matters, some conditions, such as BWS, have different surveillance guidelines depending on the genetic variation that causes the disease, adding another level of granularity to the problem [20]. There is currently no standard definition for genomic phenotypes because this remains an evolving area of research.

Uses of Genetic Data in the Electronic Health Record

Ultimately, genetic data have 3 primary purposes for being incorporated into the EHR: delivery of information

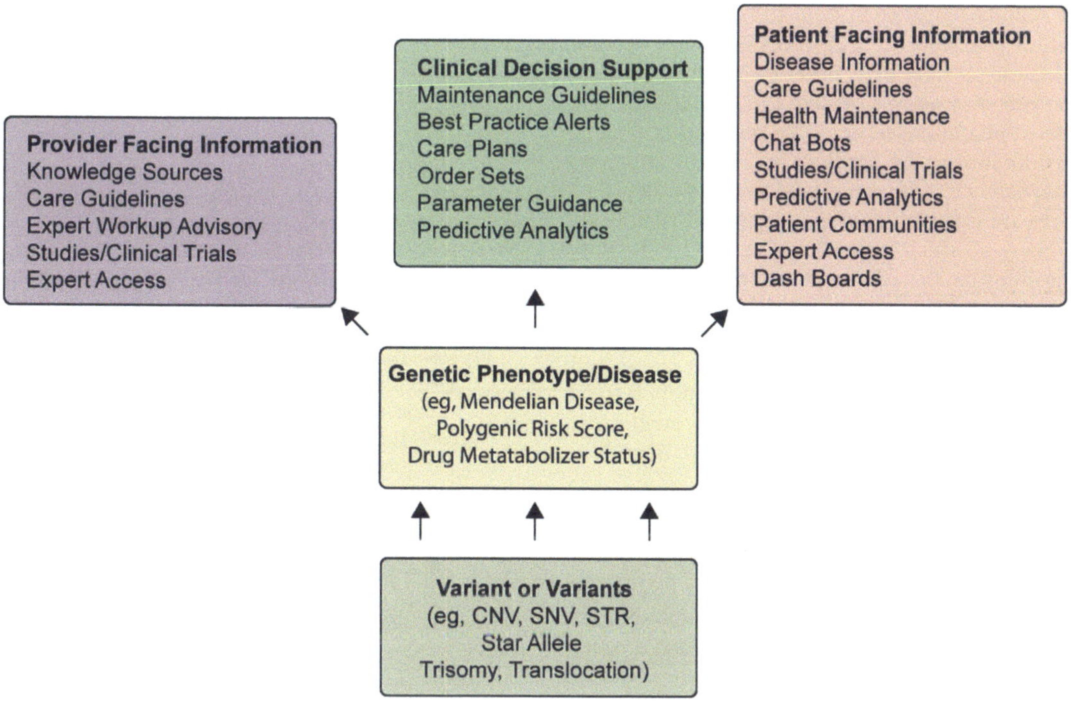

FIG. 3 Single gene variants or combinations of variants drive genetic phenotypes. These genetic phenotypes can then be utilized in the EHR to drive various forms of targeted information and clinical decision support. (*Courtesy of* Nephi Walton, MD, MS, FACMG, Forty Fort, PA.)

to providers, delivery of information to patients, and CDS to enable targeted management based on patients' genetic data and phenotypes.

Systems have been devised to deliver information to patients based on genomic data using Infobuttons as well as other proprietary technologies [89,90]. Infobuttons is a standard method of context-sensitive content delivery that has been widely implemented by EHR vendors [91,92]. Infobuttons are found next to terms on the problem list, medications, and laboratory tests. Providers can click on the Infobutton to link to resources specific to the term they are next to [91]. There are currently 2 major deficiencies that confound the delivery of standardized content: (1) there is currently no native ability in EHRs to enable Infobuttons with structured genetic data; (2) there is the lack of standardized structured resources to deliver information to patients and providers at the point of care. Similar to ancillary systems, pharmacogenomics is more mature in this realm. PharmGKB is currently the sole HL7-compliant Infobutton genomic data resource that can provide targeted information to patients and providers around genomic variants, although other resources can be used through OpenInfobuttons [93]. Efforts are underway through the eMERGE network and ClinGen to develop Infobutton-compliant genomic resources to deliver targeted information to patients and providers [94].

CDS systems are designed to use the EHR to assist in translating knowledge into appropriate clinical care. These systems, when implemented correctly, have been shown to be very effective in improving patient care [95–98]. Such improvements may be through stopping a physician from prescribing a contraindicated medication, providing tailored management guidelines, providing standardized order sets to manage a condition, or even systems that control not just effectiveness of therapy but selecting the right medication based on price [99]. CDS tools are not just for health care providers, they can also be used to assist patients in managing their health [100]. CDS has a strong role to play in precision medicine, assisting physicians in tailoring care to each patient's genetic condition without requiring excessive amounts of research on the physician's part [101]. These types of tools become exponentially more valuable as the collective knowledge of genetics and therapeutic options based on genetic data increases and the human capacity to store and synthesize this information is exceeded [102]. Most genomics decision support systems have been developed around pharmacogenomics at academic centers [9,73]. Implementing outside of pharmacogenomics has required adding genetic conditions to the problem list because structured data have only recently been available in EHRs [5].

There are many other uses for genomic data in the EHR, many of which are outlined in Fig. 3. Structured genetic information allows directing of patients and providers to studies and clinical trials based on the patient's genetic condition or predisposition. It allows patients to connect to social networks of patients with similar conditions. It also allows targeted support to patients to manage their own health care through expert access, chat bots, predictive analytics, or patient dashboards. The possibilities are endless.

Looking Ahead

Significant progress is needed to achieve a scalable integration of genomic data into the EHR. Improving the standards for genetic data and providing an adequate infrastructure to house genetic data in the EHR are two key components to achieving success in this area. A third and equally important step forward is the development of an open API to interact with and populate genetic data. EHR vendors have been soliciting input for development of genetic data systems; however, genomic data integration is in its infancy and an open architecture is needed so that the scientific community can perform the needed research and develop tools that will further inform development needs. Clinicians face many challenges, but there is great potential if they can enable this technology can be enabled and the promise of precision medicine delivered on.

REFERENCES

[1] Stark Z, Dolman L, Manolio TA, et al. Integrating genomics into healthcare: a global responsibility. Am J Hum Genet 2019;104(1):13–20.

[2] Shirts BH, Salama JS, Aronson SJ, et al. CSER and eMERGE: current and potential state of the display of genetic information in the electronic health record. J Am Med Inform Assoc 2015;22(6):1231–42.

[3] Abul-Husn NS, Kenny EE. Personalized medicine and the power of electronic health records. Cell 2019; 177(1):58–69.

[4] Tarczy-Hornoch P, Amendola L, Aronson SJ, et al. A survey of informatics approaches to whole-exome and whole-genome clinical reporting in the electronic health record. Genet Med 2013;15(10):824.

[5] Ohno-Machado L, Kim J, Gabriel RA, et al. Genomics and electronic health record systems. Hum Mol Genet 2018;27(R1):R48–55.

[6] Biesecker LG. ACMG secondary findings 2.0. Genet Med 2017;19(5):604.

[7] Sperber NR, Carpenter JS, Cavallari LH, et al. Challenges and strategies for implementing genomic services in diverse settings: experiences from the Implementing GeNomics In pracTicE (IGNITE) network. BMC Med Genomics 2017;10(1):35.

[8] Caraballo PJ, Hodge LS, Bielinski SJ, et al. Multidisciplinary model to implement pharmacogenomics at the point of care. Genet Med 2017;19(4):421.

[9] Rasmussen LV, Smith ME, Almaraz F, et al. An ancillary genomics system to support the return of pharmacogenomic results. J Am Med Inform Assoc 2019;26(4): 306–10.

[10] Patrinos GP, Giannopoulou E, Katsila T, et al. Integrating next-generation sequencing in the clinical pharmacogenomics workflow. Front Pharmacol 2019;10.

[11] Aronson SJ, Clark EH, Babb LJ, et al. The GeneInsight suite: a platform to support laboratory and provider use of DNA-based genetic testing. Hum Mutat 2011; 32(5):532–6.

[12] Furness M. Sapientia: accelerating rare disease diagnosis and treatment. Per Med 2016;13(5):415–8, Future Medicine.

[13] McCarty CA, Chisholm RL, Chute CG, et al. The eMERGE Network: a consortium of biorepositories linked to electronic medical records data for conducting genomic studies. BMC Med Genomics 2011;4(1):13.

[14] Green RC, Goddard KAB, Jarvik GP, et al. Clinical sequencing exploratory research consortium: accelerating evidence-based practice of genomic medicine. Am J Hum Genet 2016;98(6):1051–66.

[15] Weitzel KW, Alexander M, Bernhardt BA, et al. The IGNITE network: a model for genomic medicine implementation and research. BMC Med Genomics 2015;9(1):1.

[16] Levy S, Sutton G, Ng PC, et al. The diploid genome sequence of an individual human. PLoS Biol 2007; 5(10):e254.

[17] Wang L, McLeod HL, Weinshilboum RM. Genomics and drug response. N Engl J Med 2011;364(12): 1144–53.

[18] Gupta VK, Paul S, Dutta C. Geography, ethnicity or subsistence-specific variations in human microbiome composition and diversity. Front Microbiol 2017;8:1162.

[19] Feuk L, Carson AR, Scherer SW. Structural variation in the human genome. Nat Rev Genet 2006;7(2):85.

[20] Shuman C, Beckwith JB, Weksberg R. Beckwith-Wiedemann syndrome [Internet]. In: GeneReviews. Seattle (WA): University of Washington; 2016.

[21] Kim S, Misra A. SNP genotyping: technologies and biomedical applications. Annu Rev Biomed Eng 2007; 9:289–320.

[22] Piel FB, Steinberg MH, Rees DC. Sickle cell disease. N Engl J Med 2017;376(16):1561–73.

[23] Eilbeck K, Lewis SE, Mungall CJ, et al. The Sequence Ontology: a tool for the unification of genome annotations. Genome Biol 2005;6(5):R44.
[24] Sehn JK. Insertions and deletions (Indels). In: Clinical genomics. Elsevier; 2015. p. 129–50.
[25] Kumar D. Disorders of the genome architecture: a review. Genomic Med 2008;2(3–4):69–76.
[26] Lakich D, Kazazian HH, Antonarakis SE, et al. Inversions disrupting the factor VIII gene are a common cause of severe haemophilia A. Nat Genet 1993;5(3):236.
[27] Puig M, Casillas S, Villatoro S, et al. Human inversions and their functional consequences. Brief Funct Genomics 2015;14(5):369–79.
[28] Zheng J. Oncogenic chromosomal translocations and human cancer. Oncol Rep 2013;30(5):2011–9.
[29] Sankar S, Lessnick SL. Promiscuous partnerships in Ewing's sarcoma. Cancer Genet 2011;204(7):351–65.
[30] Zarrei M, MacDonald JR, Merico D, et al. A copy number variation map of the human genome. Nat Rev Genet 2015;16(3):172.
[31] Freeman JL, Perry GH, Feuk L, et al. Copy number variation: new insights in genome diversity. Genome Res 2006;16(8):949–61.
[32] Petro G, Mayr D, Hillemanns P, et al. Analysis of HER-2/neu amplification in endometrial carcinoma by chromogenic in situ hybridization. Correlation with fluorescence in situ hybridization, HER-2/neu, p53 and Ki-67 protein expression, and outcome. Mod Pathol 2004;17(3):277.
[33] Redon R, Ishikawa S, Fitch KR, et al. Global variation in copy number in the human genome. Nature 2006;444(7118):444.
[34] Shapira SK. An update on chromosome deletion and microdeletion syndromes. Curr Opin Pediatr 1998;10(6):622–7.
[35] Wilson D, Burn J, Scambler P, et al. DiGeorge syndrome: part of CATCH 22. J Med Genet 1993;30(10):852–6.
[36] Dashnow H, Lek M, Phipson B, et al. STRetch: detecting and discovering pathogenic short tandem repeat expansions. Genome Biol 2018;19(1):121.
[37] Carlson KD, Sudmant PH, Press MO, et al. MIPSTR: a method for multiplex genotyping of germline and somatic STR variation across many individuals. Genome Res 2015;25(5):750–61.
[38] O'Roak BJ, Vives L, Fu W, et al. Multiplex targeted sequencing identifies recurrently mutated genes in autism spectrum disorders. Science 2012;338(6114):1619–22.
[39] T O'Dushlaine C, Edwards RJ, Park SD, et al. Tandem repeat copy-number variation in protein-coding regions of human genes. Genome Biol 2005;6(8):R69.
[40] Gatchel JR, Zoghbi HY. Diseases of unstable repeat expansion: mechanisms and common principles. Nat Rev Genet 2005;6(10):743.
[41] Sun JH, Zhou L, Emerson DJ, et al. Disease-associated short tandem repeats co-localize with chromatin domain boundaries. Cell 2018;175(1):224–38.e15.
[42] Hannan AJ. Tandem Repeat Polymorphisms. Tandem Repeat Polymorphisms. Springer; 2012. p. 1–9.
[43] Garber KB, Visootsak J, Warren ST. Fragile X syndrome. Eur J Hum Genet 2008;16(6):666.
[44] Boland CR, Thibodeau SN, Hamilton SR, et al. A National Cancer Institute workshop on microsatellite instability for cancer detection and familial predisposition: development of international criteria for the determination of microsatellite instability in colorectal cancer. Cancer Res 1998;58(22):5248–57.
[45] Kim T-M, Laird PW, Park PJ. The landscape of microsatellite instability in colorectal and endometrial cancer genomes. Cell 2013;155(4):858–68.
[46] Cheon CK. Genetics of Prader-Willi syndrome and Prader-Will-like syndrome. Ann Pediatr Endocrinol Metab 2016;21(3):126.
[47] Bhat SA, Majid S, Rashid S. Diagnostic utility of epigenetics in breast cancer–a review. Cancer Treat Res Commun 2019;19:100125.
[48] Shariatpanahi AM, Yassi M, Nouraie M, et al. The importance of stool DNA methylation in colorectal cancer diagnosis: A meta-analysis. PLoS One 2018;13(7):e0200735.
[49] Hassold T, Hunt P. To err (meiotically) is human: the genesis of human aneuploidy. Nat Rev Genet 2001;2(4):280.
[50] Korenberg JR, Chen XN, Schipper R, et al. Down syndrome phenotypes: the consequences of chromosomal imbalance. Proc Natl Acad Sci U S A 1994;91(11):4997–5001.
[51] Shahjahani M, Hadad EH, Azizidoost S, et al. Complex karyotype in myelodysplastic syndromes: diagnostic procedure and prognostic susceptibility. Oncol Rev 2019;13(1).
[52] Rajagopalan H, Lengauer C. Aneuploidy and cancer. Nature 2004;432(7015):338.
[53] Haldeman-Englert CR, Saitta SC, Zackai EH. Chromosome disorders. In: Avery's diseases of the newborn. Elsevier; 2018. p. 211–23.e2.
[54] Palmer EE, Peters GB, Mowat D. Chromosome microarray in Australia: a guide for paediatricians. J Paediatr Child Health 2012;48(2):E59–67.
[55] Seligsohn U, Lubetsky A. Genetic susceptibility to venous thrombosis. N Engl J Med 2001;344(16):1222–31.
[56] Mostert B, Jiang Y, Sieuwerts AM, et al. KRAS and BRAF mutation status in circulating colorectal tumor cells and their correlation with primary and metastatic tumor tissue. Int J Cancer 2013;133(1):130–41.
[57] Myers KA, Johnstone D, Dyment DA. Epilepsy genetics: Current knowledge, applications, and future directions. Clin Genet 2019;95(1):95–111.
[58] Bos JM, Towbin JA, Ackerman MJ. Diagnostic, prognostic, and therapeutic implications of genetic testing for hypertrophic cardiomyopathy. J Am Coll Cardiol 2009;54(3):201–11.
[59] Relling MV, Evans WE. Pharmacogenomics in the clinic. Nature 2015;526(7573):343.

[60] Shearer AE, Smith RJ. Genetics: advances in genetic testing for deafness. Curr Opin Pediatr 2012;24(6):679.
[61] Venter JC, Adams MD, Myers EW, et al. The sequence of the human genome. Science 2001;291(5507):1304–51.
[62] Palmer EE, Schofield D, Shrestha R, et al. Integrating exome sequencing into a diagnostic pathway for epileptic encephalopathy: Evidence of clinical utility and cost effectiveness. Mol Genet Genomic Med 2018; 6(2):186–99.
[63] O'daniel JM, Lee K. Whole-genome and whole-exome sequencing in hereditary cancer: impact on genetic testing and counseling. Cancer J 2012;18(4):287–92.
[64] LaDuca H, Farwell KD, Vuong H, et al. Exome sequencing covers>98% of mutations identified on targeted next generation sequencing panels. PLoS One 2017;12(2):e0170843.
[65] Marchuk DS, Crooks K, Strande N, et al. Increasing the diagnostic yield of exome sequencing by copy number variant analysis. PLoS One 2018;13(12):e0209185.
[66] Whitford W, Lehnert K, Snell RG, et al. Evaluation of the performance of copy number variant prediction tools for the detection of deletions from whole genome sequencing data. J Biomed Inform 2019;94:103174.
[67] Hoffman-Andrews L. The known unknown: the challenges of genetic variants of uncertain significance in clinical practice. J Law Biosci 2017;4(3):648.
[68] Fereydooni A, Dardik A, Nassiri N. Molecular changes associated with vascular malformations. J Vasc Surg 2019;70(1):314–26.e1.
[69] Lalonde E, Ebrahimzadeh J, Rafferty K, et al. Molecular diagnosis of somatic overgrowth conditions: a single-center experience. Mol Genet Genomic Med 2019; 7(3):e536.
[70] Cock PJ, Fields CJ, Goto N, et al. The Sanger FASTQ file format for sequences with quality scores, and the Solexa/Illumina FASTQ variants. Nucleic Acids Res 2009; 38(6):1767–71.
[71] Li H, Handsaker B, Wysoker A, et al. The sequence alignment/map format and SAMtools. Bioinformatics 2009;25(16):2078–9.
[72] Danecek P, Auton A, Abecasis G, et al. The variant call format and VCFtools. Bioinformatics 2011;27(15): 2156–8.
[73] Dolin R, Boxwala A, Shalaby J. A pharmacogenomics clinical decision support service based on FHIR and CDS hooks. Methods Inf Med 2018;57(S 02): e115–23.
[74] Starren J, Williams MS, Bottinger EP. Crossing the omic chasm: a time for omic ancillary systems. JAMA 2013; 309(12):1237–8.
[75] Hunter JE, Irving SA, Biesecker LG, et al. A standardized, evidence-based protocol to assess clinical actionability of genetic disorders associated with genomic variation. Genet Med 2016;18(12):1258.
[76] Ramos EM, Din-Lovinescu C, Berg JS, et al. Characterizing genetic variants for clinical action. Am J Med Genet C Semin Med Genet 2014;166c(1):93–104.
[77] Harrison SM, Dolinsky JS, Johnson AEK, et al. Clinical laboratories collaborate to resolve differences in variant interpretations submitted to ClinVar. Genet Med 2017; 19(10):1096.
[78] Landrum MJ, Kattman BL. Clinvar at five years: delivering on the promise. Hum Mutat 2018;39(11): 1623–30.
[79] Harrison SM, Dolinksy JS, Chen W, et al. Scaling resolution of variant classification differences in ClinVar between 41 clinical laboratories through an outlier approach. Hum Mutat 2018;39(11):1641–9.
[80] Møller RS, Heron SE, Larsen LHG, et al. Mutations in KCNT 1 cause a spectrum of focal epilepsies. Epilepsia 2015;56(9):e114–20.
[81] Michelucci R, Pasini E, Malacrida S, et al. Low penetrance of autosomal dominant lateral temporal epilepsy in Italian families without LGI 1 mutations. Epilepsia 2013;54(7):1288–97.
[82] Mighton C, Charames GS, Wang M, et al. Variant classification changes over time in BRCA1 and BRCA2. Genet Med 2019. [Epub ahead of print].
[83] Baker SW, Murrell JR, Nesbitt AI, et al. Automated clinical exome reanalysis reveals novel diagnoses. J Mol Diagn 2019;21(1):38–48.
[84] Initiative EG, Berkovic SF, Goldstein DB, et al. The epilepsy genetics initiative: systematic reanalysis of diagnostic exomes increases yield. Epilepsia 2019;60(5): 797–806.
[85] Deignan JL, Chung WK, Kearney HM, et al. Points to consider in the reevaluation and reanalysis of genomic test results: a statement of the American College of Medical Genetics and Genomics (ACMG). Genet Med 2019;21(6):1267.
[86] Devaney S. All of us research program. New England Journal of Medicine 2019;381(7):668–76.
[87] Mascia C, Uva P, Leo S, et al. OpenEHR modeling for genomics in clinical practice. Int J Med Inform 2018; 120:147–56.
[88] Alterovitz G, Warner J, Zhang P, et al. SMART on FHIR genomics: facilitating standardized clinico-genomic apps. J Am Med Inform Assoc 2015;22(6):1173–8.
[89] Williams JL, Rahm AK, Zallen DT, et al. Impact of a patient-facing enhanced genomic results report to improve understanding, engagement, and communication. J Genet Couns 2018;27(2):358–69.
[90] Del Fiol G, Williams MS, Maram N, et al. Integrating genetic information resources with an EHR. In: AMIA annual symposium proceedings. American Medical Informatics Association; 2006.
[91] Del Fiol G, Rocha RA, Clayton PD. Infobuttons at intermountain healthcare: utilization and infrastructure. In: AMIA annual symposium proceedings. American Medical Informatics Association; 2006:180(4).
[92] Crump JK, Del Fiol G, Williams MS, et al. Prototype of a standards-based EHR and genetic test reporting tool coupled with HL7-compliant infobuttons. AMIA Jt Summits Transl Sci Proc 2018;2017:330.

[93] Heale BS, Overby CL, Del Fiol G, et al. Integrating genomic resources with electronic health records using the HL7 Infobutton standard. Appl Clin Inform 2016; 7(03):817–31.

[94] Overby CL, Rasmussen LV, Hartzler A, et al. A template for authoring and adapting genomic medicine content in the eMERGE infobutton project. In: AMIA annual symposium proceedings. American Medical Informatics Association; 2014.

[95] Blackmore CC, Mecklenburg RS, Kaplan GS. Effectiveness of clinical decision support in controlling inappropriate imaging. J Am Coll Radiol 2011;8(1): 19–25.

[96] Selby NM, Fluck RJ. Making the right decision: do clinical decision support systems for AKI improve patient outcomes? J Am Soc Nephrol 2018;29(2):352–4.

[97] Sperl-Hillen JM, Rossom RC, Kharbanda EO, et al. Priorities wizard: multisite web-based primary care clinical decision support improved chronic care outcomes with high use rates and high clinician satisfaction rates. EGEMS (Wash DC) 2019;7(1):9.

[98] Vader JM, La Rue SJ. Clinical Decision Support for Heart Failure Referral—More Work, Better Outcomes? J Card Fail 2017;23(10):727–8.

[99] Roncato R, Dal Cin L, Mezzalira S, et al. FARMAPRICE: a pharmacogenetic clinical decision support system for precise and cost-effective therapy. Genes 2019; 10(4):276.

[100] Grimmett C, Brooks C, Recio-Saucedo A, et al. Development of breast cancer choices: a decision support tool for young women with breast cancer deciding whether to have genetic testing for BRCA1/2 mutations. Support Care Cancer 2019;27(1):297–309.

[101] Krumm N, Shirts BH. Technical, biological, and systems barriers for molecular clinical decision support. Clin Lab Med 2019;39(2):281–94.

[102] Walsh S, de Jong EEC, van Timmeren JE, et al. Decision support systems in oncology. JCO Clin Cancer Inform 2019;3:1–9.

Hematopathology

Advances in Molecular Pathology 2 (2019) 35–43
ADVANCES IN MOLECULAR PATHOLOGY

Molecular Genetics in Myelodysplasia Outcomes Prognostication

Lucas H. Rifkin, MD, Eric Y. Loo, MD*
Department of Pathology and Laboratory Medicine, Dartmouth-Hitchcock Medical Center, One Medical Center Drive, Lebanon, NH 03756, USA

KEYWORDS
• Myelodysplasia • MDS • Prognostic scoring • Machine-learning • Molecular genetics • Risk-assessment

KEY POINTS

- Current prognostic scoring for myelodysplasia acceptably stratifies patients by survival, but is suboptimal for predicting response to treatment and risk of leukemic transformation.
- The genomic landscape in myelodysplasia has been fairly well-described and many independent markers of prognosis have been described, but these data have not yet been incorporated effectively into any prognostic scoring system.
- The quantity of data points and variables related to molecular genetic testing is immense, and optimal use of this information in future prognostic scoring systems may require a big-data approach with incorporation of machine-learning algorithms.

INTRODUCTION

Myelodysplastic syndromes (MDS) are a spectrum of clonal stem cell disorders, generally characterized by hematologic dyspoiesis and progressive peripheral cytopenias. These diseases exhibit broad behavioral heterogeneity, reflective of various clinical factors and the complex underlying genetics that drive pathobiology. Although the genomic landscape and chromosomal abnormalities underlying this set of diseases is being elucidated, the exact abnormalities in cellular pathways and sequence of events necessary to produce the myelodysplastic phenotype are still largely unexplained. This has been a hindrance to disease classification and prognostication, and an impediment to optimization of individual therapy.

The clinical behavior of MDS is variable. A subset of patients will have an indolent course with stable nonprogressive disease. Other MDS may behave aggressively, typified by a more rapidly progressive clinical course and genetic instability. Morbidity and mortality typically arises as a result of complications related to cytopenias or from progression to acute leukemia. Disease classification based on the morphologic evaluation of the bone marrow insufficiently stratifies disease outcomes for individual patients. In order to overcome this shortfall, clinical prognostic scoring systems have been developed as an adjunct to morphology-based disease classification.

There are currently no diagnostic tests that can fully predict the clinical behavior of MDS, but prognostic accuracy has improved with the ongoing integration of genetics into classification and scoring systems. This article outlines the evolution of prognostic modeling systems used to clinically stratify MDS. The key systems

Disclosure: The authors have nothing to disclose.

*Corresponding author, *E-mail address:* Eric.Y.Loo@hitchcock.org

https://doi.org/10.1016/j.yamp.2019.07.002
2589-4080/19/

that arose during the reiterative process are presented, and genetic drivers of the disease process are described as currently understood.

MORPHOLOGY-BASED DISEASE CLASSIFICATION AND ONSET OF PROGNOSTIC SCORING SYSTEMS

The French-American-British (FAB) working group provided the first widely accepted diagnostic criteria for MDS in 1982 [1]. The classification schema was based entirely around bone marrow morphologic data and incorporated items such as marrow blast percentage and ringed sideroblasts in delineating MDS categories. Although this FAB system laid the foundations for subsequent classification structures, there was broad variation in patient survival results. In general, the defined disease subtypes did not provide meaningful prognostic stratification for individual patient outcomes. In 1985, Foucar and colleagues [2] investigated this performance aspect of the FAB classification system, finding that the 5 morphologic subtypes stratified into only 2 groups with regard to survival. Many groups began to independently develop other methods for meaningful risk-stratification.

The Bournemouth score, published in 1985, focused on assessment of additional clinical factors and was the first of more than a dozen systems to classify and stratify risk in MDS to be developed over a relatively short time span [3–7]. None of these systems gained general acceptance, and the wide variety of proposed models and classification schemes created inconsistency in terminology and clinical practice. Growing demands for a consensus system led to the MDS Risk Analysis Workshop held at the Third International MDS Symposium in Chicago. Efforts from this project culminated in the publication of the International Prognostic Scoring System (IPSS) in 1997.

The IPSS incorporated both clinical and genetic factors, and it performed acceptably well in evaluating clinical outcomes of patients with MDS. For more than a decade, the IPSS functioned as a widely accepted risk-stratification tool, but the model had a few important limitations. Only a handful of the recurrent cytogenetic aberrancies in MDS were used by the scoring system. Additionally, the system often failed to assign an informed prognostic category, with an unacceptably high proportion of cases designated as intermediate-risk.

Shortly after the release of the IPSS, the World Health Organization (WHO) published its 2001 classification system for hematologic neoplasms, becoming the accepted successor to the FAB system. Major changes to disease classification were introduced, including a reduction in the threshold blast percentage required for a diagnosis of acute myeloid leukemia (AML) from 30% to 20% and recognition of deletion of 5q [del(5q)] as a genetically defined MDS subtype, among others. Although several recurrent genetic changes were included as AML-subtype defining, del(5q) was the sole cytogenetic abnormality that delineated an MDS entity.

The IPSS was revised in 2012 (IPSS-R). The prognostic marker categories were not altered (cytogenetics, cytopenias, and blast percentage), but assessment of markers in these categories was refined. The list of relevant cytogenetic abnormalities was expanded, the risk group tiers were increased from 3 to 5, and cytogenetic findings were given more prognostic weight. Although the presence and number of cytopenias were included in the original IPSS, the revised system provided a more nuanced assessment of cytopenia severity. Four minor variables that were not in the original system were also introduced (performance status, ferritin, lactate dehydrogenase, and beta-2 microglobulin), but these were not incorporated into the scoring calculations. The IPSS-R has endured for nearly a decade as a widely adopted prognostic system, providing a basis for treatment decisions in clinical practice.

However, the IPSS-R is most effective for cases with very high or low scores, corresponding to very poor and very good risk, respectively. Prognostic reliability suffers using the IPSS-R in cases with an intermediate prognostic score. In more recent years, technological advances have permitted the elucidation of previously unknown molecular drivers of MDS. The additional consideration of somatic gene sequence mutations has the potential to improve disease subclassification, outcomes prediction, and therapy (Fig. 1).

CLONAL HEMATOPOIESIS AND THE MOLECULAR GENETICS OF MYELODYSPLASTIC SYNDROMES

About 10% of apparently healthy persons older than the age of 65 years, and greater than 20% of those older than the age of 90 years, have been found to harbor recurrent harbor somatic mutations in myeloid malignancy-associated genes [8,9]. Presence of acquired mutations in myeloid neoplasm-related genes before the onset of disease has been termed clonal hematopoiesis of indeterminate potential (CHIP). Identification of CHIP confers a modest increase in risk for the development of a subsequent hematologic cancer, estimated at

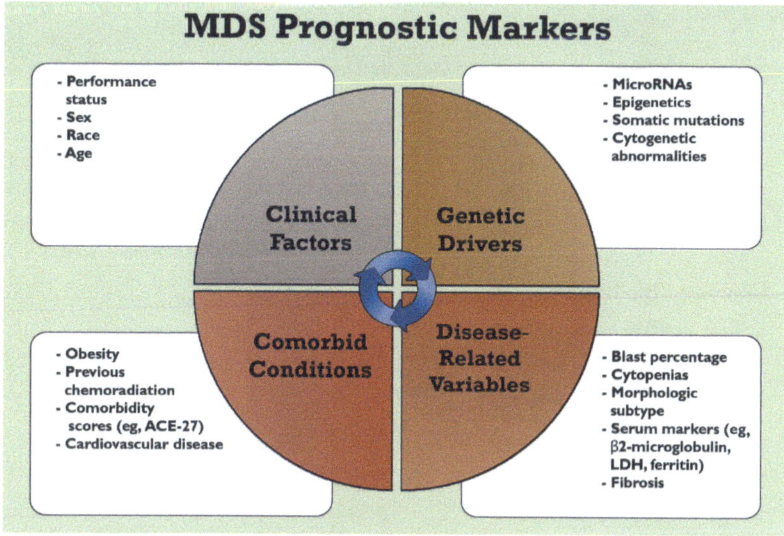

FIG. 1 Markers that have been used for risk prognostication in myelodysplasia.

about 1% per year [8,9]. The founding clonal event in MDS is thought to generally arise in myeloid-lineage committed stem cells, though lymphoid cancers have been found to carry gene mutations typical of age-related clonal hematopoiesis, suggesting that the initiating event may also occur in early common hematopoietic stem cells [10–13].

Disease behavior and clinical outcomes do correlate with these molecular sequence aberrancies. In persons who develop MDS, it has been found that a stable clinical course is associated with mutational stability, whereas cases with progression to AML typically show mutational instability [14]. Current prognostic scoring models are largely founded on underlying cytogenetic abnormalities, and there has been difficulty in synthesizing the extensive amount of molecular genetic data into a clinically accessible model for outcomes prognostication. Before 2005, only the *TP53*, *NRAS*, *KRAS*, *RUNX1*, and *ATRX* genes were known to be recurrently mutated in MDS, but variants were present in less than 10% of cases [15]. Bejar and colleagues [16] provided an early attempt at incorporating molecular data into MDS prognostic scoring in 2011. This study showed that somatic point mutations in a small selection of genes (*TP53*, enhancer of zeste 2 polycomb repressive complex 2 subunit [*EZH2*], ETS variant 6 [*ETV6*], *RUNX1*, and ASXL transcriptional regulator 1 [*ASXL1*]) were predictors of poor overall survival; IPSS-stratified MDS cases were shown to follow the survival curves of the next-highest IPSS risk group if they were found to carry mutations in 1 or more of these genes.

Currently, more than 40 genes have been found to be recurrently mutated in myelodysplasia. The frequency of involvement of most of these genes rarely exceeds 10%, and the variety of potential sequence aberrations is broad. However, nearly 90% of MDS patients will be found to have at least 1 somatic mutation in standard myeloid-gene sequencing panels commercially available today [17]. Unfortunately, there is presently no widely accepted prognostic model available for MDS that has successfully incorporated molecular genetic aberrations.

Some studies have demonstrated independent prognostic significance for various genes, and other studies have shown outcome correlations for several genes within a common general functional group [18]. Table 1 includes a synopsis of some commonly mutated genes in MDS and their prognostic impact.

SPLICEOSOME GENE MUTATIONS

The spliceosome is a multimegadalton ribonucleoprotein complex that functions to remove introns from transcribed pre-mRNA to generate mature mRNA. Splicing pathway gene mutations are common in MDS and collectively are found in more than half of all cases [19–21]. Splicing factor 3b subunit 1 (*SF3B1*), serine and arginine rich splicing factor 2 (*SRSF2*), U2 small nuclear RNA auxiliary factor 1

TABLE 1
Commonly Mutated Genes in Myelodysplasia

Functional Group	Gene	Frequency	Prognostic Effect	Notes
Spliceosome	SF3B1	20%–30%	Favorable	Associated with ring-sideroblast formation; currently the only gene that may influence WHO-subtype MDS assignment
	SRSF2	5%–15%	Adverse	Highly associated with TET2 mutations in chronic myelomonocytic leukemia (CMML)
	U2AF1	12%–16%	Adverse	—
	ZRSR2	~5%	Unclear	—
Tumor suppressor	TP53	5%–10%	Adverse	Associated with complex karyotypes
Cohesin complex	STAG2	5%–7%	Adverse	—
	RAD21	~2%	Adverse	Found more in secondary AML (s-AML)
	SMC3	~2%	Adverse	Found more in s-AML
DNA methylation	TET2	20%–30%	Unclear	Potential early event in MDS, common mutation in CHIP
	DNMT3A	~10%	Adverse	Potential early event in MDS, common mutation in CHIP
	IDH1/2	~5%	Unclear	—
Histone modification	ASXL1	15%–20%	Adverse	Potential early event in MDS, common mutation in CHIP
	EZH2	5%–10%	Adverse	—
Transcription factor	RUNX1	~10%	Adverse	May be acquired at disease progression
Cell signaling	NRAS	~5%	Adverse	Often found in cases with normal karyotypes
	CBL	~5%	Adverse	—

Abbreviations: CMML, chronic myelomonocytic leukemia; s-AML, secondary AML.

(*U2AF1*), and zinc finger CCCH-type (*ZRSR2*) are the most commonly affected genes, with alternative 3′ splice site usage, retained introns, and exon skipping being the most common resultant abnormal splicing events [20]. Despite the variety of affected genes and sequence aberrancies, these mutations result in common dysregulation of RNA splicing, protein synthesis, and mitochondrial dysfunction, which are mechanisms that are likely of etiologic importance in MDS [20]. However, the prognostic implications of mutations in this functional group differ depending on the affected gene.

SF3B1 is among most commonly mutated genes in MDS, found in 20% to 30% of all cases, and has generally been associated with a favorable prognosis [22]. Mutation of *SF3B1* is closely associated with ring-sideroblast formation; 60% to 80% of MDS with ring sideroblasts harbor mutated *SF3B1*, which is also common in the crossover entity myelodysplastic/myeloproliferative neoplasm with ringed sideroblasts and thrombocytosis [22]. *SF3B1* mutations tend to be mutually exclusive of other splicing factor mutations and other genetic abnormalities in MDS, with notable exceptions being DNA methyltransferase 3 alpha (*DNMT3A*) and tet methylcytosine dioxygenase 2 (*TET2*). [23] Mutation of other splicing factor genes, such as *U2AF1* and *SRSF2*, are found in less than 10% of MDS with ring sideroblasts; these generally demonstrate poor overall survival and not the favorable prognosis typical of *SF3B1*-mutated cases [24].

Though some overlap is observed, the aberrantly spliced genes associated with each mutated splicing factor have been found to be different, and this may contribute to disparities in disease phenotype and outcomes [20]. Mutations of U2AF1 are present in 12% to 16% of MDS cases and have been associated with anemia, thrombocytopenia, and worse survival in low-risk and high-risk MDS [25,26]. *SFSF2* mutations are found in approximately 5% to 15% of MDS overall, but are seen in about half of chronic myelomonocytic leukemia cases with comutation of *TET2*. [21,26] Mutated *SRSF2* has been reported as an independent poor-risk marker for overall survival and more frequent progression to AML [27,28]. *ZRSR2* is mutated in approximately 5% of MDS, and other splicing factors are mutated at lower frequencies, thus there is less certainty about their associations with disease behavior [19,28]. Some groups have found inferior overall survival and a higher rate of AML transformation in cases with *ZRSR2* mutation and wild type *TET2* [29].

Positive and negative relationships have been found with genes in other functional groups and with some conventional cytogenetic lesions. Cases with mutant (mut)-*U2AF1* have been found to be enriched for comutation of *ASXL1* and isolated trisomy 8, and inversely related to mut-*TP53* and complex karyotypes [25,28]. *SRSF2* mutations are found to functionally reduce protein expression of EZH2 through aberrant splicing but are also generally found to be mutually exclusive of *EZH2* gene sequence mutations [21,30]. *SRSF2* mutations do tend to show cooccurrence with mutations in isocitrate dehydrogenase [NADP(+)] 1, cytosolic (*IDH1*) or IDH 2, mitochondrial (*IDH1/2*), *TET2*, *RUNX1*, *ASXL1*, and stromal antigen (*STAG*)-*2*.

TP53 TUMOR SUPPRESSOR GENE MUTATIONS

In the setting of MDS, mutation and loss of the *TP53* tumor suppressor gene is associated with complex karyotype abnormalities and an unfavorable clinical course. Additional clinical features of MDS with *TP53* mutation include a lower median platelet count, higher bone marrow blast percentage, and relatively quick relapse after various forms of treatment [31]. This study also found that *TP53* mutations had an independent impact on prognosis as significant as having severe anemia and greater than having a bone marrow blast proportion of 10% to 29% (blast amounts equivalent to MDS with excess blasts-2 and oligoblastic AML), and that the impact of harboring a mutation was pronounced, even in patients assigned to the IPSS-R very-high-risk group [31]. Mutations of *TP53* were also strongly associated with poor outcomes after hematopoietic stem cell transplantation in MDS, predicting decreased over all survival and progression-free survival in univariate analysis [32].

About 20% of the myelodysplasia subtype MDS with isolated del(5q) harbor *TP53* mutations, and the WHO specifically identifies these cases as having an increased risk for leukemic progression and a poor response to lenalidomide. *TP53* is also the most commonly mutated gene in therapy-related MDS, found in 30% to 40% of cases. The selective pressure of cytotoxic therapy is thought to influence leukemogenesis through the preferential expansion of therapy-resistant background *TP53*-mutant positive clonal hematopoietic stem cell populations [33]. This quality of the early or founding clone is postulated to contribute to the frequent cytogenetic abnormalities and poor response to subsequent therapy typical of therapy-related MDS [33].

Patients with MDS and a complex karyotype generally harbor fewer mutations in genes other than *TP53* when compared with cases with noncomplex cytogenetics [16,31]. Additionally, cases with mut-*TP53* are found to carry fewer mutations in *ASXL1*, *U2AF1*, and *RUNX1* compared with wild-type (wt)-*TP53* cases. However, these cases are enriched for high-complexity cytogenetics, including monosomal karyotype, del(5q), monosomy 7, and abnormalities of chromosome 17; with abnormalities of chromosome 17 suggesting abrogation of wt-*TP53* activity [31].

COHESIN COMPLEX MUTATIONS

Cohesin is a multisubunit chromosome-associated protein complex that is critical for chromosome separation during cell division. The cohesin complex also participates in repair of DNA damage and regulation of gene expression through formation of large-scale chromatin structures. Genes encoding portions of this complex are mutated in about 10% to 15% of MDS cases, including structural maintenance of chromosomes (SMC)-1A, *SMC3*, RAD21 cohesin complex component (*RAD21*), *STAG1*, and *STAG2* [34]. Most variants are heterozygous nonsense and frameshift events, anticipated to cause protein truncation and loss of function. Similar to spliceosome mutations, variants affecting cohesin pathway genes tend to be exclusive of each other. Defects in cohesin are associated with poor overall survival in MDS, and are found at higher frequency in cases with excess blasts than in lower-grade disease [35]. The *STAG2* gene has specifically been identified as an independent marker of high-risk disease, and *RAD21* and *SMC3* mutations are more often found in secondary AML [35].

Chromatin modifiers (*ASXL1*) and transcriptional regulators (*RUNX1*, Ras-family genes, and BCL6 corepressor [*BCOR*]) have been described as frequently comutated, and cohesin may have a cooperative role in epigenetic regulation given reports of a higher response rate to hypomethylating agents in cohesin-mutated MDS [35]. Although cohesin dysfunction could theoretically lead to chromosomal instability given its role in cellular replication, this does not seem to bear out as a cause for progression or transformation in MDS because mutations have not been associated with aneuploidy or complex cytogenetics in AML [36].

MUTATIONS IN EPIGENETIC REGULATORS

Methylation of DNA and histone or chromatin modification are important ways through which gene expression can be epigenetically regulated, and genes affecting these processes are mutated in as many as 60% to 70% of MDS cases [37]. Variants in the *TET2*, *DNMT3A*, and *ASXL1* genes are commonly identified in age-related clonal hematopoiesis, and likely represent early events in the development of myelodysplasia [8,10]. The *IDH1*, *IDH2*, and *EZH2* genes are also commonly affected and typically grouped into the same functional categories, but their mechanisms of causing disease and prognostic significance are quite disparate.

TET2 and *DNMT3A* both have critical roles in DNA methylation; mutations occur in about 20% to 30% and approximately 10% of MDS cases, respectively. Despite the high prevalence and early acquisition in CHIP and MDS, the prognostic impact of *TET2* variants is uncertain owing to conflicting data [24]. Variants in *DNMT3A* are also early acquisitions in disease pathogenesis that are not usually acquired during disease progression; these have been found to be independent markers of poor prognosis and associated with both a higher risk of leukemic transformation and worse overall survival [38]. Detecting a pathogenic variant in either of these genes has been associated with better therapeutic responses to hypomethylating agents [39].

IDH-1 and *IDH-2* encode critical enzymes of the citric acid cycle, catalyzing the decarboxylation of isocitrate to α-ketoglutarate. They are generally included under the DNA methylation gene group because their metabolic product affects the function of some epigenetic regulators. The TET and KDM protein families, for example, functionally depend on α-ketoglutarate but are inhibited by 2-hydroxyglutarate, which is an abnormal oncometabolite produced as a result of mut-*IDH1/2*. Somatic variants are found in approximately 5% of MDS cases, but their prognostic impact is uncertain owing to conflicting data [24]. Although targeted IDH1/2 inhibitors are available, they are currently US Food and Drug Administration (FDA)-approved only for use in relapsed or refractory AML; evaluation is ongoing for utility in other cancer types.

ASXL1 is a key regulator of chromatin remodeling and gene activity. This gene is among most frequently affected across multiple myeloid neoplasms, and mutation has uniformly been associated with poor prognosis across the spectrum of malignant myeloid diseases [40]. Pathogenic mutations are typically nonsense or frameshift types, causing a C-terminus truncation. Alterations in function include overexpression of various genes such as *FOS* and PR/SET domain 16 (*PRDM16*) through an abnormal gain-of-function [41]. *ASXL1* variants are prevalent in CHIP and idiopathic cytopenia of undetermined significance may be found in about 15% to 20% of MDS cases, and they are independently predictive of poor survival [42,43]. *EZH2* is another gene involved in histone modification that may be mutated in 5% to 10% of MDS cases. Mutations of *EZH2* have also been shown to independently predict poor overall survival in MDS, in the context of both early and late-stage disease acquisition [44].

MUTATIONS AFFECTING TRANSCRIPTION FACTORS AND CELL SIGNALING PATHWAYS

Transcription factors and cell-signaling proteins are another heterogeneous category of recurrently mutated genes in MDS. Some of the more common examples include *RUNX1*, Cbl proto-oncogene (*CBL*), *NRAS*, and *BCOR*; though all of these are generally only found at a frequency of 5% to 10% or less [24]. Generally, mutation of these genes has been associated with adverse prognostic risk in MDS [24]. Mutations are most frequently found in *RUNX1*, which encodes the α-subunit of the core binding factor complex, a critical regulator of normal hematopoiesis. Across studies, *RUNX1* mutations predict poor overall survival and secondary acute leukemia transformation whether they occur as an early or late event [16,45].

NEW APPROACHES AND FUTURE DIRECTIONS FOR PROGNOSTIC MODELING

Accurate prognostic risk modeling in patients with MDS is crucial for the provision of correct risk-adapted treatment, with strategies ranging from observation to allogeneic stem cell transplantation. Azanucleoside therapy was first FDA-approved for use in MDS in 2004 and has been shown to prolong survival, improve quality of life, and delay progression to acute leukemia in 40% to 60% of patients [46–49]. However, the treatment is not curative, many patients with high-risk MDS fail to have an objective clinical response, and most patients who initially respond often become refractory to therapy within a few years. Significant effort has been invested in improving prognostication for myelodysplasia. The IPSS scoring system, published in 1997, was the first widely used system. Since then, several other models have been put forward for contemporary use, including the WHO Prognostic Scoring System (WPSS) in 2007, the MD Anderson Prognostic Scoring System (MDAPSS) in 2008, the French Prognostic Scoring System in 2011, and the IPSS-R in 2012. Comparative evaluations have shown that these systems are all able to stratify patients well by overall survival, but none of these prognostic tools are able to predict the probability of objective response to azanucleoside therapy [50].

Numerous gene sequence mutations are known to have independent prognostic significance in MDS (see previous discussion). This has generated significant interest in using mutational data to develop better tools for prediction of disease behavior [51]. Although gene mutations affecting DNA methylation pathways have been found to predict a better response to azanucleoside hypomethylating therapy, the practical application of these data has been limited. No method is able to reliably predict a poor-enough therapeutic response to warrant withholding hypomethylating agent treatment. Notably, commonly used predictive models were typically restricted to de novo disease, and the lack of post-treatment and secondary or therapy-related MDS cases may account for some of the discrepancies in behavioral predictions. However, there is ongoing effort to create new models that can reliably recognize those patients who would be better candidates for alternative and/or aggressive therapies.

Second-generation sequencing (so-called next-gen sequencing) techniques have led to a better understanding of the genomic landscape underlying the pathogenesis of MDS. Several attempts have been made to supplement existing prognostic modeling systems with molecular data to enhance their predictive power. In 2011, Bejar and colleagues [16] were able to use molecular markers of poor-outcome to improve outcome projections generated with the IPSS model. However, many subsequent attempts at refining contemporary scoring systems have produced inconsistent results; the prognostic significance of mutated genes is dissimilar, and their impact on survival seems to change depending on the clinical context [52–54]. It has generally been difficult to show added clinical value for inclusion of molecular markers in cases already categorized at high-risk or very-high-risk, but added value has been described in lower risk MDS in which allogeneic stem cell transplantation was being considered [53]. Regardless, it seems that integration of molecular data into any of the major established prognostic scoring systems can improve predictive power; Al-Issa and colleagues [55] demonstrated this for the IPSS, WPSS, MDAPSS, and IPSS-R in a cohort that included post-treatment MDS patients. After adjusting for model score and age, they found prognostic significance for the *EZH2*, *SF3B1*, and *TP53* genes. In all models, incorporation of these 3 genes and the patient's age showed appropriate upstaging or downstaging into a more appropriate risk category.

A variety of additional variables have complicated integration of molecular data into prognostic scoring, including variant allele frequency, mutation location, mutation type (missense vs other), and potential interactions with comutated genes. Sole focus on overall survival may be insufficient, and assessment of leukemic transformation risk will likely be a provision in newer prognostic tools. However, a simple formula for risk-calculation is unrealistic given the mass of variables under consideration. Although this potentially limits clinical practicability, some groups are attempting to overcome the challenge of incorporating big-data into personalized risk modeling with the aid of machine-learning algorithms.

A collaborative team from Cleveland Clinic and Munich Leukemia Laboratory used this approach to process genomic and clinical data and create a trainable prognostic assessment system; the trained and validated system was subsequently translated into a Web application to aid in generation of survival probabilities. Nearly 2 dozen markers are used, and ranked from most to least impactful on overall survival include cytogenetic risk categories by IPSS-R: platelets, mutation number, hemoglobin, bone marrow blasts percentage, 2008 WHO diagnosis, white blood count, age, absolute neutrophil count, absolute lymphocyte count, *TP53*, *RUNX1*, *STAG2*, *ASXL1*, absolute monocyte counts, *SF3B1*, *SRSF2*, *RAD21*, secondary versus de novo MDS, *NRAS*, nucleophosmin 1 (*NPM1*), *TET2*, and *EZH2*. Presented at the 2018 annual conference of the American Society for Hematology, the system outperformed all contemporary models in predicting overall survival and leukemic transformation, including the IPSS, IPSS-R, WPSS, and MDAPSS. Although the use of such of technology for risk modeling may be in its infancy, the performance of this model presented by Nazha and colleagues [56] demonstrates great potential to enhance personalized clinical care.

No single MDS risk-stratification tool has yet achieved general consensus usage for clinical care. An overwhelming amount of molecular prognostic markers for MDS have been described, and the use of machine-learning algorithms is probably necessary for development of future integrated models for predicting clinical behavior. Although these tools will probably look markedly different from those in common use today, the benefits for patient care are certain.

REFERENCES

[1] Bennett JM, Catovsky D, Daniel MT, et al. Proposals for the classification of the myelodysplastic syndromes. Br J Haematol 1982;51(2):189–99.

[2] Foucar K, Langdon RM 2nd, Armitage JO, et al. Myelodysplastic syndromes. A clinical and pathologic analysis of 109 cases. Cancer 1985;56(3):553–61.

[3] Mufti GJ, Stevens JR, Oscier DG, et al. Myelodysplastic syndromes: a scoring system with prognostic significance. Br J Haematol 1985;59(3):425–33.

[4] Steensma DP. The changing classification of myelodysplastic syndromes: what's in a name? Hematology 2009;2009:645–55.

[5] Sanz GF, Sanz MA, Vallespí T, et al. Two regression models and a scoring system for predicting survival and planning treatment in myelodysplastic syndromes: a multivariate analysis of prognostic factors in 370 patients. Blood 1989;74(1):395–408.

[6] Aul C, Gattermann N, Heyll A, et al. Primary myelodysplastic syndromes: analysis of prognostic factors in 235 patients and proposals for an improved scoring system. Leukemia 1992;6(1):52–9.

[7] Morel P, Declercq C, Hebbar M, et al. Prognostic factors in myelodysplastic syndromes: critical analysis of the impact of age and gender and failure to identify a very-low-risk group using standard mortality ratio techniques. Br J Haematol 1996;94(1):116–9.

[8] Steensma DP, Bejar R, Jaiswal S, et al. Clonal hematopoiesis of indeterminate potential and its distinction from myelodysplastic syndromes. Blood 2015;126(1): 9–16.

[9] Genovese G, Kähler AK, Handsaker RE, et al. Clonal hematopoiesis and blood-cancer risk inferred from blood DNA sequence. N Engl J Med 2014;371(26): 2477–87.

[10] Jaiswal S, Fontanillas P, Flannick J, et al. Age-related clonal hematopoiesis associated with adverse outcomes. N Engl J Med 2014;371(26):2488–98.

[11] Quivoron C, Couronné L, Della Valle V, et al. TET2 inactivation results in pleiotropic hematopoietic abnormalities in mouse and is a recurrent event during human lymphomagenesis. Cancer Cell 2011;20(1):25–38.

[12] Yoda S, Nakanishi K, Tano A, et al. Diagnostic value of automated quantification of nuclear cardiology in Japanese patients with single vessel coronary artery disease: comparison between Japanese and American normal databases. J Cardiol 2013;62(4):224–9.

[13] Couronné L, Bastard C, Bernard OA. TET2 and DNMT3A mutations in human T-cell lymphoma. N Engl J Med 2012;366(1):95–6.

[14] Woll PS, Kjällquist U, Chowdhury O, et al. Myelodysplastic syndromes are propagated by rare and distinct human cancer stem cells in vivo. Cancer Cell 2014;25(6): 794–808.

[15] Look AT. Molecular pathogenesis of MDS. Hematology Am Soc Hematol Educ Program 2005;156–60.

[16] Bejar R, Stevenson K, Abdel-Wahab O, et al. Clinical effect of point mutations in myelodysplastic syndromes. N Engl J Med 2011;364(26):2496–506.

[17] Lee E, Podoltsev N, Gore SD, et al. The evolving field of prognostication and risk stratification in MDS : Recent developments and future directions. Blood Rev 2016; 30(1):1–10.

[18] Lindsley RC, Mar BG, Mazzola E, et al. Acute myeloid leukemia ontogeny is defined by distinct somatic mutations. Blood 2015;125(9):1367–76.

[19] Yoshida K, Sanada M, Shiraishi Y, et al. Frequent pathway mutations of splicing machinery in myelodysplasia. Nature 2011;478:64–9.

[20] Pellagatti A, Armstrong RN, Steeples V, et al. Impact of spliceosome mutations on RNA splicing in myelodysplasia: dysregulated genes/pathways and clinical associations. Blood 2018;132(12):1225–40.

[21] Saez B, Walter MJ, Graubert TA. Splicing factor gene mutations in hematologic malignancies. Blood 2017; 129(10):1260–9.

[22] Visconte V, Rogers HJ, Singh J, et al. SF3B1 haploinsufficiency leads to formation of ring sideroblasts in myelodysplastic syndromes. Blood 2012;120(16): 3173–86.

[23] Malcovati L, Karimi M, Papaemmanuil E, et al. SF3B1 mutation identifies a distinct subset of myelodysplastic syndrome with ring sideroblasts. Blood 2015;126(2):233–41.

[24] Hasserjian RP, Orazi A, Brunning RD, et al. Myelodysplastic syndromes: overview. In: Swerdlow SH, Campo E, Harris NL, Jaffe ES, Pileri SA, et al, editors. WHO classification of tumours of haematopoietic and lymphoid tissues, revised. 4th edition. Lyon (France): IARC; 2017. p. 98–106.

[25] Li B, Liu J, Jia Y, et al. Clinical features and biological implications of different U2AF1 mutation types in myelodysplastic syndromes. Genes Chromosomes Cancer 2018;57(2):80–8.

[26] Makishima H, Visconte V, Sakaguchi H, et al. Mutations in the spliceosome machinery, a novel and ubiquitous pathway in leukemogenesis. Blood 2012;119(14): 3203–10.

[27] Zheng X, Zhan Z, Naren D, et al. Prognostic value of SRSF2 mutations in patients with de novo myelodysplastic syndromes: a meta-analysis. PLoS One 2017;12(9): e0185053.

[28] Thol F, Kade S, Schlarmann C, et al. Frequency and prognostic impact of mutations in SRSF2, U2AF1, and ZRSR2 in patients with myelodysplastic syndromes. Blood 2012;119(15):3578–84.

[29] Damm F, Kosmider O, Gelsi-Boyer V, et al. Mutations affecting mRNA splicing define distinct

clinical phenotypes and correlate with patient outcome in myelodysplastic syndromes. Blood 2012; 119(14):3211–8.
[30] Kim E, Ilagan JO, Liang Y, et al. SRSF2 mutations contribute to myelodysplasia by mutant-specific effects on exon recognition. Cancer Cell 2015;27(5):617–30.
[31] Haase D, Stevenson KE, Neuberg D, et al. TP53 mutation status divides myelodysplastic syndromes with complex karyotypes into distinct prognostic subgroups. Leukemia 2019;33(7):1747–58.
[32] Bejar R, Stevenson KE, Caughey B, et al. Somatic mutations predict poor outcome in patients with myelodysplastic syndrome after hematopoietic stem-cell transplantation. J Clin Oncol 2014;32(25):2691–8.
[33] Wong TN, Ramsingh G, Young AL, et al. Role of TP53 mutations in the origin and evolution of therapy-related acute myeloid leukaemia. Nature 2015;518(7540):552–5.
[34] Kon A, Shih LY, Minamino M, et al. Recurrent mutations in multiple components of the cohesin complex in myeloid neoplasms. Nat Genet 2013;45(10):1232–7.
[35] Thota S, Viny AD, Makishima H, et al. Genetic alterations of the cohesin complex genes in myeloid malignancies. Blood 2014;124(11):1790–8.
[36] Thol F, Bollin R, Gehlhaar M, et al. Mutations in the cohesin complex in acute myeloid leukemia: clinical and prognostic implications. Blood 2014;123(6): 914–20.
[37] Ogawa S. Genetics of MDS. Blood 2019;133(10):1049–59.
[38] Lin ME, Hou HA, Tsai CH, et al. Dynamics of DNMT3A mutation and prognostic relevance in patients with primary myelodysplastic syndrome. Clin Epigenetics 2018; 10:42.
[39] Traina F, Visconte V, Elson P, et al. Impact of molecular mutations on treatment response to DNMT inhibitors in myelodysplasia and related neoplasms. Leukemia 2014; 28(1):78–87.
[40] Gelsi-Boyer V, Brecqueville M, Devillier R, et al. Mutations in ASXL1 are associated with poor prognosis across the spectrum of malignant myeloid diseases. J Hematol Oncol 2012;5:12.
[41] Yang H, Kurtenbach S, Guo Y, et al. Gain of function of ASXL1 truncating protein in the pathogenesis of myeloid malignancies. Blood 2018;131(3):328–41.
[42] Shin DY, Park JK, Kim SM, et al. ASXL1 is a molecular predictor in idiopathic cytopenia of undetermined significance. Leuk Lymphoma 2019;60(3):756–63.
[43] Mangaonkar AA, Gangat N, Al-Kali A, et al. Prognostic impact of ASXL1 mutations in patients with myelodysplastic syndromes and multilineage dysplasia with or without ring sideroblasts. Leuk Res 2018;71:60–2.
[44] Bejar R, Stevenson KE, Caughey BA, et al. Validation of a prognostic model and the impact of mutations in patients with lower-risk myelodysplastic syndromes. J Clin Oncol 2012;30(27):3376–82.
[45] Tsai SC, Shih LY, Liang ST, et al. Biological activities of runx1 mutants predict secondary acute leukemia transformation from chronic myelomonocytic leukemia and myelodysplastic syndromes. Clin Cancer Res 2015; 21(15):3541–51.
[46] Fenaux P, Mufti GJ, Hellstrom-Lindberg E, et al. Efficacy of azacitidine compared with that of conventional care regimens in the treatment of higher-risk myelodysplastic syndromes: a randomised, open-label, phase III study. Lancet Oncol 2009;10(3):223–32.
[47] Silverman LR, Demakos EP, Peterson BL, et al. Randomized controlled trial of azacitidine in patients with the myelodysplastic syndrome: a study of the cancer and leukemia group B. J Clin Oncol 2002;20(10):2429–40.
[48] Kornblith AB, Herndon JE 2nd, Silverman LR, et al. Impact of azacytidine on the quality of life of patients with myelodysplastic syndrome treated in a randomized phase III trial: a Cancer and Leukemia Group B study. J Clin Oncol 2002;20(10):2441–52.
[49] Lübbert M, Suciu S, Baila L, et al. Low-dose decitabine versus best supportive care in elderly patients with intermediate- or high-risk myelodysplastic syndrome (MDS) ineligible for intensive chemotherapy: final results of the randomized phase III study of the European Organisation for Research and Treatment of Cancer Leukemia Group and the German MDS Study Group. J Clin Oncol 2011;29(15):1987–96.
[50] Zeidan AM, Sekeres MA, Garcia-Manero G, et al. Comparison of risk stratification tools in predicting outcomes of patients with higher-risk myelodysplastic syndromes treated with azanucleosides. Leukemia 2016;30(3): 649–57.
[51] Lee EJ, Zeidan AM. Genome sequencing in myelodysplastic syndromes: can molecular mutations predict benefit from hypomethylating agent therapy? Expert Rev Hematol 2015;8(2):155–8.
[52] Bejar R, Papaemmanuil E, Haferlach T, et al. Somatic mutations in MDS patients are associated with clinical features and predict prognosis independent of the IPSS-R: analysis of combined datasets from the international working group for prognosis in MDS-molecular committee. Blood 2015;126(23):907.
[53] Tefferi A, Lasho TL, Patnaik MM, et al. Targeted next-generation sequencing in myelodysplastic syndromes and prognostic interaction between mutations and IPSS-R. Am J Hematol 2017;92(12):1311–7.
[54] Gangat N, Mudireddy M, Lasho TL, et al. Mutations and prognosis in myelodysplastic syndromes: karyotype-adjusted analysis of targeted sequencing in 300 consecutive cases and development of a genetic risk model. Am J Hematol 2018;93(5):691–7.
[55] Al-Issa K, Zarzour A, Radivoyevitch T, et al. Incorporation of molecular data into the current prognostic models in treated patients with myelodysplastic syndromes: which model is the best. Blood 2016;128(22):50.
[56] Nazha A, Komrokji RS, Meggendorfer M, et al. A personalized prediction model to risk stratify patients with myelodysplastic syndromes. [Abstract: #793]. Presented at The 2018 ASH Annual Meeting, December 3, 2018; San Diego, CA.

Advances in Molecular Pathology 2 (2019) 45–58
ADVANCES IN MOLECULAR PATHOLOGY

Assessing Measurable Residual Disease in Acute Myeloid Leukemia

Daniel L. Duncan, MD[a], Joshua F. Zeidner, MD[b], Nathan D. Montgomery, MD, PhD[c,*]
[a]Foundation Medicine, 7010 Kit Creek Road, Morrisville, NC 27560, USA; [b]Division of Hematology/Oncology, The University of North Carolina at Chapel Hill, CB #7305, Chapel Hill, NC 27599-7305, USA; [c]Department of Pathology and Laboratory Medicine, The University of North Carolina at Chapel Hill, CB #7525, Chapel Hill, NC 27599-7525, USA

KEYWORDS
• Acute myeloid leukemia • Measurable residual disease • Minimal residual disease • Monitoring • Prognosis • Next-generation sequencing • Quantitative PCR

KEY POINTS
- Although 70% to 80% of patients with acute myeloid leukemia (AML) achieve a complete morphologic remission with intensive induction chemotherapy, more than half relapse, indicating that clinically meaningful residual disease is undetectable by morphologic methods.
- The depth of response to therapy, quantified as measurable residual disease (MRD), predicts outcomes in patients with AML, independent of pretreatment genetic features.
- Informative molecular markers for disease monitoring should be stably present in founder clones but absent from preleukemic cells.
- Historically, the most important molecular method for molecular MRD monitoring has been quantitative real-time polymerase chain reaction directed at recurrent fusion transcripts and the common *NPM1* indel mutations.
- Next-generation sequencing–based methods are rapidly expanding the list of driver mutations that can be monitored in AML.

INTRODUCTION

Acute myeloid leukemia (AML) is an aggressive malignancy, characterized by a monotonous proliferation of immature myeloid cells, called blasts. In younger patients who are healthy enough to tolerate aggressive regimens, AML treatment has been largely unchanged for several decades: typically 1 or 2 cycles of intensive induction chemotherapy with regimens that include cytarabine and an anthracycline with or without additional targeted agents, followed by less intensive consolidation therapy. Although outcomes vary based on AML subtype and patient age, approximately 70% to 80% of patients treated with standard induction regimens achieve morphologic complete remission (CR) [1], which is defined by fewer than 5% blasts in a manual differential count performed on a stained bone marrow aspirate smear (Table 1). However, more than half of these patients achieving morphologic

Disclosure: The authors have no disclosures relevant to subject matter in this article. Unrelated to this review, D.L. Duncan is a former employee of Cancer Genetics, Inc. and a current employee at Foundation Medicine. J.F. Zeidner has received honoraria from Celgene, Tolero, and Agios; has served as a consultant for Celgene and AsystBio Laboratories; and has received research funding from Merck, Takeda, and Tolero.

*Corresponding author, *E-mail address:* nathan.montgomery@unchealth.unc.edu

https://doi.org/10.1016/j.yamp.2019.07.003
2589-4080/19/

TABLE 1
Important Terminology in Measurable Residual Disease Testing

Term	Definition
Morphologic complete remission	<5% blasts in a manual differential of a bone marrow aspirate smear
MRD (minimal residual disease)	The presence of leukemic cells below the limit of detection by traditional, microscopy-based methods
CRMRD−	2 successive MRD-negative samples at least 4 wk apart (assay sensitivity at least 10^{-3})
Molecular persistence at low copy numbers	(1) Morphologic complete remission, (2) <2% VAF or target/reference gene ratio, (3) absence of a 1-log increase in all successive measurements
Molecular progression	≥1-log increase in MRD copy number in 2 consecutive positive samples
Molecular relapse	(1) Patient previously CRMRD−, (2) first positive result should be confirmed with a second positive result 4+ wk later, (3) copy number must increase by ≥1 log in the 2 consecutive positive samples

Abbreviations: CRMRD−, complete molecular remission measurable residual disease negative; MRD, measurable residual disease; VAF, variant allele fraction.

CR subsequently relapse, indicating that clinically meaningful residual disease frequently goes undetected by morphologic methods [1].

Accurate risk stratification is critical in AML to distinguish patients who may be cured by chemotherapy alone from those likely to benefit from allogeneic hematopoietic stem cell transplantation (allo-HSCT). Although allo-HSCT is a potentially curative intervention, it is also associated with significant morbidity and mortality. As such, selection of patients likely to benefit from allo-HSCT is a difficult risk/reward assessment, dependent on best estimates of an individual patient's relapse risk and ability to tolerate transplant.

Several baseline factors help to predict relapse risk, including clinical variables (eg, age, prior chemotherapy/radiation, and whether the patient's AML arose secondarily from a lower-grade myeloid neoplasm) and pretreatment disease-associated genetic features. The latter have become particularly important in recent decades, because increasingly granular genetic subtypes of AML have been defined [2]. For instance, the 2016 World Health Organization classification includes 11 categories of AML with recurrent genetic anomalies, and the 2017 European LeukemiaNet (ELN) risk stratification system is even more granular, recognizing 18 distinct genetic subtypes of AML distributed between favorable, intermediate, and adverse risk categories [3,4]. Although a detailed understanding of pretreatment genetic features has improved relapse risk prediction, patient outcomes remain variable, even within ELN-recognized risk groups. For this reason, additional tools are sought to better identify patients likely to be cured by standard chemotherapy and those patients likely to benefit from additional treatment and/or allo-HSCT.

Increasingly, it is appreciated that one of the strongest independent predictors of AML outcome is the depth of response to therapy [5–9]. Measurable residual disease (MRD), also referred to historically as minimal residual disease, is the presence of leukemic cells below the limit of detection by traditional microscopy-based methods. Presence of MRD after therapy is associated with increased relapse risk and shorter survival [5,10–13]. In some genetic subtypes of AML, quantification of disease response by MRD methods may help to better select patients likely to benefit from allo-HSCT [14,15]. In addition, detection of MRD in previously negative patients generally predicts imminent relapse [16–18].

This article first summarizes characteristics of informative molecular MRD markers, highlighting the limitations of both preleukemic and subclonal mutations. Next, it reviews the AML categories and mutations with high-level evidence for molecular monitoring. Then, it introduces important molecular methods used for MRD testing, focusing primarily on the established role of quantitative polymerase chain reaction (PCR), before considering the emerging role of next-generation sequencing (NGS) in assessing mutational clearance and, in the future, for sensitive MRD detection. Current recommendations regarding the performance, interpretation, and timing of MRD assays are also reviewed.

MEASURABLE RESIDUAL DISEASE DETECTION BY NONMOLECULAR METHODS: THE ROLE OF MULTIPARAMETER FLOW CYTOMETRY

MRD testing, albeit not standardized across institutions, has historically been performed predominantly by multiparameter flow cytometry (MFC). MRD detection by MFC is not emphasized in this molecular-focused review. However, much of the literature showing the value of

MRD detection in AML was generated using MFC-based methods. In addition, MFC continues to have potential advantages and is recommended as the preferred method of MRD detection by ELN, except in patients with AML characterized by *NPM1* mutation or *PML-RARA*, *CBFβ-MYH11*, or *RUNX1-RUNX1T1* gene fusion [5].

The major advantage of MFC-based assays for MRD detection is their broad applicability to nearly all cases of AML, unlike fusion-specific or mutation-specific molecular assays, which individually are applicable only to particular AML subtypes [5]. In addition, MFC MRD detection does not require batching, which may lead to more rapid turnaround times compared with molecular MRD assays that may be run only once or twice a week at many centers [9]. In contrast, MRD detection by MFC has certain shortcomings, including the need for specialized expertise, which may not be available even at some university-based cancer centers. In addition, flow cytometry–based assays are challenging to standardize across centers, are frequently less sensitive than quantitative PCR (qPCR), and can be affected by antigenic shifts in the immunophenotype of leukemic blasts.

FEATURES OF INFORMATIVE MOLECULAR MEASURABLE RESIDUAL DISEASE MARKERS

AML is characterized by a complex hierarchy of mutations, which can be temporally defined as (1) preleukemic mutations, (2) leukemia-initiating mutations, and (3) subclonal mutations arising after leukemia initiation (Fig. 1). Important driver mutations that affect disease behavior and inform prognosis may arise at any of these steps. However, only mutations arising in temporal proximity to the leukemia-initiating event function as reliable MRD markers.

Preleukemic mutations may arise years before development of AML, often representing a premalignant clonal proliferation referred to as clonal hematopoiesis of indeterminate potential (CHIP) or, alternatively, age-related clonal hematopoiesis (see Fig. 1B) [19,20]. The most common CHIP mutations are in the epigenetic modifiers *DNMT3A*, *TET2*, and *ASXL1* [21,22]. Individuals bearing CHIP clones are predisposed to malignancy, but acquisition of additional cooperative and later leukemia-initiating mutations is necessary for progression.

After therapy, clones harboring preleukemic mutations may persist in patients who remain in morphologic remission for more than a decade [23]. In a recently published retrospective analysis of 482 patients with AML monitored using a 54-gene NGS panel, persistence of *DNMT3A*, *TET2*, and *ASXL1* mutations, called *DTA* mutations, had no impact on survival in patients with AML in morphologic CR, unlike persistence of mutations in other driver genes (called non-*DTA* mutations) [24]. In some patients in continued CR, these preleukemic *DTA* mutations were found at variant allele fractions (VAFs) approaching 50%, suggesting that the preleukemic clone can dominate posttherapy hematopoiesis [24]. Hence, monitoring preleukemic mutations results in false-positive MRD results in many cases, with poor predictive value for risk of relapse (see Fig. 1F). One exception to this rule may be the posttransplant setting, in which detection of even preleukemic clones suggests persistence of a disease-related population, which may place patients at increased risk of relapse.

Although preleukemic mutations lack adequate specificity as MRD markers, subclonal mutations have insufficient sensitivity. Cooperating driver mutations in *FLT3*, *RAS* family members, and *KIT* (among other genes) typically arise after the leukemia-initiating event and are not reliably found at relapse. As such, mutational clearance in these cases may lead to false-negative MRD results (see Fig. 1E). However, monitoring subclonal mutations may still be valuable; for instance, to assess mutational persistence in patients receiving targeted therapies such as midostaurin (for *FLT3*-mutated AML). However, given their absence in the founding leukemia clone, these mutations do not serve as sensitive markers of persistent disease.

In contrast with preleukemic and subclonal mutations, the ideal MRD marker (1) is reliably present at relapse, meaning that it either was the leukemia-initiating mutation or arose in close proximity to that event; and (2) was not present in preleukemic cells. Mutations fulfilling these requirements could theoretically be identified in any new AML. However, the molecular markers used to date are a small number of recurrent genetic anomalies with well-defined performance characteristics in the context of MRD. The evidence-based utility of 4 specific markers is best established: *NPM1* C-terminal frameshift mutations and *PML-RARA*, *CBFβ-MYH11*, and *RUNX1-RUNX1T1* gene fusions. Both the ELN and the National Comprehensive Cancer Network (NCCN) endorse molecular MRD monitoring in patients with AML harboring these mutations [5,25].

EVIDENCE FOR CLINICAL UTILITY OF MOLECULAR MEASURABLE RESIDUAL DISEASE MONITORING

Nucleophosmin 1

Mutations in *Nucleophosmin 1* (*NPM1*) are found in approximately 20% to 35% of cases of AML and in nearly half of AML cases with normal cytogenetics [2,26–29].

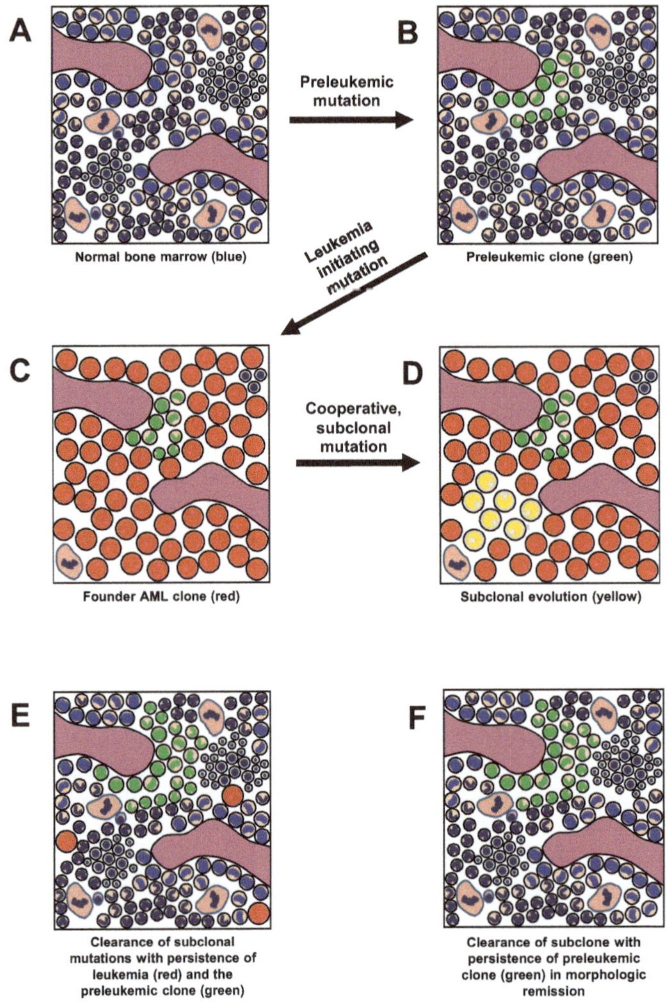

FIG. 1 Mutational hierarchy of AML. (**A**) The normal bone marrow contains a heterogeneous mixture of hematopoietic cells showing a full range of maturation (normal cells are shown with blue nuclei). (**B**) The earliest events in leukemogenesis occur on acquisition of preleukemic mutations in genes such as *DNMT3A*, *TET2*, and *ASXL1* (preleukemic clones shown in green). (**C**) Preleukemic clones progress to AML after acquiring additional, leukemia-initiating mutations (leukemic cells of the founder AML clone shown in red). (**D**) After progression to AML, molecular evolution continues with cooperative mutations producing diverse subclones (leukemic cells with a subclonal mutation are shown in yellow). (**E**) Subclonal mutations are insensitive MRD markers because they may be cleared despite persistence of leukemic cells of the founder AML clone or of distinct subclones. (**F**) Preleukemic mutations are nonspecific MRD markers because they may persist even in long-standing remission.

Nearly all of these *NPM1* mutations are 4-base insertions at the 3′ end of the gene. The altered reading frame creates an ectopic nuclear export signal, resulting in aberrant localization of the NPM1 protein to the cytoplasm. The canonical type A mutation (c.860_863dupTCTG, p.Trp288fs*12) is most common, representing approximately 80% of all *NPM1* mutations [16].

Although *NPM1* mutations are often considered favorable molecular alterations, outcomes are not uniform. Prognosis is modified by the presence of other pretreatment mutations, such as *FLT3* internal tandem duplication, as well as the depth of response to therapy using NPM1 mutant transcript level as an MRD marker. Over the last decade, several studies have established the predictive value of *NPM1* mutation monitoring, typically using reverse transcriptase qPCR methods [11,12,14,16,29,30]. Given variations in AML therapy between the United States and Europe, extrapolation of results to centers with divergent treatment protocols must be undertaken cautiously. However, certain themes have proved consistent, with NPM1 mutant transcript monitoring proving valuable both for refining progress and predicting imminent relapse.

Several studies, predominantly conducted in Europe, where 2 rounds of induction chemotherapy are standard, have shown that both the log reduction in NPM1 mutant transcript level and the NPM1 mutant transcript/ABL1 transcript ratio after double induction are associated with outcome. However, predictive thresholds may vary between bone marrow and peripheral blood samples. For instance, multiple studies have suggested that failing to achieve a 3-log reduction in NPM1 mutant transcript level in bone marrow after double-induction therapy is an informative predictor of relapse, with sensitivity of 50% and specificity of 81% in one German study [16,30]. In the same cohort, end-of-treatment NPM1 mutant transcript/ABL1 transcript ratios greater than 0.01 were also associated with a 78% 2-year cumulative incidence rate of relapse [30]. More recent publications have suggested that peripheral blood may be equally or even more discriminatory. A French study supported a 4-log reduction as prognostic in blood, with potential utility in identifying patients likely to benefit from allo-HCT [14]. Similarly, Ivey and colleagues [12] showed that persistence of NPM1 mutant transcripts in blood after second induction is associated with increased risk of relapse in the next 3 years (82% vs 30%) and worse survival (24% vs 75%). These data should be interpreted cautiously in patients receiving 1 cycle of conventional 7 + 3-like induction therapy, because these analyses were conducted in the context of double-induction regimens and the intensity of initial treatment may affect NPM1 MRD levels.

Increasing NPM1 transcript level in patients previously in molecular remission is also informative. Multiple data suggest that an increasing NPM1 transcript level in patients who previously had no evidence of NPM1 MRD is a harbinger of imminent hematologic relapse [12,16]. In their seminal publication on NPM1 mutant transcript monitoring, Schnittger and colleagues [16] showed that a 1-log or greater increase in bone marrow NPM1 mutant transcript level preceded relapse in more than half of cases, an observation that has been confirmed in subsequent studies in both bone marrow and peripheral blood [12].

PML-RARA

Acute promyelocytic leukemia with *PML-RARA* fusion is an aggressive form of AML that was historically associated with devastating coagulopathy and rapid death. However, outcomes are now excellent in patients treated with all-*trans* retinoic acid (ATRA), typically in combination with arsenic trioxide or cytotoxic chemotherapy. PML-RARA fusion transcripts are sensitive and specific markers of leukemic cells in acute promyelocytic leukemia and are typically detected by reverse transcriptase qPCR methods.

During therapy, PML-RARA results may correlate with response but should not affect management [5]. ATRA induces differentiation rather than death of leukemic promyelocytes. As a result, PML-RARA fusion transcripts persist in maturing granulocytic cells without leukemic potential during therapy. In contrast, achieving molecular remission after therapy is a critical MRD benchmark associated with very low risk of relapse [17]. Moreover, in patients successfully achieving PCR negativity, subsequent detection of PML-RARA fusion transcripts heralds imminent relapse [17].

Markers in Core Binding Factor Acute Myeloid Leukemia: *CBFβ-MYH11* and *RUNX1-RUNX1T1*

Core binding factor (CBF) is a transcription factor involved in regulation of hematopoiesis. Translocations involving CBF components are found in 2 forms of AML with recurrent gene fusions: AML with t(8;21)(q22;q22.1); *RUNX1-RUNX1T1*, and AML with inv(16)(p13.1;q22) or t(16;16) (p13.1;q22); *CBFβ-MYH11*. Both forms of AML are associated with favorable prognosis, although relapse still occurs in approximately 30% to 40% of patients [7,31].

Similar to AML with *NPM1* mutation, risk of relapse in CBF AML is affected by other pretreatment mutations, most notably exon 17 *KIT* mutations [32–35]. However, depth of response to therapy is ultimately the most informative marker of outcome in these patients. MRD detection in CBF AML involves detection of either *RUNX1-RUNX1T1* or *CBFβ-MYH11* fusion transcript using reverse transcriptase qPCR assays [13,36–39]. For both gene fusions, a less than 3-log reduction in the level of the fusion transcript is a strong predictor of relapse risk, and transcript levels are more informative than *KIT* mutation status in AML with *RUNX1-RUNX1T1* [15,37,39].

In both AML with *RUNX1-RUNX1T1* and AML with *CBFβ-MYH11*, approximately one-third of patients in long-standing morphologic CR continue to have low positive fusion transcript detection [13,18]. These results reiterate that 3-fold reduction rather than molecular remission is the target end point in these diseases. However, for patients with AML with *RUNX1-RUNX1T1* or *CBFβ-MYH11* who do achieve molecular remission, subsequent conversion from PCR negativity to PCR positivity is associated with a very high risk of relapse in the next 6 months and decreased overall survival [18,37].

In addition, CBF AML provides one of the few examples for which there are data supporting improvement in outcomes resulting from MRD-directed treatment decisions. In a study of 86 patients with AML with *CBFβ-MYH11*, Qin and colleagues [15] showed that allogeneic transplant decreased the cumulative incidence of relapse and improved overall survival in high-risk patients who failed to achieve a 3-log reduction in transcript level after therapy. Similar benefit was not seen in patients with a greater than 3-log reduction in *CBFβ-MYH11*.

METHODS OF MOLECULAR MEASURABLE RESIDUAL DISEASE DETECTION

To reliably detect and quantify low levels of residual disease, molecular assays used for MRD detection must achieve several basic performance characteristics:

1. Excellent analytical sensitivity (low limit of detection)
2. Accurate distinction of mutant and wild-type alleles or transcripts
3. Linearity across the analytical measurement range

Most assays achieving these requirements have involved mutant transcript detection by qPCR, although some other methods, such as detection of AML-related gene expression abnormalities, have also shown at least modest utility. More recently, new methods such as droplet digital PCR (ddPCR) and deep sequencing by NGS diversified the list of modalities used for MRD monitoring. These methods are reviewed later, with emphasis on the well-established role of qPCR assays and the exciting emerging role of NGS-based methods.

Quantitative Polymerase Chain Reaction

For more than a decade, qPCR has been used for clinical-grade MRD assays and is recommended by the ELN and the NCCN as an important method for monitoring AML with either mutated *NPM1* or with recurrent *PML-RARA*, *CBFβ-MYH11*, or *RUNX1-RUNX1T1* fusions [5,25]. Most qPCR assays offer exquisite analytical sensitivity, achieving limits of detection between 1 in 10^{-4} to 1 in 10^{-6}, representing a 10-fold to 100-fold improved sensitivity relative to MFC in some cases.

Either DNA or RNA can be used as the template in qPCR assays. However, 2 advantages make RNA the generally preferred analyte, despite being the more labile nucleic acid. The first advantage of RNA is added analytical sensitivity. Most driver mutations are present as a single DNA copy, meaning as a heterozygous mutation, in AML. In contrast there are often many mutant transcripts in that same cell, providing greater signal for detection. However, because expression levels may be variable between cells or even at different points in therapy, there is imperfect correlation between transcript level and absolute number of leukemic cells. The second advantage of RNA is fusion detection. Common AML fusions, such as *PML-RARA*, *CBFβ-MYH11*, and *RUNX1-RUNX1T1*, arise from diverse genomic breakpoints. As such, DNA-based qPCR MRD assays would need to be patient specific. With RNA, this genomic diversity is irrelevant because the varied breakpoints tend to result in common fusion transcripts. Nearly all patients with a recurrent fusion can therefore be monitored with a small number of primer pairs or even a single primer with RNA-based assays. For instance, RUNX1-RUNX1T1 fusion transcripts can be detected with a single primer pair, whereas CBFβ-MYH11 detection requires 3 different reverse primers and a single forward primer to capture the full diversity of observed breakpoints [9].

Detailed discussion of qPCR methods is beyond the scope of this review. However, TaqMan qPCR assays are briefly reviewed because of their popularity. These assays offer additional specificity through incorporation of a hydrolysis probe that hybridizes to the target amplicon during the annealing phase of PCR. At the 5′ end of the hydrolysis probe, there is a reporter fluorochrome, and at the 3′ end, there is a quencher molecule (Fig. 2A). During elongation, the hydrolysis probe is cleaved by Taq polymerase's intrinsic exonuclease activity, which frees the reporter fluorochrome from the quencher molecule. Fluorescence is then measured at the end of the elongation step of each PCR cycle, with the amount of fluorescence being proportional to the number of product molecules generated in each cycle. A fluorescence threshold is established within the exponential phase of amplification, and the number of cycles required to cross that threshold (cycle threshold [CT] value) is determined for the target transcript (Fig. 2B). In qPCR assays, detection of the mutant transcript must be normalized to a housekeeping transcript, typically ABL1. This normalization corrects for variation in cellularity and RNA yield between different samples. Ultimately, mutant transcripts are reported as

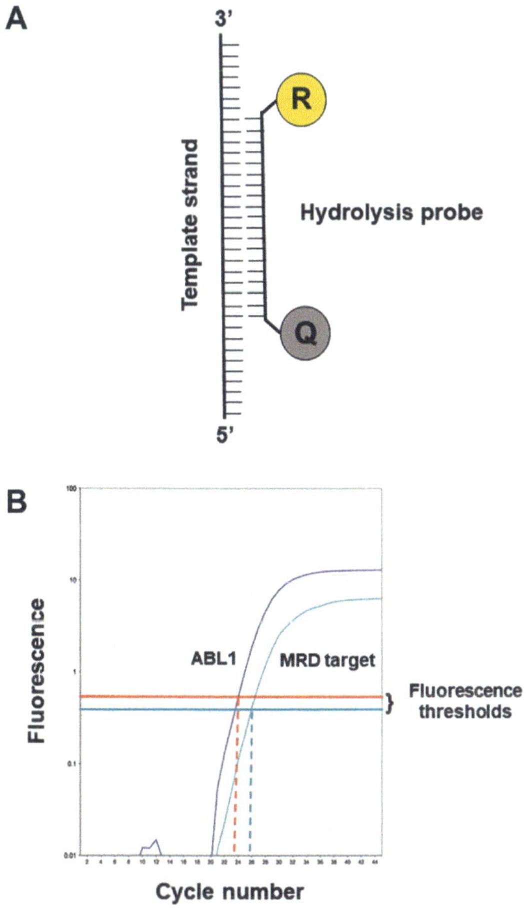

FIG. 2 Quantitative PCR with fluorescent hydrolysis probes (TaqMan). (**A**) Hydrolysis probes used in qPCR hybridize within the amplicon of the MRD target or housekeeping control target. The 5′ end of the probe contains a fluorescent reporter. When the probe is intact, reporter fluorescence is quenched by a 3′ quencher molecule. The reporter is freed from the quencher with Taq polymerases and intrinsic exonuclease activity hydrolyzes the probe. (**B**) An example of qPCR results for an MRD transcript target (*aqua curve, right*) and an ABL1 housekeeping control (*blue curve, left*). The red horizontal line indicates the fluorescence threshold for determination of the ABL1 cycle threshold (CT) value (24 cycles), and the teal horizontal line indicates the fluorescence threshold for determination of the MRD target CT value (26 cycles).

percentage of the MRD target transcript copy number normalized to the housekeeping transcript copy number or, in some laboratories, as the number of mutant transcripts per 10,000 to 100,000 cell equivalents.

The primary technical limitation of qPCR methods is that they require generation of a standard curve spanning the analytical measurement range, which should be established with each run. However, in clinical practice, the more important limitation of qPCR-based methods is that the utility is well established only for *NPM1* mutations, the *PML-RARA* fusion seen in acute promyelocytic leukemia, and the *CBFβ-MYH11* and *RUNX1-RUNX1T1* fusions defining core binding factor AML. As such, fewer than half of all patients with AML can be monitored using widely available qPCR methods, including a particularly small percentage of older patients with AML [9].

WT1 Overexpression

The transcription factor *WT1* is overexpressed in most cases of AML, with transcript levels as much as 1000-fold higher in bone marrow and up to 100,000-fold higher in the peripheral blood leukocytes of patients with newly diagnosed AML compared with normal individuals [40]. For this reason, WT1 transcript monitoring has been proposed as a potential MRD assay, again using quantitative reverse transcriptase PCR methods.

In practice, fewer than half of AMLs express WT1 at a high enough level to be able to appreciate even a 2-log reduction in disease burden, which even then is a less than 1-log improvement compared with traditional morphology [41]. In addition, some *WT1* mutations lead to false-negative results by disrupting primer binding sites [41]. As such, WT1 expression monitoring is not widely used, nor is it endorsed in the ELN or NCCN guidelines [5,25].

Droplet Digital Polymerase Chain Reaction

In recent years, ddPCR has emerged as a powerful competing method to traditional qPCR assays for MRD detection. In ddPCR, nucleic acid templates are partitioned into thousands of nanoliter-sized water-in-oil droplets, with amplification reagents and fluorescent probes similar to those described for qPCR (Fig. 3) [42]. Amplification and fluorescence detection are performed with primers and probes specific to both a control target and the mutation of interest. At the end of each reaction, the number of droplets with fluorescence above a defined threshold is determined for both the targeted mutation and the control. In addition, statistical corrections are performed to account for the presence of multiple targets in some positive droplets. This method allows the accurate determination of the number of both targets and the ratio of the mutant target to the control target.

ddPCR assays can achieve analytical sensitivities of approximately 10^{-5} for gene fusions and indel mutations and 10^{-3} or better for single nucleotide variants

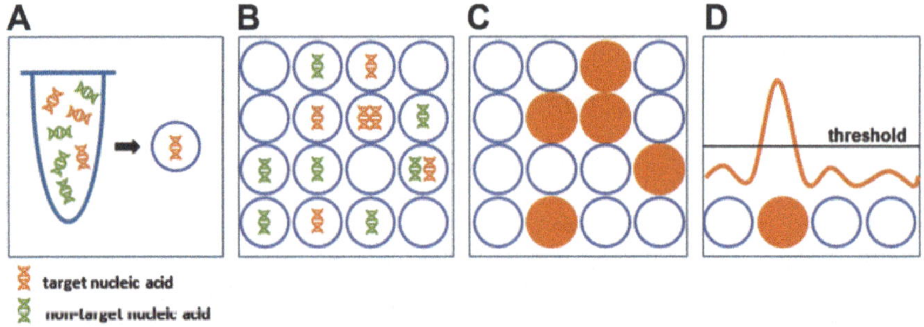

FIG. 3 ddPCR. (A) Nucleic acid is partitioned into thousands of droplets each containing reagents for an individual PCR and fluorescence detection. (B) Nucleic acids are randomly distributed throughout the population of droplets. (C) PCR proceeds with each droplet generating fluorescence if the target nucleic acid is present. (D) In the analysis step, droplets are analyzed individually for fluorescence (above or below a quantitative threshold) for more precise quantitation of input material. The number of positive droplets is proportional to the amount of target input.

[6]. Although this performance is comparable with qPCR assays, ddPCR has some practical advantages. First, because targets are measured more directly than in qPCR, a standard curve is not necessary on every run [6]. In addition, at least for some targets, ddPCR seems to have superior precision [9].

Next-Generation Sequencing

As discussed, the most common clinically implemented molecular techniques for MRD detection are mutation specific and depend on single, recurrent, molecular driver mutations. However, *NPM1* mutations and the recurrent gene fusions discussed earlier are found in only 55% of cases of AML in young adults and in just 30% of cases in patients more than 60 years of age [43]. As such, molecular MRD monitoring has not been possible in most patients historically. Creating patient-specific custom-designed PCR-based assays for disease monitoring provides some hope for overcoming the genetic diversity of AML. However, this approach requires intensive laboratory development and validation work for each new diagnosis. Furthermore, identifying a single, informative MRD marker in a given individual's AML may not be possible, because numerous genomically distinct subclones often occur within a leukemia [44,45]. In addition, the predominant driving genetic event may change over the natural disease course or in response to therapeutic intervention [46]. As such, there is a limit to the utility of single mutation molecular MRD assays, despite the exquisite sensitivity and quantitative nature of these tests.

The desire for a one-size-fits-all molecular MRD test is therefore great. The increase of clinical NGS techniques offers hope for a multitarget AML sequencing assay suitable for MRD detection and monitoring. Traditional NGS assays are not acceptable for MRD testing because of limitations of sensitivity [47,48]. The advent of larger sequencers allowing increased depth of coverage has increased NGS sensitivity. However, with this increase in sensitivity comes an increase in false-positive variant calls caused by sequencing error rates inherent to the technologies used as well as other artifacts introduced into samples, such as oxidative DNA damage [49,50]. Although dependent on the details of library preparation and downstream analysis, the error rate of most commonly used NGS processes is between 0.1% and 1%. Therefore, achieving clinically reportable levels of sensitivity that are relevant to MRD detection is a challenge with traditional NGS approaches.

Several techniques have been developed to tackle this problem by reducing false-positive variant calls and effectively increasing sensitivity in NGS tests. These techniques leverage the interaction of assay chemistry and bioinformatic analysis and are based on adding a molecular barcode or unique molecular identifier (UMI) during the wet laboratory phase of sequencing, and subsequently performing bioinformatic deduplication and error correction before variant calling.

Calling low-frequency variants with unique molecular identifiers

UMIs are random oligonucleotides incorporated into fragments of sample nucleic acid during library preparation for NGS. The goal of tagging sample nucleic acid fragments is to provide a means of identifying sequencing reads belonging to unique parent molecules during bioinformatic analysis [51]. UMIs can greatly assist in confidently calling low-frequency variants in broad DNA-based NGS panels. This ability is appealing for MRD detection, in which identifying small clonal populations is of primary concern.

There are several published and commercially available wet bench approaches to incorporating UMIs during library preparation [52–54]. However, the fundamental components are similar: particularly, UMIs are always added before PCR steps to allow for elimination of amplification bias (Fig. 4). For most applications, UMIs are incorporated as part of a target enrichment process and are often coupled with universal adapters during initial ligation immediately after sample fragmentation. After sequencing, the bioinformatic pipeline can take advantage of the UMI-harboring libraries to perform basic error correction, which is done by first creating consensus reads by grouping all sequencing reads bearing the same UMI. This deduplication step reduces the total number of sequencing reads to a subset of read families (see Fig. 4D) [55].

Once reads are grouped into single molecule–associated families, true variants are identified for reporting and artifactual variants are removed in the error correction process (see Fig. 4E). A true variant should be present in all reads tied to a single UMI, because each of these reads is tied to 1 starting molecule. In contrast, an artifactual variant will be present in some but not all of the reads harboring the same UMI [56]. So, at the most basic level, error correction tools remove any variant not present in all members of a UMI consensus family and allow variant calls to be made on any variant represented in the totality of a consensus family. These rules may be changed depending on the desired characteristics of the assay to allow for less stringent inclusion or exclusion criteria. Furthermore, a minimum family size requirement may be implemented to increase specificity beyond error correction alone [55,57].

There are a host of bioinformatic tools for assisting with error correction using UMIs. Many are available free from either the developers or as part of larger NGS analysis packages such as Genome Analysis Toolkit. An incomplete list of tools, including some not explicitly mentioned in other references, follows:

- Aryee-Lab: https://github.com/aryeelab/umi
- DuNovo: https://github.com/galaxyproject/dunovo
- DuplexSeq: https://github.com/loeblab/Duplex-Sequencing
- Genome Analysis Toolkit: https://software.broadinstitute.org/gatk/
- Presto: https://bitbucket.org/kleinstein/presto/src
- Strand: http://www.strand-ngs.com
- UMI-tools: https://github.com/CGATOxford/UMI-tools

By implementing these tools in conjunction with the addition of UMIs in the wet bench workflow, the high sensitivity of deep sequencing can be preserved without

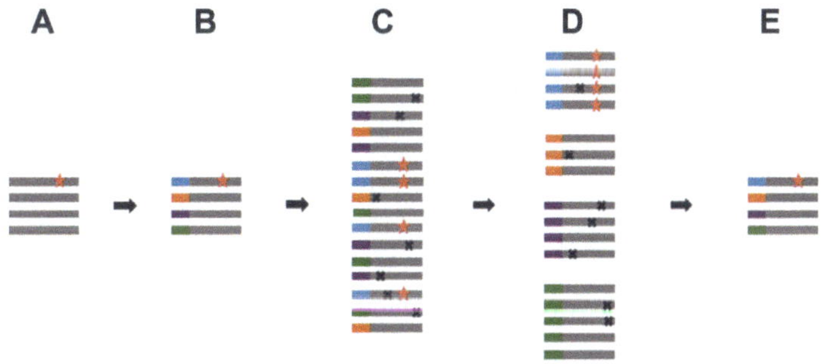

FIG. 4 Using UMIs to accurately detect and quantify MRD in NGS. (**A**) Initial population. In the context of MRD testing, the starting material contains only a minority of DNA fragments harboring true leukemia-specific variants (indicated by a *red star*). (**B**) UMIs are used to tag individual fragments of DNA in the starting material. Importantly, UMIs are added as early in the work flow as possible to control for as many potential errors as possible. (**C**) PCR amplification. The starting material proceeds through library preparation, including PCR steps to yield populations of related molecules, each harboring a shared UMI. Errors accrue during this process (represented by *black Xs*). (**D**) Family creation. Once sequencing of the library is complete, reads are grouped into families of molecules sharing the same UMI. (**E**) Consensus. Family members are compared with one another using predefined thresholds for acceptance to generate a consensus read. In general, variants that are present in every family member are considered true variants and are thus included in the resulting consensus, whereas variants appearing in some but not all family members are considered to be artifactual (arising after addition of the UMI) and are not included in the consensus read.

sacrificing positive predictive value. This ability allows confidence in reporting results to very low limits of detection. The described UMI methods can reduce error rates using traditional NGS technology to 10^{-5} under ideal conditions [55]. Thus, error correction using UMIs in traditional NGS workflows may yield sequencing results sufficiently sensitive for clinical implementation in the MRD setting. However, there is an additional NGS work flow known as duplex sequencing, capable of generating sequencing data with still a lower false-positive rate.

Duplex Sequencing with Unique Molecular Identifiers. Duplex sequencing is a library preparation method that employs a duplex tag UMI. Duplex tags are created by first affixing a standard UMI to target DNA and then using DNA polymerase to synthesize the opposite strand. This process generates 2 complementary tags on duplex DNA. After the duplex tags are affixed, both strands of the sample DNA are sequenced. Consensus sequence families are generated for all reads of the same strand, as with other typical UMI-based workflows. However, there may still be errors introduced during the initial PCR cycle that are common to all consensus members and therefore not removed during error correction. So, in a step unique to duplex sequencing, the consensus sequences from the 2 complementary strands are compared with one another. Any variant identified in 1 strand but not shared by its complement can be removed as an artifact. The variants remaining in the resultant duplex consensus sequences therefore have a higher confidence because of the additional level of stringency for variant calling [58].

The theorized false-positive rate for variant calling from duplex sequencing data is 10^{-7} based on expected artifactual calls from DNA damage compared with data generated in the original studies [59]. One subsequent study has used this number to conservatively report variants at allelic fractions less than 0.001 [60]. Duplex sequencing could therefore dramatically improve the lower limit of detection for clinical NGS assays. The tradeoff for superior confidence in low-frequency variant calls is in sequencing throughput. Duplex sequencing necessarily requires sequencing duplex strands of target DNA, and therefore has effectively half the per-run sequencing capacity of more common single-strand NGS workflows [55]. However, the sacrifice in throughput may be worthwhile in the context of MRD testing when there is clear clinical advantage to reporting low-frequency variants.

CURRENT RECOMMENDATIONS FOR THE TIMING AND INTERPRETATION OF MEASURABLE RESIDUAL DISEASE ASSAYS

At present, the ELN guidelines provide the most granular recommendations on timing and actionability of MRD testing [5]. However, as noted earlier, these recommendations are based on European treatment paradigms that have not been globally adopted. Nevertheless, many of the ELN's best practice recommendations can be extrapolated to other settings, and, in some cases, similar guidelines are endorsed by the NCCN [25]. Most importantly, the ELN endorses MRD monitoring as part of the standard of care for all patients with AML [5]. This recommendation raises several questions, including what assays should be run, when MRD testing should be performed, and how MRD results should be interpreted.

Sample and Assay Requirements

The ELN guidelines include helpful guidance to laboratories regarding (1) sample requirements, (2) necessary limits of detection, and (3) best practices for defining positive results.

MRD assays can be performed on either peripheral blood or bone marrow, with distinct performance characteristics for each sample type. When bone marrow aspirates are performed, material is often procured for multiple assays, including morphologic assessment, flow cytometry, cytogenetics, and molecular studies. With skilled operators, the initial aspirate pull typically is representative of marrow cellularity. However, after the initial aspirate pull, the needle track begins to bleed, and subsequent pulls are increasingly diluted by peripheral blood (termed hemodilution). To maximize sensitivity and uniformity, the ELN recommends that the first aspirate pull be used for MRD assays, and the NCCN similarly recommends a first or early pull for this testing [5,25]. At centers opting instead to send first-pull aspirates for morphology and subsequent pulls for MRD testing, it is important to recognize the limitations inherent to testing hemodilute bone marrow samples, particularly when bone marrow–specific MRD benchmarks are used for clinical decision making.

Although MRD is defined as the presence of leukemic cells below the 5% limit of detection of microscopy-based methods, the ELN recommends a minimum limit of detection of 10^{-3} for clinical MRD assays [5]. In laboratories using qPCR assays, standards should be included on each run that cover the range of patient results to ensure linearity [5]. In addition, laboratories are encouraged to run molecular MRD assays in triplicate, with results considered positive only if the target is detected in at least 2 of 3 replicates [5].

Important Measurable Residual Disease Definitions

The ELN guidelines define several important terms that are helpful in describing MRD results (see Table 1). The first 2 terms recognize molecular MRD milestones that identify patients at lower risk of relapse. The more stringent of these ELN-recognized categories is Complete Molecular Remission MRD negative (CRMRD−), which is defined by 2 successive MRD-negative samples obtained at least 4 weeks apart using an assay with a sensitivity of at least 10^{-3} [5]. Because low-level persistence of molecular MRD may not be associated with high relapse risk in all cases, the ELN also defines a category of patients in molecular persistence at low copy numbers. This milestone is less stringent and is defined by (1) morphologic complete response, (2) less than 2% VAF or target/reference gene ratio, and (3) absence of a 1-log increase in all successive measurements [5]. Importantly, these definitions must be interpreted in the broader context of the ELN guidelines, which currently recommend molecular MRD testing only for AML with mutated *NPM1* or *PML-RARA*, *CBFβ-MYH11*, or *RUNX1-RUNX1T1* fusions. As the breadth of mutations that can be accurately monitored increases with NGS-based assays, these definitions will require revision and additional nuance.

The ELN also has provided evidence-based definitions for molecular progression and molecular relapse, which are important concepts for identifying patients at imminent risk of disease progression and hematologic relapse. Molecular progression is defined as a 1-log (10-fold) increase in MRD copy number in 2 consecutive positive samples [5]. Molecular relapse is a similar concept in patients who had previously achieved CRMRD− [5]. To meet the definition of molecular relapse, the ELN guidelines require that the first positive result be confirmed by a second positive result 4 weeks or more after the patient converted from negative to positive. Moreover, the MRD copy number must increase by at least 1 log in those consecutive positive samples. For the most accurate comparison of sequential qPCR results, the ELN recommends that initial negative-to-positive sample be included in the same run as the repeat, to allow direct comparison of the fold increase within a single run.

Timing

Evidence-based guidance on timing of MRD assessment is generally lacking in the current literature. Recommendations for current best practices are largely based on expert opinion. Although the ELN guidelines are based on European treatment paradigms, the underlying tenets are broadly applicable. These recommendations can be broadly broken into testing (1) during treatment, (2) after therapy is completed (eg, during posttreatment remission), and (3) before and after transplant.

During treatment, the ELN recommends MRD measurements be performed at diagnosis to establish baseline disease burden, after induction, and on completion of therapy. At these time points, the ELN recommends that both peripheral blood and bone marrow be tested to facilitate future comparison. After treatment, the ELN recommends continued MRD monitoring for 2 years. Testing is recommended every 3 months in bone marrow or every 4 to 6 weeks in peripheral blood. Although the periodicity of testing may vary between centers, these recommendations provide a helpful benchmark for reasonable use.

MRD testing should also be performed no more than 4 weeks before allo-HSCT. The significance of MRD at the last pretransplant time point is well established for MFC-based flow assays, in which MRD depth is strongly correlated with posttransplant outcome [61]. The relationship between pretransplant molecular MRD and outcomes is not as well established and is certain to be variable between targets and assays. However, establishing the depth of response before transplant is likely to refine relapse risk. Posttransplant monitoring is also informative in conjunction with engraftment assays.

Of note, NCCN guidelines similarly recommend MRD testing on completion of initial induction and before transplant. However, NCCN recommendations are more ambiguous at other time points, noting simply that testing should be guided by therapeutic regimen [25].

SUMMARY AND FUTURE DIRECTIONS

Minimal residual disease testing is now an important part of standard care for patients with AML. The presence of MRD at key time points is associated with increased risk of relapse and shorter survival. Although not all pretreatment somatic mutations are specific or reliably sensitive markers of disease, excellent predictive value has been established for several recurrent mutations. The advent of new technologies such as ddPCR and NGS is improving the precision of MRD testing and increasing the breadth of molecular targets that can be monitored, respectively. These developments predict an expanded role for posttreatment molecular MRD monitoring in the future.

Although the ability to detect low levels of residual disease will continue to improve, the critical next step is to translate detection into meaningful intervention. The predictive power of MRD assessment is established, but there are disappointingly few trials showing that early intervention affects outcome. Here too, NGS-based MRD assays may prove valuable, offering the potential to both quantify persistent disease and identify targetable mutations for maintenance or salvage therapy. These developments suggest increased importance for molecular laboratories as mutations become not just variables for risk stratification but also the measurable unit of disease and the target of intervention.

REFERENCES

[1] Mrozek K, Marcucci G, Nicolet D, et al. Prognostic significance of the European LeukemiaNet standardized system for reporting cytogenetic and molecular alterations in adults with acute myeloid leukemia. J Clin Oncol 2012;30(36):4515–23.

[2] Papaemmanuil E, Gerstung M, Bullinger L, et al. Genomic classification and prognosis in acute myeloid leukemia. N Engl J Med 2016;374(23):2209–21.

[3] Swerdlow SH, Campo E, Harris NL, et al, editors. WHO classification of tumours of haematopoietic and lymphoid tissues, vol. 2, Revised 4th edition. Lyon (France): IARC; 2017.

[4] Dohner H, Estey E, Grimwade D, et al. Diagnosis and management of AML in adults: 2017 ELN recommendations from an international expert panel. Blood 2017; 129(4):424–47.

[5] Schuurhuis GJ, Heuser M, Freeman S, et al. Minimal/measurable residual disease in AML: a consensus document from the European LeukemiaNet MRD Working Party. Blood 2018;131(12):1275–91.

[6] Zhou Y, Wood BL. Methods of detection of measurable residual disease in AML. Curr Hematol Malig Rep 2017;12(6):557–67.

[7] Moors I, Vandepoele K, Philippe J, et al. Clinical implications of measurable residual disease in AML: Review of current evidence. Crit Rev Oncol Hematol 2019;133:142–8.

[8] Roug AS, Ommen HB. Clinical use of measurable residual disease in acute myeloid leukemia. Curr Treat Options Oncol 2019;20(4):28.

[9] Selim AG, Moore AS. Molecular minimal residual disease monitoring in acute myeloid leukemia: challenges and future directions. J Mol Diagn 2018;20(4):389–97.

[10] Chen X, Xie H, Wood BL, et al. Relation of clinical response and minimal residual disease and their prognostic impact on outcome in acute myeloid leukemia. J Clin Oncol 2015;33(11):1258–64.

[11] Kronke J, Schlenk RF, Jensen KO, et al. Monitoring of minimal residual disease in NPM1-mutated acute myeloid leukemia: a study from the German-Austrian acute myeloid leukemia study group. J Clin Oncol 2011;29(19):2709–16.

[12] Ivey A, Hills RK, Simpson MA, et al. Assessment of minimal residual disease in standard-risk AML. N Engl J Med 2016;374(5):422–33.

[13] Corbacioglu A, Scholl C, Schlenk RF, et al. Prognostic impact of minimal residual disease in CBFB-MYH11-positive acute myeloid leukemia. J Clin Oncol 2010; 28(23):3724–9.

[14] Balsat M, Renneville A, Thomas X, et al. Postinduction minimal residual disease predicts outcome and benefit from allogeneic stem cell transplantation in acute myeloid leukemia with NPM1 mutation: a study by the acute leukemia French Association Group. J Clin Oncol 2017;35(2):185–93.

[15] Qin YZ, Xu LP, Chen H, et al. Allogeneic stem cell transplant may improve the outcome of adult patients with inv(16) acute myeloid leukemia in first complete remission with poor molecular responses to chemotherapy. Leuk Lymphoma 2015;56(11):3116–23.

[16] Schnittger S, Kern W, Tschulik C, et al. Minimal residual disease levels assessed by NPM1 mutation-specific RQ-PCR provide important prognostic information in AML. Blood 2009;114(11):2220–31.

[17] Grimwade D, Jovanovic JV, Hills RK, et al. Prospective minimal residual disease monitoring to predict relapse of acute promyelocytic leukemia and to direct pre-emptive arsenic trioxide therapy. J Clin Oncol 2009; 27(22):3650–8.

[18] Yin JA, O'Brien MA, Hills RK, et al. Minimal residual disease monitoring by quantitative RT-PCR in core binding factor AML allows risk stratification and predicts relapse: results of the United Kingdom MRC AML-15 trial. Blood 2012;120(14):2826–35.

[19] Steensma DP, Bejar R, Jaiswal S, et al. Clonal hematopoiesis of indeterminate potential and its distinction from myelodysplastic syndromes. Blood 2015;126(1):9–16.

[20] Shlush LI. Age-related clonal hematopoiesis. Blood 2018; 131(5):496–504.

[21] Genovese G, Kahler AK, Handsaker RE, et al. Clonal hematopoiesis and blood-cancer risk inferred from blood DNA sequence. N Engl J Med 2014;371(26):2477–87.

[22] Jaiswal S, Fontanillas P, Flannick J, et al. Age-related clonal hematopoiesis associated with adverse outcomes. N Engl J Med 2014;371(26):2488–98.

[23] Ploen GG, Nederby L, Guldberg P, et al. Persistence of DNMT3A mutations at long-term remission in adult patients with AML. Br J Haematol 2014;167(4):478–86.

[24] Jongen-Lavrencic M, Grob T, Hanekamp D, et al. Molecular minimal residual disease in acute myeloid leukemia. N Engl J Med 2018;378(13):1189–99.

[25] Network NCC. Acute myeloid leukemia (Version 2.2019). Available at: https://www.nccn.org/professionals/physician_gls/pdf/aml.pdf. Accessed April 1, 2019.

[26] Suzuki T, Kiyoi H, Ozeki K, et al. Clinical characteristics and prognostic implications of NPM1 mutations in acute myeloid leukemia. Blood 2005;106(8):2854–61.

[27] Falini B, Mecucci C, Tiacci E, et al. Cytoplasmic nucleophosmin in acute myelogenous leukemia with a normal karyotype. N Engl J Med 2005;352(3):254–66.

[28] Chou WC, Tang JL, Lin LI, et al. Nucleophosmin mutations in de novo acute myeloid leukemia: the

age-dependent incidences and the stability during disease evolution. Cancer Res 2006;66(6):3310–6.
[29] Thiede C, Koch S, Creutzig E, et al. Prevalence and prognostic impact of NPM1 mutations in 1485 adult patients with acute myeloid leukemia (AML). Blood 2006; 107(10):4011–20.
[30] Hubmann M, Kohnke T, Hoster E, et al. Molecular response assessment by quantitative real-time polymerase chain reaction after induction therapy in NPM1-mutated patients identifies those at high risk of relapse. Haematologica 2014;99(8):1317–25.
[31] Grimwade D, Walker H, Oliver F, et al. The importance of diagnostic cytogenetics on outcome in AML: analysis of 1,612 patients entered into the MRC AML 10 trial. The medical research council adult and children's leukaemia working parties. Blood 1998;92(7):2322–33.
[32] Shimada A, Taki T, Tabuchi K, et al. KIT mutations, and not FLT3 internal tandem duplication, are strongly associated with a poor prognosis in pediatric acute myeloid leukemia with t(8;21): a study of the Japanese Childhood AML Cooperative Study Group. Blood 2006; 107(5):1806–9.
[33] Cairoli R, Beghini A, Grillo G, et al. Prognostic impact of c-KIT mutations in core binding factor leukemias: an Italian retrospective study. Blood 2006;107(9):3463–8.
[34] Kim HJ, Ahn HK, Jung CW, et al. KIT D816 mutation associates with adverse outcomes in core binding factor acute myeloid leukemia, especially in the subgroup with RUNX1/RUNX1T1 rearrangement. Ann Hematol 2013;92(2):163–71.
[35] Ayatollahi H, Shajiei A, Sadeghian MH, et al. Prognostic importance of C-KIT mutations in core binding factor acute myeloid leukemia: a systematic review. Hematol Oncol Stem Cell Ther 2017;10(1):1–7.
[36] Perea G, Lasa A, Aventin A, et al. Prognostic value of minimal residual disease (MRD) in acute myeloid leukemia (AML) with favorable cytogenetics [t(8;21) and inv(16)]. Leukemia 2006;20(1):87–94.
[37] Jourdan E, Boissel N, Chevret S, et al. Prospective evaluation of gene mutations and minimal residual disease in patients with core binding factor acute myeloid leukemia. Blood 2013;121(12):2213–23.
[38] Willekens C, Blanchet O, Renneville A, et al. Prospective long-term minimal residual disease monitoring using RQ-PCR in RUNX1-RUNX1T1-positive acute myeloid leukemia: results of the French CBF 2006 trial. Haematologica 2016;101(3):328–35.
[39] Wang Y, Wu DP, Liu QF, et al. In adults with t(8;21) AML, posttransplant RUNX1/RUNX1T1-based MRD monitoring, rather than c KIT mutations, allows further risk stratification. Blood 2014;124(12):1880–6.
[40] Inoue K, Sugiyama H, Ogawa H, et al. WT1 as a new prognostic factor and a new marker for the detection of minimal residual disease in acute leukemia. Blood 1994;84(9):3071–9.
[41] Cilloni D, Renneville A, Hermitte F, et al. Real-time quantitative polymerase chain reaction detection of minimal residual disease by standardized WT1 assay to enhance risk stratification in acute myeloid leukemia: a European LeukemiaNet study. J Clin Oncol 2009; 27(31):5195–201.
[42] Huggett JF, Cowen S, Foy CA. Considerations for digital PCR as an accurate molecular diagnostic tool. Clin Chem 2015;61(1):79–88.
[43] Grimwade D, Freeman SD. Defining minimal residual disease in acute myeloid leukemia: which platforms are ready for "prime time"? Blood 2014;124(23):3345–55.
[44] Grimwade D, Ivey A, Huntly BJ. Molecular landscape of acute myeloid leukemia in younger adults and its clinical relevance. Blood 2016;127(1):29–41.
[45] Klco JM, Spencer DH, Miller CA, et al. Functional heterogeneity of genetically defined subclones in acute myeloid leukemia. Cancer Cell 2014;25(3):379–92.
[46] Ding L, Ley TJ, Larson DE, et al. Clonal evolution in relapsed acute myeloid leukaemia revealed by whole-genome sequencing. Nature 2012;481(7382):506–10.
[47] Ommen HB. Monitoring minimal residual disease in acute myeloid leukaemia: a review of the current evolving strategies. Ther Adv Hematol 2016;7(1):3–16.
[48] Hourigan CS, Gale RP, Gormley NJ, et al. Measurable residual disease testing in acute myeloid leukaemia. Leukemia 2017;31(7):1482–90.
[49] Fox EJ, Reid-Bayliss KS, Emond MJ, et al. Accuracy of next generation sequencing platforms. Next Gener Seq Appl 2014;1 [pii:1000106].
[50] Costello M, Pugh TJ, Fennell TJ, et al. Discovery and characterization of artifactual mutations in deep coverage targeted capture sequencing data due to oxidative DNA damage during sample preparation. Nucleic Acids Res 2013;41(6):e67.
[51] Hiatt JB, Patwardhan RP, Turner EH, et al. Parallel, tag-directed assembly of locally derived short sequence reads. Nat Methods 2010;7(2):119–22.
[52] Kinde I, Wu J, Papadopoulos N, et al. Detection and quantification of rare mutations with massively parallel sequencing. Proc Natl Acad Sci U S A 2011;108(23): 9530–5.
[53] Hiatt JB, Pritchard CC, Salipante SJ, et al. Single molecule molecular inversion probes for targeted, high-accuracy detection of low-frequency variation. Genome Res 2013;23(5):843–54.
[54] Gregory MT, Bertout JA, Ericson NG, et al. Targeted single molecule mutation detection with massively parallel sequencing. Nucleic Acids Res 2016;44(3):e22.
[55] Salk JJ, Schmitt MW, Loeb LA. Enhancing the accuracy of next-generation sequencing for detecting rare and subclonal mutations. Nat Rev Genet 2018;19(5):269–85.
[56] Young AL, Wong TN, Hughes AE, et al. Quantifying ultra-rare pre-leukemic clones via targeted error-corrected sequencing. Leukemia 2015;29(7):1608–11.
[57] Smith T, Heger A, Sudbery I. UMI-tools: modeling sequencing errors in Unique Molecular Identifiers to improve quantification accuracy. Genome Res 2017; 27(3):491–9.

[58] Schmitt MW, Kennedy SR, Salk JJ, et al. Detection of ultra-rare mutations by next-generation sequencing. Proc Natl Acad Sci U S A 2012;109(36):14508–13.

[59] Kennedy SR, Schmitt MW, Fox EJ, et al. Detecting ultralow-frequency mutations by Duplex Sequencing. Nat Protoc 2014;9(11):2586–606.

[60] Krimmel JD, Schmitt MW, Harrell MI, et al. Ultra-deep sequencing detects ovarian cancer cells in peritoneal fluid and reveals somatic TP53 mutations in noncancerous tissues. Proc Natl Acad Sci U S A 2016;113(21):6005–10.

[61] Araki D, Wood BL, Othus M, et al. Allogeneic hematopoietic cell transplantation for acute myeloid leukemia: time to move toward a minimal residual disease-based definition of complete remission? J Clin Oncol 2016;34(4):329–36.

Advances in Molecular Pathology 2 (2019) 59–64
ADVANCES IN MOLECULAR PATHOLOGY

Philadelphia-Like Lymphoblastic Leukemia

Approach to Testing in Clinical Laboratories for Diagnosis, Prognosis, and Therapeutic Risk Assessment

Michelle Afkhami, MD
Clinical Molecular Diagnostic Laboratory, Department of Pathology, City of Hope National Cancer Center, 1500 N. Duarte Road, Room 2287D, Duarte, CA 91010, USA

KEYWORDS
• Philadelphia-like acute lymphoblastic leukemia • BCR-ABL1-like ALL • B-ALL rearrangements • Low-density array (LDA) • Next-generation sequencing (NGS) • RNA sequencing (RNAseq) • Whole-exome sequencing (WES) • Whole-genome sequencing (WGS)

KEY POINTS
- The genomic landscape of the Philadelphia (Ph)-like acute lymphoblastic leukemia (ALL) has been defined in detail by advances in sequencing techniques, but classification by the gene expression profile still remains the mainstay of defining this entity.
- Gene expression classifiers have been well described for childhood Ph-like ALLs; however, many of these were not reproducible between different studies.
- Although Ph-like ALL has been associated with a poor outcome, detecting kinase gene fusions and *JAK/STAT* mutations shows promise for targeted therapies.

INTRODUCTION

B-cell acute lymphoblastic leukemia (B-ALL)/lymphoblastic lymphoma is a clonal disorder of lymphoid progenitors in the peripheral blood, bone marrow, or tissue. This disease is characterized by arrest of maturation and rapid proliferation of lymphoblasts, a type of early hematopoietic precursor cell. B-ALL is one of the most common childhood malignancies, representing about 25% of all cancers diagnosed in children younger than 14 years old, and 80% of all childhood leukemias. In adults, B-ALL is also a significant disease, accounting for 20% of all acute leukemias [1].

Some genetic and environmental factors that predispose to ALL have been reported. These include certain risk factors, such as age, race/ethnicity (more common in Caucasians than African Americans), gender (slight male predominance), radiation exposure, chemical exposure (including benzene or chemotherapy), specific viruses, and certain genetic syndromes (such as Down, Klinefelter, Bloom, and Li Fraumeni syndromes, Fanconi anemia, ataxia-telangiectasia, and neurofibromatosis). The American Cancer Society estimates the number of new ALL cases in the United States in 2019 at approximately 5930 (3280 male cases and 2650 female cases), with about 1500 deaths (850 male deaths and 650 female deaths) [2].

One of the most frequent cytogenetic alterations in B-ALL is *BCR-ABL1* t(9;22), also known as the

Disclosure: Michelle Afkhami receives research support from department of pathology at City of Hope.
E-mail address: mahtaafk@hotmail.com

https://doi.org/10.1016/j.yamp.2019.07.004
2589-4080/19/

Philadelphia (Ph) chromosome. This genetic abnormality occurs in 25% of adult and about 4% of childhood B-ALL cases. Rearrangement involving the major breakpoint in the *BCR* gene results in a 210-kDa protein, which is detected in 20% to 30% of adult cases and less commonly in pediatric ALLs. The minor breakpoint encodes a 190-kDa protein that is more prevalent in both adult and pediatric cases, 70% to 80% and 90%, respectively. Multiple signaling pathways are activated owing to upregulation of this oncogenic fusion, including RAS/MEK/ERK (activation of transcription factors, including NF-kB), PI-3 kinase/AKT (cell growth, cell survival, and inhibition of apoptosis), and JAK-STAT (cell growth and survival) [3,4].

Markers of high-risk status at the time of diagnosis include age $\geq$10 years and/or initial white blood cell count $\geq$50,000/μL. The prognosis for B-ALL has been better characterized because of recent insights into the molecular genomic pathways of this disease. Long-term disease-free survival is achieved in greater than 90% of pediatric patients after treatment, and in around 40% to 45% of adults [5–7].

Greater accessibility and use of genomic technologies led to the discovery of a new subgroup of B-ALL in 2009, lacking BCR-ABL1 fusions but harboring a kinase-activated gene expression profile similar to Ph-positive ALLs. This entity was called Ph-like or *BCR-ABL1*-like ALL and was associated with an unfavorable outcome. It is characterized by distinct gene expression profiles, chromosomal rearrangements, and both gene copy number alterations (CNAs) and sequence mutations that affect lymphoid development, tumor suppression, cytokine receptors, kinases, and other signaling pathways [8–19]. This subtype also has activation of constitutive signal transduction pathways, often owing to tyrosine kinase (TK) fusions other than *BCR-ABL1* [20]. Ph-like ALL comprises 20% to 25% of B-ALL in adolescents and young adults and is associated with worse survival rates; however, the frequency and biology of this in older populations (>65) are not clearly known. Age-related differences may be due to disease-related factors such as a higher frequency of unfavorable genomic abnormalities in adults, and patient-related factors including decreased tolerance to chemotherapy or other medical conditions; however, this needs to be better defined with more precise risk criteria [16,17,21–25].

B-ACUTE LYMPHOBLASTIC LEUKEMIA GENOMIC CLASSIFICATION

The 2016 World Health Organization classification of tumors of the hematopoietic and lymphoid tissues currently recognizes Ph-like ALL as a provisional entity under ALL with known cytogenetic abnormalities [26,27] (Box 1).

The Ph-like subgroup has a diversity of potential abnormalities, and no single system for identification of this subtype has yet achieved general acceptance. Genomic alterations that can help with identification of this subgroup are listed later in this discussion.

GENE EXPRESSION

The Ph-like expression classifiers were first described about a decade ago by the Dutch Childhood Oncology Group (DCOG) using array-based techniques of hierarchical clustering, consisting of 110 probe sets (Affymetrix) [8,11]. In the DCOG study, the cases were characterized by comparative genomic hybridization arrays and molecular cytogenetics. Genomic loss and gain were defined as having a minimum of 3 adjacent probes deviating beyond the threshold of 0.8 for single copy loss and 1.8 for biallelic loss [12].

Around the same time, the St. Jude Children's Research Hospital Childhood Oncology Group (COG) also described a Ph-like gene expression profile using a prediction analysis of microarray classifiers consisting of 257 probe sets by Affymetrix. These 2 methods only had 9 probe sets in common. However, both groups detected *IKZF1* and *VPREB1* deletion, in addition or amplification of a portion of chromosome 21 (iAMP21) [12].

BOX 1
World Health Organization 2016 Classification of B-Cell Acute Lymphoblastic Leukemia

B lymphoblastic leukemia/lymphoma, not otherwise specified

B lymphoblastic leukemia/lymphoma with recurrent genetic abnormalities

- Hypodiploidy
- Hyperdiploidy
- *BCR-ABL*1, t(9;22) (q34;q11.2)
- *KMT2A (MLL)* rearranged, t(v;11q23)
- *ETV6-RUNX1*, t(12;21)(p13;q22)
- *TCF3-PBX1*, t(1;19)(q23;p13.3)
- *IL3-IGH*, t(5;14)(q31;q32)
- iAMP21, intrachromosomal amplification of chromosome 21
- *BCR-ABL1*-like or Ph-like, translocations involving tyrosine kinase or cytokine receptors

Based on a low-density array (LDA) with a 15-gene classifier, introduced by Harvey and colleagues [13,16], Roberts and colleagues [17,18,20,28] developed an 8-gene assay consisting of *JCHAIN, SPATS2L, CA6, NRXN3, MUC4, CRLF2, ADGRF1*, and *BMPR1B*.

Sadras and colleagues [29] used a 9-gene signature, including *BMPR1B, CA6, CHN2, GPR110, JCHAIN, MUC4, NRXN3, SPATS2L, TP53INP1*, and *EEF2* as a housekeeping gene. The *CRLF2* expression was detected by Taqman LDA and flow cytometry study. The *CRLF2, KRAS, NRAS, JAK1, JAK2*, and *IL7Rα* mutations were detected by Sanger sequencing, and *IKZF1* deletions were detected by multiplex ligation-dependent probe amplification (MLPA), which is a multiplex PCR method detecting abnormal copy numbers of different genomic DNA or RNA sequences (RNAseq). While this assay is able to distinguish sequences differing in only 1 nucleotide. Then, messenger RNAseq was performed to detect fusions. They classified most of their *CRLF2*-rearranged patients as Ph-like, characterized by significantly higher expression levels of *MUC4, GPR110*, and *IL2RA/CD25*.

Chiaretti and colleagues [30,31] recently identified 9 genes commonly overexpressed by Ph-like ALLs, including *SOCS2, IFITM1, CD99, TP53INP1, IFITM2, JCHAIN, NUDT4, CD97*, and *SEMA6A*. In addition to their gene expression classifier, they used reverse transcriptase-polymerase chain reaction (RT-PCR) for *CRLF2* transcript quantification.

COPY NUMBER LOSS

IKZF1 encodes IKAROS, a zinc finger protein that plays important roles in hematopoiesis, regulation of cellular adhesion and migration, and as a tumor suppressor. *IKZF1* deletions have been identified in both *BCR-ABL1*-positive and *BCR-ABL1*-negative ALLs, in about 15% and 30% of pediatric and adult ALL cases, and more than 70% of adult Ph-like ALLs. About 40% to 50% of *CRLF2*-rearranged B-ALLs have concurrent *IKZF1* deletion. In addition, Sadras and colleagues [29] showed that more than 60% of *CRLF2*-rearranged cases with a Ph-like gene expression profile also had *IKZF1* deletion. However, recent studies have not clearly shown an independent inferior prognostic value for this latter alteration.

Other frequently deleted genes are cyclin-dependent kinase (CDK) inhibitors 2A and 2B (*CDKN2A/2B*) located on chromosome 9p21, which encode P16 and P15, respectively. *CDKN2A* and *CDKN2B* inhibit CDK4 and CDK6 and control cellular proliferation by preventing entry into the S phase of the cell cycle, and their inactivation may contribute to uncontrolled growth in human cancers. The frequency of *CDKN2A/2B* deletion in *KMT2A*-rearranged cell lines was significantly lower than that in non-*KMT2A*-rearranged cell lines. *CDKN2A/2B* gene deletion has been reported in about 50% of Ph-like ALLs and is more commonly seen in cases that are negative for tyrosine kinase (TK) rearrangement.

Deletion of the *EBF1* and *BTG1* genes is seen in about 30% of Ph-like ALLs and has been associated with a poor prognosis. In a study for the Spanish PETHEMA Group and the Spanish Society of Hematology, deletions of *EBF1, IKZF1*, and *CDKN2A/B* were reported to have an independent adverse prognosis in adolescents and adults with B-ALL. This suggests that these CNAs should be included in the initial risk assessment of ALL. A recent in vitro study showed the frequencies of *IKZF1, CDKN2A/2B, BTG1*, and *PAX5* deletion were significantly higher in *BCR-ABL1*-positive than those in Ph-negative B-ALL cell lines. Multiple studies used MLPA methods for detection of copy number variation in up to 12 genes in B-ALL patients [12,30,32,33].

Deletion of *VPREB1* (V-set pre-B-cell surrogate light chain 1), along with *IKZF1*, has been reported initially by both the DCOG and COG studies in childhood B-ALL [8,11,12]. This deletion is not specific to Ph-like cases and can happen in a variety of subtypes of ALL, such as *ETV6-RNX1* translocation or Down syndrome–related B-ALL. Focal deletion of the *VPREB1* has been associated with lower disease-free survival and overall survival [34].

REARRANGEMENTS

Patients with *ETV6-RUNX1* translocation or chromosomal hyperdiploidy have been reported to have a better prognosis in both childhood and adult ALLs. On the other hand, hypodiploidy, *KMT2A* (*MLL*), *BCR-ABL1, TCF3-HLF*, and *E2A-HLF* translocations are described as prognostic biomarkers for high-risk disease. The Ph-like ALL subtype has been associated with a wide variety of rearrangements.

Some recent studies propose dividing this subtype into 2 groups based on cytokine receptor-like factor 2 (*CRLF2*) rearrangement or overexpression, and fusions that cause TK pathway activation. These fusions can be detected by interphase fluorescence in situ hybridization (FISH) analysis or RNAseq. Expression levels can be assessed by flow cytometry, low density array (LDA), or RNAseq studies. The first group is marked by overexpression of *CRLF2*, which is seen in around 50% of cases of Ph-like B-ALLs [15,20,21]. Often this overexpression is driven by fusions involving the *CRLF2* gene, including *P2RY8-CRLF2* and *IGH-CRLF2* fusions. These cases also commonly have JAK-STAT mutations, with the *JAK2* R683G mutation being the most common. These mutations result in JAK-STAT pathway activation, and therapies involving JAK inhibition should be considered [21].

The second major group of Ph-like ALLs includes fusions that activate TK pathways affecting kinases, such as *ABL1*, *ABL2*, *CSF1R*, *PDGFRB*, *EBF1*, and *NTRK3*, which could be treated with ABL-type TK inhibitors [15,20,21,25,32–35].

In children, adolescents, and young adults, approximately 50% of Ph-like ALLs activate JAK-STAT and PI3K/mTOR signaling via rearrangement of cytokine receptor-like factor 2 (*CRLF2-R*) with common co-occurrence of *JAK2* or *JAK1* point mutations. An additional 10% to 15% of Ph-like ALL harbor *JAK2* or *EPOR* rearrangements, whereas another 15% to 20% have translocations or fusions involving *ABL1*, *ABL2*, *CSF1R*, or *PDGFRB* (*ABL*-class lesions) [35].

MUTATIONS

In the COSMIC/TCGA databases, the most common mutations in B-ALLs are in *IKZF1*, *KRAS*, *PAX5*, *NRAS*, *JAK1*, *JAK2*, *PTPN11*, *FLT3*, *P53*, *IL7R*, *CREBBP*, *CRLF2*, *SETD2*, *NT5C2*, *KDM6A*, *SH2B3*, *NF1*, *KMT2D*, *EPF1*, and *NCOR1* genes.

Investigation of the loci with recurrent CNA determined that approximately 40% of B-ALL cases demonstrate mutations in B-lineage specification genes, most frequently *PAX5*, *EBF1*, and *IKZF1* [12,13,36–38]. A follow-up study identified mutation of *IKZF1* as a near-obligate event, occurring in 84% of cases, in *BCR-ABL1*-positive B-ALL, and as a mutation acquired during the progression from chronic phase chronic myeloid leukemia to lymphoid blast crisis.

Mutations in transcriptional coactivators *CREBBP* and *NCOR1*, the transcription factors *ERG*, *SPI1*, *TCF4*, and *TCF7L2*, components of the Ras signaling pathway, and histone genes have been found in relapsed ALLs. A resequencing study of matched diagnosis and relapse samples identified *CREBBP* as a gene mutated in 18% of B-ALL cases that relapsed, but was essentially always unmutated in cases that did not relapse [39].

A recent study by Feng and colleagues [40] found that *FAT1* was the most commonly mutated gene in B-ALL (about 11%), followed by *SF1*, *CRLF2*, *TET2*, *PTPN11*, *NRAS*, *CREBBP*, *JAK2*, *DIS3*, *MPL*, and *KML2D* (>5% of the cases). In Ph-positive B-ALL, *FAT1*, *CRLF2*, *SF1*, *EP300*, and *CREBBP* genes appear to be mutated at higher incidences. However, *PTPN11*, *SF1*, *TET2*, *NRAS*, *JAK2*, *DIS3*, and *FAT1* gene mutations have also been described in Ph-negative ALLs. Germline mutations of *GATA3* have been found to increase the risk of relapse in Ph-like childhood ALLs [41].

SUMMARY

The National Comprehensive Cancer Network guideline for ALL version 2.2019 recommends molecular characterization of ALL to include G-banded chromosome analysis, FISH studies for the major recurrent genetic abnormalities, and RT-PCR for *BCR-ABL1* (p190 and p210). Furthermore, additional testing is encouraged for gene fusions and other mutations if a case is found to be *BCR-ABL1* negative. Additional optional tests include Array comparative genomic hybridization (array CGH) in cases of aneuploidy or failed karyotype [42].

FISH studies are more readily available to most laboratories and can be highly specific for selected rearrangements, such as *IGH*. However, this method may not be practical for general screening in ALL cases because of the broad variety of rearrangements. To expedite a diagnosis and facilitate the most-appropriate therapy for the patient, DNA next-generation sequencing (NGS) and RNAseq assays represent the most optimal option.

Many laboratories that perform genetic analysis of leukemias in-house now have test panels of variable size, ranging between 20 genes to a WES. These assays are mainly designed to detect mutations and fusions and may use PCR, Sanger, RT-PCR, and NGS methods. Gene expression assays are not commonly available in-house for many laboratories; however, some LDA assays are commercially available.

Chiaretti and colleagues [31] recently summarized the testing strategies different groups have taken to identify Ph-like cases. These assays include assorted combinations of various methods, including FISH, LDA, RT-PCR, NGS (RNAseq, WES, WGS) [17,20] or more simplified approaches, including RT-PCR for known fusion transcripts, *JAK2* mutations, and *CRLF2* rearrangement [35].

Roberts and colleagues [28] recently described reduced frequency of Ph-like ALL and targetable alterations in standard-risk ALL compared to patients with high-risk disease. They started with an 8-gene TaqMan LDA by PCR assay upfront for identification of Ph-Like ALL. In cases with high *CRLF2* expression, the *CRLF2* rearrangement status was assessed by FISH analysis, and JAK1 or JAK2 mutation status by Sanger sequencing. The remaining cases with low expression of *CRLF2* were tested with an RT-PCR assay for 41 known kinase fusions involving *ABL1*, *ABL2*, *CSF1R*, *JAK2*, *NTRK3*, and *PDGFRB* genes. If no *CRLF2* or kinase fusions were identified, then whole transcriptome sequencing was pursued.

Benefits of proceeding with a stepwise testing algorithm for this entity are cost saving in cases that are negative for Ph-like ALL by an initial LDA assay. However, for cases that are found to be Ph-like, the subsequent reflexive testing steps would be clinically time consuming and run the risk of incomplete testing owing to sample depletion.

At the author's facility, most of the B-ALL cases are in adults, and a combination of cytogenetics, RT-PCR, DNAseq, and RNAseq NGS studies are performed on all initial and relapsed B-ALL cases. These assays were designed in consideration of the frequency of the alterations found in the population seen at the author's cancer center. As reviewed above, most of the determinants for diagnosis were established in childhood cohorts. Those at the author's facility are currently validating their own gene expression assay with respect to an adult patient cohort, which will be published separately.

The author's cancer center RNAseq assay was designed to assess the most common and recently described targetable kinase gene fusions in Ph-like ALLs. However, they found that FISH studies for *IGH* rearrangement were necessary because *IGH-CRLF2* and *IGH-EPOR* translocations could be missed because of a lack of a fusion transcript product, or rearrangements involving regions outside of primer coverage. To increase the odds of detecting *CRLF2* rearrangement, especially for cases with potential *JAK1* or *JAK2* mutations, they evaluate the *CRLF2* expression level and reflex to *IGH* FISH testing in cases with high expression.

Several advantages have been found by doing comprehensive testing upfront for these patients. The most obvious advantage is a significantly shortened turnaround time. Next, only 1 DNA and 1 RNA extraction need to be performed from the EDTA bone marrow aspirate or peripheral blood tubes. A third benefit is that only small amounts of DNA (10 ng)/RNA (150 ng) are required for testing of all the relevant alterations. Fourth, the assay is performed in-house from original DNA/RNA extraction material, which decreases the risk of preanalytical and postanalytical errors. A final benefit is having all the alterations comprehensively issued in 1 integrated report. However, this approach would only be cost-effective for Ph-like ALL cases.

The genomic heterogeneity in Ph-like ALL is broad, and many of the findings have unclear relevance across age groups and additional research is necessary. Understanding the evolution of this disease with comparison between the initial and relapse clones may help with the development of minimal residual disease assays, and optimize the treatment of these patients.

REFERENCES

[1] Redaelli A, Laskin BL, Stephens JM, et al. A systematic literature review of the clinical and epidemiological burden of acute lymphoblastic leukaemia (ALL). Eur J Cancer Care (Engl) 2005;14(1):53–62.

[2] Available at: https://www.cancer.org/cancer/acute-lymphocytic-leukemia.

[3] Van rhee F, Hochhaus A, Lin F, et al. p190 BCR-ABL mRNA is expressed at low levels in p210-positive chronic myeloid and acute lymphoblastic leukemias. Blood 1996;87(12):5213–7.

[4] Melo JV. The diversity of BCR-ABL fusion proteins and their relationship to leukemia phenotype. Blood 1996; 88(7):2375–84.

[5] Rowe JM, Buck G, Burnett AK, et al. Induction therapy for adults with acute lymphoblastic leukemia: results of more than 1500 patients from the International ALL Trial: MRC UKALL XII/ECOG E2993. Blood 2005;106:3760–7.

[6] Hunger SP, Mullighan CG. Acute lymphoblastic leukemia in children. N Engl J Med 2015;373(16):1541–52.

[7] Liu X, Zou Y, Wang H, et al. Treatment outcome of childhood standard-risk and median-risk acute lymphoblastic leukemia with CCLG-2008 protocol. Zhonghua Er Ke Za Zhi 2014;52(6):449–54 [in Chinese].

[8] Pullarkat V, Slovak ML, Kopecky KJ, et al. Impact of cytogenetics on the outcome of adult acute lymphoblastic leukemia: results of Southwest Oncology Group 9400 study. Blood 2008;111(5):2563–72.

[9] Ravandi F, O'brien S, Thomas D, et al. First report of phase 2 study of dasatinib with hyper-CVAD for the frontline treatment of patients with Philadelphia chromosome-positive (Ph+) acute lymphoblastic leukemia. Blood 2010;116(12):2070–7.

[10] Rowe JM. Optimal management of adults with ALL. Br J Haematol 2009;144(4):468–83.

[11] Den Boer ML, van Slegtenhorst M, De Menezes RX, et al. A subtype of childhood acute lymphoblastic leukaemia with poor treatment outcome: a genome-wide classification study. Lancet Oncol 2009;10:125–34.

[12] Mullighan CG, Su X, Zhang J, et al. Deletion of IKZF1 and prognosis in acute lymphoblastic leukemia. N Engl J Med 2009;360(5):470–80.

[13] Harvey RC, Mullighan CG, Chen IM, et al. Rearrangement of CRLF2 is associated with mutation of JAK kinases, alteration of IKZF1, Hispanic/Latino ethnicity, and a poor outcome in pediatric B-progenitor acute lymphoblastic leukemia. Blood 2010;115(26):5312–21.

[14] Kang H, Chen IM, Wilson CS, et al. Gene expression classifiers for relapse-free survival and minimal residual disease improve risk classification and outcome prediction in pediatric B-precursor acute lymphoblastic leukemia. Blood 2010;115(7):1394–405.
[15] Tasian SK, Doral MY, Borowitz MJ, et al. Aberrant STAT5 and PI3K/mTOR pathway signaling occurs in human CRLF2-rearranged B-precursor acute lymphoblastic leukemia. Blood 2012;120(4):833–42.
[16] Harvey RC, Kang H, Roberts KG, et al. Development and validation of a highly sensitive and specific gene expression classifier to prospectively screen and identify B-precursor acute lymphoblastic leukemia (ALL) patients with a Philadelphia chromosome-like signature for therapeutic targeting and clinical intervention. Blood 2013; 123(21):ASH annual meeting abstract #826.
[17] Roberts KG, Gu Z, Payne-Turner D, et al. High frequency and poor outcome of Philadelphia chromosome-like acute lymphoblastic leukemia in adults. J Clin Oncol 2017;35:394–401.
[18] Jain N, Roberts KG, Jabbour E, et al. Ph-like acute lymphoblastic leukemia: a high-risk subtype in adults. Blood 2017;129:572–81.
[19] Wells J, Jain N, Konopleva M. Philadelphia chromosome-like acute lymphoblastic leukemia: progress in a new cancer subtype. Clin Adv Hematol Oncol 2017;15(7):554–61.
[20] Roberts KG, Li Y, Payne-turner D, et al. Targetable kinase-activating lesions in Ph-like acute lymphoblastic leukemia. N Engl J Med 2014;371(11):1005–15.
[21] Reshmi SC, Harvey RC, Roberts KG, et al. Targetable kinase gene fusions in high-risk B-ALL: a study from the Children's Oncology Group. Blood 2017;129(25):3352–61.
[22] Iacobucci I, Li Y, Roberts KG, et al. Truncating erythropoietin receptor rearrangements in acute lymphoblastic leukemia. Cancer Cell 2016;29(2):186–200.
[23] Tasian SK, Hurtz C, Wertheim GB, et al. High incidence of Philadelphia chromosome-like acute lymphoblastic leukemia in older adults with B-ALL. Leukemia 2017;31:981–4.
[24] Boer JM, Den boer ML. BCR-ABL1-like acute lymphoblastic leukaemia: from bench to bedside. Eur J Cancer 2017;82:203–18.
[25] Tasian SK, Teachey DT, Li Y, et al. Potent efficacy of combined PI3K/mTOR and JAK or ABL inhibition in murine xenograft models of Ph-like acute lymphoblastic leukemia. Blood 2017;129(2):177–87.
[26] Arber DA, Orazi A, Hasserjian R, et al. The 2016 revision to the World Health Organization classification of myeloid neoplasms and acute leukemia. Blood 2016; 127:2391–405.
[27] Inthal A, Zeitlhofer P, Zeginigg M, et al. CREBBP HAT domain mutations prevail in relapse cases of high hyperdiploid childhood acute lymphoblastic leukemia. Leukemia 2012;26:1797–803.
[28] Roberts KG, Reshmi SC, Harvey RC, et al. Genomic and outcome analyses of Ph-like ALL in NCI standard-risk patients: a report from the Children's Oncology Group. Blood 2018;132:815–24.
[29] Sadras T, Heatley SL, Kok CH, et al. Differential expression of MUC4, GPR110 and IL2RA defines two groups of CRLF2-rearranged acute lymphoblastic leukemia patients with distinct secondary lesions. Cancer Lett 2017;408:92–101.
[30] Chiaretti S, Messina M, Grammatico S, et al. Rapid identification of BCR/ABL1-like acute lymphoblastic leukaemia patients using a predictive statistical model based on quantitative real time-polymerase chain reaction: clinical, prognostic and therapeutic implications. Br J Haematol 2018;181:642–52.
[31] Chiaretti S, Messina M, Foà R. BCR/ABL1-like acute lymphoblastic leukemia: how to diagnose and treat? Cancer 2019;125(2):194–204.
[32] Ruiz-delgado GJ, Cantero-fortiz Y, León-peña AA, et al. IKAROS gene deleted B-cell acute lymphoblastic leukemia in Mexican Mestizos: observations in seven patients and a short review of the literature. Rev Invest Clin 2016; 68(4):210–4.
[33] Ribera J, Morgades M, Zamora L, et al. Prognostic significance of copy number alterations in adolescent and adult patients with precursor B acute lymphoblastic leukemia enrolled in PETHEMA protocols. Cancer 2015; 121(21):3809–17.
[34] Mangum DS, Downie J, Mason CC, et al. VPREB1 deletions occur independent of lambda light chain rearrangement in childhood acute lymphoblastic leukemia. Leukemia 2014;28(1):216–20.
[35] Herold T, Schneider S, Metzeler KH, et al. Adults with Philadelphia chromosome-like acute lymphoblastic leukemia frequently have IGH-CRLF2 and JAK2 mutations, persistence of minimal residual disease and poor prognosis. Haematologica 2017;102(1):130–8.
[36] Russell LJ, Capasso M, Vater I, et al. Deregulated expression of cytokine receptor gene, CRLF2, is involved in lymphoid transformation in B-cell precursor acute lymphoblastic leukemia. Blood 2009;114(13):2688–98.
[37] Mullighan CG, Goorha S, Radtke I, et al. Genome-wide analysis of genetic alterations in acute lymphoblastic leukaemia. Nature 2007;446:758–64.
[38] Maude SL, Tasian SK, Vincent T, et al. Targeting JAK1/2 and mTOR in murine xenograft models of Ph-like acute lymphoblastic leukemia. Blood 2012;120(17):3510–8.
[39] Mullighan CG, Zhang J, Kasper LH, et al. CREBBP mutations in relapsed acute lymphoblastic leukeamia. Nature 2011;471:235–9.
[40] Feng J, Li Y, Jia Y, et al. Spectrum of somatic mutations detected by targeted next generation sequencing and their prognostic significance in adult patients with acute lymphoblastic leukemia. J Hematol Oncol 2017;10(1):61.
[41] Perez-Andreu V, Roberts KG, Harvey RC, et al. Inherited GATA3 variants are associated with Ph-like childhood acute lymphoblastic leukemia and risk of relapse. Nat Genet 2013;45(12):1494–8.
[42] NCCN Guidelines® for Acute Lymphoblastic Leukemia V.2.2019 © National Comprehensive Cancer Network, Inc. 2019. All rights reserved. Available at: www.NCCN.org. Accessed May 15, 2019.

Advances in Molecular Pathology 2 (2019) 65–75
ADVANCES IN MOLECULAR PATHOLOGY

Myeloid Gene Panel Testing with Correlation to Updated Clinical Practice Guidelines

Laura N. Toth, DO, MPH*, Daniel Babu, MD
Department of Pathology, University of New Mexico Health Sciences Center, MSC08 4640, 1 University of New Mexico, Albuquerque, NM 87131, USA

KEYWORDS
• AML • MDS • MPN • Molecular • Panel • Diagnosis • Risk • Treatment

KEY POINTS
- Readers will understand the need for multigene testing for myeloid neoplasms.
- Readers will understand how the findings of molecular testing affect diagnosis, risk stratification, and treatment of patients with myeloid neoplasms in terms of current practice guidelines.
- Readers will understand the limitations of large panel testing for myeloid neoplasms.

INTRODUCTION

Myeloid neoplasms are a broad category of hematopoietic diseases including myelodysplastic syndrome (MDS); myeloproliferative neoplasms (MPNs) with subtypes including polycythemia vera (PV), essential thrombocythemia (ET), and primary myelofibrosis (PMF); myelodysplastic neoplasm (MDS)/myeloproliferative neoplasm (MPN); and acute myeloid leukemia (AML). Diagnosis and evaluation of these entities is a multifaceted process that includes cytomorphologic, cytogenetic, flow cytometric, and molecular evaluation. As next-generation sequencing (NGS) has become increasingly accessible, several variants have been shown to carry prognostic significance, in addition to aiding in diagnosis and providing options for targeted therapy. Numerous guideline-producing entities including, but not limited to, the World Health Organization (WHO), the National Comprehensive Cancer Network (NCCN), European LeukemiaNet (ELN), the College of American Pathologists (CAP), the Association for Molecular Pathology (AMP), and the American Society of Hematology (ASH) have designated a large number of variants as clinically significant or frequently mutated in myeloid neoplasms. Because of this, large panel testing strategies have become increasingly popular.

This article reviews the diagnostic and clinical significance of myeloid gene panel testing, the integration of molecular findings into clinical practice guidelines, and the inherent limitations of large panel testing.

SIGNIFICANCE

Diagnosis

MDS remains one of the most difficult diagnoses to establish because many of the morphologic features described as dysplastic may be associated with nonneoplastic causes, including nutritional deficiencies, medication effects, and toxic exposures.

Disclosure: The authors have nothing to disclose.

*Corresponding author, *E-mail address:* laura.n.toth@gmail.com

https://doi.org/10.1016/j.yamp.2019.07.005
2589-4080/19/

Although molecular findings have not been formally incorporated into the diagnostic classification of MDS, the identification of certain variants may aid in establishing the presence of a neoplastic clone. The NCCN has released a list of genes that have been described in the literature as frequently associated with MDS. In addition, the AMP has developed a list of genes recommended for inclusion in myeloid gene panel testing [1]. It must be noted that certain variants (*TET2*, *DNMT3A*, and *ASXL1*) have previously been described in association with clonal hematopoiesis of indeterminate potential (CHIP) and clonal cytopenias of undetermined significance (CCUS) [2–4]. Also the detection of certain variants (eg, *SF3B1*) lowers the previous threshold of ring sideroblasts from greater than or equal to 15% to greater than or equal to 5% in the diagnosis of MDS with ring sideroblasts (MDS-RS) [5].

In the latest revision of the WHO Classification of Tumors of Haematopoietic and Lymphoid Tissues (2017), the category of AML with recurrent genetic abnormalities has expanded with new mutational subgroups. AML with mutated *NPM1* and AML with biallelic mutations of *CEBPA*, previously considered provisional entities, are now formally recognized [5,6]. In addition, the revision now includes the provisional entity of AML with mutated *RUNX1* [5]. The CAP and the ASH have strongly recommended testing for *FLT3*-internal tandem duplication (ITD), *NPM1*, *CEBPA*, and *RUNX1* for the initial diagnostic work-up of AML without recurrent cytogenetic abnormalities or myelodysplasia-related changes [7].

In contrast with AML classification, there are no mutation-defined subcategories of BCR-ABL1–negative myeloproliferative neoplasms. However, presence of particular variants, namely *JAK2*, *CALR*, and *MPL*, signals a clonal process and helps fulfill diagnostic criteria, even if the variants are not specific [5]. Specific variants are also not definitional for entities under the general WHO category of MDS/MPN either; however, variant identification may aid in establishing a primary diagnosis. For example, the diagnosis of chronic myelomonocytic leukemia (CMML) may be challenging if duration of monocytosis is unknown and if myelodysplasia and cytogenetic abnormalities are lacking. Detection of CMML-associated variants, such as *TET2*, *SRSF2*, *ASXL1*, and *SETBP1*, may fulfill a criterion for diagnosis [5,8]. In addition, among high-grade myelomonocytic neoplasms, distinction between high-grade CMML and AML with monocytic differentiation can be difficult because of morphologic subjectivity of monocytic blast equivalents. The constellation of detected variants may help differentiate these entities because *ASXL1*, *EZH2*, *NRAS*, *CBL*, *NF1*, *SETBP1*, and *BCOR* are more frequently detected in CMML, whereas *NPM1* variants have more commonly been described in AML with monocytic differentiation (Table 1), although, formally, blast percentage is the final discriminator between the two entities [5,21,22,28,36,39,55,56].

Prognostication

Prognostication for clinical decision making in patients with myeloid neoplasms seems to be the arena where molecular testing currently holds the most value. Because MDS is considered a preleukemic state, particular variants have been shown to be associated with poor prognosis, as defined by shorter time to leukemic development and decreased overall survival, and identification of these variants can aid clinicians in determining the need for medical intervention. Based on current literature, the NCCN and AMP have identified several prognostically significant or frequently mutated genes in MDS (see Table 1).

The NCCN and ELN now incorporate molecular findings into their AML risk stratification models. In both risk models the presence of a biallelic *CEBPA* or *NPM1* mutation, in the absence of recurrent cytogenetic abnormalities and *FLT3*-ITD mutation, is associated with a favorable prognosis [57–59]. Per the ELN risk model, AML with concurrent mutations of *NPM1* and *FLT3*-ITD are stratified into an intermediate risk category, with all other *FLT3*-ITD cases being in the adverse category [57]. The ELN stratification model also includes mutated *RUNX1*, *ASXL1*, and *TP53* as independent poor prognostic indicators [57]. The NCCN guidelines separately include *IDH1/2* and *DNMT3A* variants as possibly poor prognostic indicators [60–63].

Core-binding factor (CBF) AMLs, which include AML with t(8;21) and AML with inv(16), are associated with favorable prognosis [5]. However, a concurrent KIT mutation in these cytogenetic subtypes is associated with increased risk of relapse and decreased overall survival [41,42]. Per the ELN guidelines, the presence of a concurrent *KIT* mutation in t(8;21) AML should not alter risk stratification, but, per NCCN guidelines, *KIT*-mutated t(8;21) AML should not be classified as favorable-risk AML based on currently published data [41,57]. Given that a *KIT* mutation may abrogate the favorable prognosis of t(8:21) and inv(16), the CAP and the ASH strongly recommend testing for *KIT* mutation in patients with CBF AMLs [7]. However, the data for AML inv(16) are not as consistent as those for AML (8;21) because some studies suggest that *KIT* mutations have no clear prognostic effect on AML with inv(16) [43,44].

TABLE 1
Clinically Relevant Genes, Their Prognostic Significance, and Prevalence in Myeloid Neoplasms

Gene Function	Gene	Clinical Significance in MDS and AML [9–15]	Clinical Significance in MPN [14,16–20]	Clinical Significance in MDS/MPN [21–24]
DNA methylation	*TET2*[a,b]	Associated with normal karyotypes. May be seen in CHIP/CCUS. (20%–25% in MDS, up to 40% of AML cases)	Uncertain prognostic significance (~20% overall)	May be associated with shorter survival in CMML (20%–60%)
	DNMT3A[a,b]	Can be seen in CHIP and CCUS. Typically a negative prognostic indicator with shortened DFS and OS in AML and MDS, especially in younger patients [25]. (12%–18% in MDS, 18%–30% of AML)	Uncertain prognostic significance (up to 15% in PV, 6% in ET, <5% in PV)	NA
	IDH1[a,b]	More commonly associated with AML. No significant effect on DFS, OS, CRR, or ORR. Therapeutic target. (<5% of MDS, 6%–10% of AML)	Independent poor prognostic indicator in PV. Associated with decreased leukemia-free survival in PMF. (<5% overall)	NA
	IDH2[a,b]	More commonly associated with AML. Poor prognostic indicator. Therapeutic target (<5% in MDS, 8%–14% of AML)	Independent poor prognostic indicator in PV and ET. Associated with decreased leukemia-free survival in PMF (<5% overall)	NA
Myeloid transcription factors	*RUNX1*[a,b]	Seen in both AML and MDS. Associated with worse prognosis in MDS and AML. (10%–15%)	Poor prognostic indicator in PMF. (<5% overall)	May be associated with higher white blood cell count at presentation (up to 40%)
	ETV6[a,b]	Associated with a poor prognosis (<5%)	NA	NA
	CEBPA[a,b]	New diagnostic category of AML. If mutation is biallelic it is associated with a better prognosis in the absence of *FLT3-ITD or NPM1* variants. If single mutation is detected it is associated with lower CRR, shorter DFS, and shorter OS. (7%–11%)	Poor prognostic indicator in PMF. (<10% overall)	NA

(continued on next page)

TABLE 1
(continued)

Gene Function	Gene	Clinical Significance in MDS and AML [9–15]	Clinical Significance in MPN [14,16–20]	Clinical Significance in MDS/MPN [21–24]
	GATA2[b]	Germline variant associated with myeloid malignancy with a worse prognosis. (NA)	NA	NA
Epigenetic regulators	*ASXL1*[a,b]	Associated with a poor prognosis in MDS and AML [26]. (~20% in MDS, 10% in AML)	Independent poor prognostic indicator in PV and PMF [27]. (Up to 35% in PMF, <15% in PV and ET)	Poor prognostic indicator (up to 40%)
	BCOR[a,b]	Associated with poor prognosis [28]. (<5% in MDS, 5%–8% in AML)	NA	Prognostic significance unclear [28]. (~7%)
	BCORL1[a]	Favorable prognostic indicator. (1%–3% in MDS)	NA	NA
	EZH2[a,b]	Associated with poor prognosis in MDS. (5%–10%)	Independent poor prognostic indicator in ET and PMF (~5% in PMF, <5% in ET and PV)	Increased risk of adverse outcomes (~6%)
Tumor suppressor genes	*TP53*[a,b]	Poor prognostic indicator. More commonly associated with complex karyotypes and del(5q) [29–31]. (8%–12% overall, but up to 45% of complex karyotype cases)	Poor prognostic indicator in PV, ET, and PMF with increased risk to leukemic transformation [32]. (<5%)	NA
	PHF6[a,b]	No prognostic influence, but more frequently associated with MDS with increased blasts. (<5%)	NA	NA
	DDX41 [33],[b]	Germline variant associated with adult-onset MDS/AML [34]. (NA)	NA	NA
	WT1[b]	Associated with a poor prognosis (<15%) [35]	NA	NA
	NF1[a,b]	–	NA	Germline variant more commonly associated with CMML or JMML. (<5%)

Splicing factors	*SRSF2*[a,b]	Poor prognostic indicator (10%–15% overall)	Poor prognostic indicator in PMF and PV (18% in PMF, <5% in PV and ET)	Prognostic significance unclear, possibly favorable [36]. (up to 45%)
	U2AF1[a,b]	Associated with poor prognosis in MDS [37]. (8%–12% in MDS, <5% in AML)	Independent poor prognostic indicator in ET. The Q157 variant is associated with decreased overall survival in younger patients with PMF [38]. (~15% of PMF, <5% of ET)	Prognostic significance unclear (~10%)
	SF3B1[a,b]	Associated with ring sideroblasts and may influence diagnosis of MDS-RS. Favorable prognostic indicator in MDS [39,40]. (20%–30%)	Independent poor prognostic indicator in ET (<5% in ET and PV)	Prognostic significance unclear, possibly favorable (~5%)
	ZRSR2[a,b]	Poor prognostic indicator in MDS. (5%–10%)	NA	NA
Cell signaling	*NRAS*[a,b]	Poor prognostic indicator in MDS. (5%–10% in MDS, up to 20% of AML)	NA	Prognostic significance unclear (20%–30%)
	KRAS[a]	Poor prognostic indicator in MDS. (1%–12%)	NA	Can be seen in CMML, prognostic significance unclear. (7%–12%)
	KIT[a,b]	Poor prognostic indicator in t(8;21) associated AML. Unclear significant impact on prognosis in AML associated with inv(16) or t(16;16) [41–44]. (20% of core binding factor AML cases)	Poor prognostic indicator in PMF. (<5% overall)	NA
	CBL [45],[a,b]	No significant prognostic impact. (<5% overall)	Poor prognostic indicator in PMF. (~5% in PMF, <5% in PV and ET)	Prognostic significance unclear (~10%)
	JAK2[a,b]	More commonly associated with MDS/MPN. (<5% overall but can be in up to 50% of MDS/MPN)	V617F is a disease-defining mutation in PV (95%). Exon 12 variant associated with younger age of presentation without significant prognostic impact in PV (<5% of PV). V617F is an intermediate prognostic indicator with higher risk of thrombosis compared with *CALR*-mutated PMF (50% in ET and PMF)	NA

(*continued on next page*)

TABLE 1
(*continued*)

Gene Function	Gene	Clinical Significance in MDS and AML [9–15]	Clinical Significance in MPN [14,16–20]	Clinical Significance in MDS/MPN [21–24]
	CALR[a,b]	NA	Improved survival and decreased risk of thrombosis compared with *JAK2*-mutated ET and PMF [46–48]. (20%–30% of ET and PMF)	NA
	STAT3 [49],[b]	Associated with large granular leukemia associated with a concurrent MDS. Can be associated with bone marrow failure [50]. (<5%)	NA	NA
	PPM1D [51],[a,b]	Can be seen in CHIP and CCUS. Associated with therapy-related MDS. (5%)	NA	NA
	MPL[a,b]	NA	Intermediate prognosis with increased risk of thrombosis compared with *CALR*-mutated PMF. (3% of ET, 10% in PMF)	NA
	PTPN11[a]	Poor prognostic indicator in MDS. (1%–2%)	NA	Can be seen in CMML, prognostic significance unclear (1%)
	CSF3R[a,b]	NA	Associated with chronic neutrophilic leukemia, prognostic significance unclear. (NA)	NA

Cohesin complex	*RAD21*[a]	Clinical significance unclear. (<1% of MDS)	NA	NA
	SMC3[a]	Clinical significance unclear (1% of MDS)	NA	NA
	STAG2[a]	Poor prognostic indicator (5%–15% of MDS)	NA	Can be seen in CMML, prognostic significance unclear (10%)
Multifunctional	*NPM1*[a,b]	Poor prognostic indicator in MDS. Favorable prognostic indicator in AML in the absence of *FLT3-ITD.* (28%–35% of AML)	NA	Rarely associated with MDS/MPN; poor prognostic indicator in CMML (<10%) [5,52,53]
	SETBP1[a,b]	Poor prognostic indicator in MDS [54]. (<5% overall)	NA	Prognostic significance unclear. (up to 12%) [54,55]
	FLT3[a,b]	Poor prognostic indicator in MDS and AML. (up to 40% of AML cases)	NA	NA

Abbreviations: CFR, complete response rate; DFS, disease-free survival; JMML, juvenile myelomonocytic leukemia; NA, not available; ORR, overall response rate; OS, overall survival

[a] Genes recommended for testing by the Association for Molecular Pathology.

[b] Genes described as clinically significant or commonly mutated in myeloid neoplasms by the NCCN.

Correlations between MPN molecular profiles and prognosis have been studied more recently but include many of the same variants described in association with AML and MDS, in addition to those mutations considered as disease defining (*JAK2, CALR, MPL*). In patients with PV, the identification of an *ASXL1*, *SRSF2*, and/or *IDH1/2* variant is a poor prognostic indicator with decreased overall survival [16]. For patients with PMF, mutations associated with a poor prognosis and/or increased risk of leukemic transformation include *ASXL1*, *EZH2*, *IDH1/2*, *SRSF2*, *TP53*, and *U2AF1* Q157 variant [16,17,27,38]. In addition, in patients with ET, clinically significant variants associated with poor prognosis include *TP53*, *IDH2*, *U2AF1*, *EZH2*, and *SF3B1* [16,32].

Targeted therapy

As molecular testing has been become increasingly informative in prognostic stratification of myeloid neoplasms, targeted therapies for AML have opened new avenues for first-line or second-line treatment in AML [64]. In addition to its role in AML subclassification, identification of a *FLT3*-ITD offers a therapeutic target. There are 2 types of *FLT3* inhibitors based on their mechanism of *FLT3* interaction, designated as type I and type II. The most commonly used are midostaurin (type I), sorafenib (type II), and newer agents including gilteritinib (type I), quizartinib (type II), and crenolanib (type I) [64,65]. Secondary resistance to FLT3 inhibitor therapy may develop, most commonly caused by a mutation of the tyrosine kinase domain at position D835 that confers resistance to type II FLT3 inhibitors [65].

New therapies targeting *IDH1* and *IDH2* variants have recently become US Food and Drug Administration approved as second-line therapy in relapsed/refractory AML [64]. Ivosidenib, an oral chemotherapeutic agent that targets *IDH1*-mutated AML, has been associated with a response rate of 41% with complete remission in 21% of patients [66]. Enasidenib is an *IDH2*-targeted drug that in clinical trials has resulted in a response rate of about 40% with complete remission seen in slightly less than 20% of patients, prolonging survival in those patients by almost 20 months [67].

Challenges in Next-Generation Sequencing Panel Testing and Alternative Testing Strategies

Myeloid gene panel testing is performed using NGS technology, which allows simultaneous sequencing of multiple gene targets from multiple patients on a single microchip. This sequencing is accomplished by fragmenting the DNA, amplifying the resulting small fragments, aligning the amplified fragments to known sequences using computer software, and then identifying changes in the amplified sequences compared with the known genome [68]. Thus, single base pair changes and small insertions or deletions can be easily identified. There are 2 commercially available sequencing platforms, Illumina and Ion Torrent, whose sequencing methodologies vary biochemically. Technical limitations, both analytical and postanalytical, do exist in NGS sequencing of certain genes, but, because various practice guidelines assign significant diagnostic, prognostic, and therapeutic relevance to variants of these genes, alternative single-gene testing strategies are often necessary to supplement multigene NGS testing.

For example, fragment size analysis may be required to detect large insertions or deletions in certain clinically relevant genes. These variants significantly alter sequence length and potentially impede accurate sequence alignment to reference genome by NGS analysis [68]. This technical limitation can be resolved by fragment size analysis with polymerase chain reaction followed by capillary electrophoresis, a method particularly used for large *FLT3*-ITD insertions [68,69]. *CALR* deletion variants can also be determined by fragment size analysis but high-resolution melting curve analysis may also be used and seems to be a more reliable and sensitive detection methodology [70].

Single-gene Sanger sequencing is also frequently used, particularly for genes that are less amenable to NGS testing because of high mutational complexity and atypical base pair composition. For instance, the high GC base pair–rich content of *CEBPA* may hamper amplification efficiency and result in poor amplicon coverage by NGS. To overcome this technical limitation, Sanger sequencing–based assays for *CEBPA* have been optimized to detect these variants including biallelic mutations, which hold the most clinical relevance [71]. Despite having lower analytical sensitivity than other methods, *CEBPA* mutation analysis by this method is usually sufficient given its select relevance to normal karyotype AML cases, which have at least 20% blasts by definition [60,71].

Sanger sequencing has also been investigated as an alternative methodology for analysis of genes with repetitive mononucleotide sequences. These specific sequences may not accurately amplify because of slipped strand mispairing. Thus, a detected variant within these sequences may represent a true somatic alteration or a false-positive caused by technical artifact [72], particularly for the *ASXL1* c.1934dupG variant, which results in an guanine (G) insertion within a

8G repeat sequence [73]. To resolve this genotyping error, some investigators have optimized a directed Sanger sequencing method followed by fragment size analysis to more confidently identify this mutation in several cases [73]. The significance of this variant is yet to be determined, but many investigators argue that it may be associated with neoplasia [74].

Two postanalytical challenges exist independently of the testing process. First, because of the complexity and multistep preparation process, the turnaround time for NGS panels is lengthy, typically 2 weeks or more. Specimen preparation for NGS usually spans 3 days, followed by a day for sequencing, and then the process of interpretation. This delay can be problematic for critically ill patients if results must be used for treatment determination. In these cases, single-gene assays should be considered.

The second problem is a lack of uniformity of reporting across laboratories. All variants detected must be classified according to the degree of clinical significance, because many identified variants may represent benign single nucleotide polymorphisms compared with multiple genetic databases. In addition, each variant must be investigated to determine whether it has been described in the diagnosed neoplasm and whether it holds clinical relevance. Even after each variant has been characterized, there seems to be universal difficulty in producing a uniform reporting structure that is easy interpreted clinically. In an effort to remedy this problem, the AMP, the CAP, and the American Society of Clinical Oncology released guidelines for the interpretation and reporting of sequence variants in January 2017. The guidelines proposed a 4-tiered system for variant classification with tier I being variants of strong clinical significance, tier II variants of potential clinical significance, tier III variants of unknown significance, and tier IV benign or likely benign variants [5]. Although this tiered system seems logical, its implementation in clinical reports has been difficult because many institutions have previously established reporting structures.

SUMMARY

As NGS technologies have become more accessible, molecular research attempting to characterize myeloid neoplasms has blossomed, identifying a multitude of potentially significant gene mutations. Because of this, various guideline-producing entities have attempted to identify which genes are considered clinically relevant and should be included as part of the routine work-up. Nearly 40 are variants specifically described by the NCCN and/or AMP as clinically significant or commonly associated with myeloid neoplasms. Because many of these variants have been incorporated into the diagnosis, prognostication, and treatment plan for myeloid neoplasms, large panel testing has become increasingly popular.

Extensive NGS panels provide a convenient manner for identifying multiple variants with a single assay, simplifying the molecular evaluation of myeloid neoplasms. However, this technology is not perfect, and clinicians and laboratorians must be aware of the inherent challenges to ensure appropriate testing is performed.

REFERENCES

[1] McClure RF, Ewalt MD, Crow J, et al. Clinical significance of DNA variants in chronic myeloid neoplasms (CMNs): a report of the association for molecular pathology. J Mol Diagn 2018;20(6):717–37.

[2] Busque L, Patel JP, Figueroa ME, et al. Recurrent somatic TET2 mutations in normal elderly individuals with clonal hematopoiesis. Nat Genet 2012;44:1179.

[3] Kwok B, Hall JM, Witte JS, et al. MDS-associated somatic mutations and clonal hematopoiesis are common in idiopathic cytopenias of undetermined significance. Blood 2015;126(21):2355.

[4] Young AL, Challen GA, Birmann BM, et al. Clonal haematopoiesis harbouring AML-associated mutations is ubiquitous in healthy adults. Nat Commun 2016;7:12484.

[5] Steven H, Swerdlow EC, Lee Harris N, et al, editors. WHO classification of tumours of haematopoietic and lymphoid tissues. 4th edition. Lyon (France): International Agency for Research on Cancer (IARC); 2017 World Health Organization Classification of Tumours.

[6] Vardiman JW, Thiele J, Arber DA, et al. The 2008 revision of the World Health Organization (WHO) classification of myeloid neoplasms and acute leukemia: rationale and important changes. Blood 2009;114(5):937.

[7] Arber DA, Borowitz MJ, Cessna M, et al. Initial Diagnostic Workup of Acute Leukemia: guideline from the college of american pathologists and the American Society of Hematology. Arch Pathol Lab Med 2017;141(10):1342–93.

[8] Arber DA, Orazi A. Update on the pathologic diagnosis of chronic myelomonocytic leukemia. Mod Pathol 2019;32(6):732–40.

[9] Papaemmanuil E, Gerstung M, Bullinger L, et al. Genomic classification and prognosis in acute myeloid leukemia. N Engl J Med 2016;374(23):2209–21.

[10] Papaemmanuil E, Gerstung M, Malcovati L, et al. Clinical and biological implications of driver mutations in myelodysplastic syndromes. Blood 2013;122(22):3616.

[11] Haferlach T, Nagata Y, Grossmann V, et al. Landscape of genetic lesions in 944 patients with myelodysplastic syndromes. Leukemia 2013;28:241.

[12] Naoe T, Kiyoi H. Gene mutations of acute myeloid leukemia in the genome era. Int J Hematol 2013;97(2):165–74.

[13] Metzeler KH, Herold T, Rothenberg-Thurley M, et al. Spectrum and prognostic relevance of driver gene mutations in acute myeloid leukemia. Blood 2016;128(5):686.

[14] Bartels S, Schipper E, Hasemeier B, et al. Routine clinical mutation profiling using next generation sequencing and a customized gene panel improves diagnostic precision in myeloid neoplasms. Oncotarget 2016;7(21):30084–93.

[15] Cazzola M, Della Porta MG, Malcovati L. The genetic basis of myelodysplasia and its clinical relevance. Blood 2013;122(25):4021–34.

[16] Tefferi A, Lasho TL, Finke CM, et al. Targeted deep sequencing in primary myelofibrosis. Blood Adv 2016;1(2):105.

[17] Guglielmelli P, Lasho TL, Rotunno G, et al. The number of prognostically detrimental mutations and prognosis in primary myelofibrosis: an international study of 797 patients. Leukemia 2014;28(9):1804.

[18] Viny AD, Levine RL. Genetics of myeloproliferative neoplasms. Cancer J 2014;20(1):61.

[19] Rumi E, Pietra D, Pascutto C, et al. Clinical effect of driver mutations of JAK2, CALR, or MPL in primary myelofibrosis. Blood 2014;124(7):1062–9.

[20] Tefferi A, Guglielmelli P, Larson DR, et al. Long-term survival and blast transformation in molecularly annotated essential thrombocythemia, polycythemia vera, and myelofibrosis. Blood 2014;124(16):2507–13.

[21] Mughal TI, Cross NCP, Padron E, et al. An International MDS/MPN Working Group's perspective and recommendations on molecular pathogenesis, diagnosis and clinical characterization of myelodysplastic/myeloproliferative neoplasms. Haematologica 2015;100(9):1117–30.

[22] Patnaik MM, Lasho TL, Finke CM, et al. Spliceosome mutations involving SRSF2, SF3B1, and U2AF35 in chronic myelomonocytic leukemia: Prevalence, clinical correlates, and prognostic relevance. Am J Hematol 2013;88(3):201–6.

[23] Reiter A, Invernizzi R, Cross NCP, et al. Molecular basis of myelodysplastic/myeloproliferative neoplasms. Haematologica 2009;94(12):1634.

[24] Itzykson R, Kosmider O, Renneville A, et al. Prognostic score including gene mutations in chronic myelomonocytic leukemia. J Clin Oncol 2013;31(19):2428–36.

[25] Walter MJ, Ding L, Shen D, et al. Recurrent DNMT3A mutations in patients with myelodysplastic syndromes. Leukemia 2011;25(7):1153.

[26] Thol F, Friesen I, Damm F, et al. Prognostic significance of ASXL1 mutations in patients with myelodysplastic syndromes. J Clin Oncol 2011;29(18):2499–506.

[27] Tefferi A, Guglielmelli P, Lasho TL, et al. CALR and ASXL1 mutations-based molecular prognostication in primary myelofibrosis: an international study of 570 patients. Leukemia 2014;(28):1494–500.

[28] Damm F, Chesnais V, Nagata Y, et al. BCOR and BCORL1 mutations in myelodysplastic syndromes and related disorders. Blood 2013;122(18):3169.

[29] Jädersten M, Saft L, Smith A, et al. TP53 mutations in low-risk myelodysplastic syndromes with del (5q) predict disease progression. J Clin Oncol 2011;29(15):1971–9.

[30] Kaneko H, Misawa S, Horiike S, et al. TP53 mutations emerge at early phase of myelodysplastic syndrome and are associated with complex chromosomal abnormalities. Blood 1995;85(8):2189–93.

[31] Sebaa A, Ades L, Baran-Marzack F, et al. Incidence of 17p deletions and TP53 mutation in myelodysplastic syndrome and acute myeloid leukemia with 5q deletion. Genes Chromosomes Cancer 2012;51(12):1086–92.

[32] Rampal R, Ahn J, Abdel-Wahab O, et al. Genomic and functional analysis of leukemic transformation of myeloproliferative neoplasms. Proc Natl Acad Sci U S A 2014;111(50):E5401–10.

[33] Jiang Y, Zhu Y, Liu Z-J, et al. The emerging roles of the DDX41 protein in immunity and diseases. Protein Cell 2017;8(2):83–9.

[34] Polprasert C, Schulze I, Sekeres Mikkael A, et al. Inherited and somatic defects in DDX41 in myeloid neoplasms. Cancer Cell 2015;27(5):658–70.

[35] Rosenfeld C, Cheever MA, Gaiger A. WT1 in acute leukemia, chronic myelogenous leukemia and myelodysplastic syndrome: therapeutic potential of WT1 targeted therapies. Leukemia 2003;17:1301.

[36] Meggendorfer M, Roller A, Haferlach T, et al. SRSF2 mutations in 275 cases with chronic myelomonocytic leukemia (CMML). Blood 2012;120(15):3080–8.

[37] Graubert TA, Shen D, Ding L, et al. Recurrent mutations in the U2AF1 splicing factor in myelodysplastic syndromes. Nat Genet 2012;44(1):53.

[38] Tefferi A, Finke CM, Lasho TL, et al. U2AF1 mutation types in primary myelofibrosis: phenotypic and prognostic distinctions. Leukemia 2018;32(10):2274–8.

[39] Malcovati L, Papaemmanuil E, Bowen DT, et al. Clinical significance of SF3B1 mutations in myelodysplastic syndromes and myelodysplastic/myeloproliferative neoplasms. Blood 2011;118(24):6239–46.

[40] Patnaik MM, Lasho TL, Hodnefield JM, et al. SF3B1 mutations are prevalent in myelodysplastic syndromes with ring sideroblasts but do not hold independent prognostic value. Blood 2012;119(2):569–72.

[41] Duployez N, Marceau-Renaut A, Boissel N, et al. Comprehensive mutational profiling of core binding factor acute myeloid leukemia. Blood 2016;127(20):2451.

[42] Paschka P, Marcucci G, Ruppert AS, et al. Adverse prognostic significance of KIT mutations in adult acute myeloid leukemia with inv(16) and t(8;21): a cancer and leukemia group B study. J Clin Oncol 2006;24(24):3904–11.

[43] Boissel LH, Brethon B, Philippe N, et al, Acute Leukemia French Association (ALFA); Leucémies Aiguës Myéloblastiques de l'Enfant (LAME) Cooperative

Groups. Incidence and prognostic impact of c-Kit, FLT3, and Ras gene mutations in core binding factor acute myeloid leukemia (CBF-AML). Leukemia 2006;20(6):965–70.

[44] Park SH, Chi HS, Min SK, et al. Prognostic impact of c-KIT mutations in core binding factor acute myeloid leukemia. Leuk Res 2011;35(10):1376–83.

[45] Schmidt MHH, Dikic I. The Cbl interactome and its functions. Nat Rev Mol Cell Biol 2005;6:907.

[46] Rumi E, Harutyunyan AS, Pietra D, et al. CALR exon 9 mutations are somatically acquired events in familial cases of essential thrombocythemia or primary myelofibrosis. Blood 2014;123(15):2416.

[47] Tefferi A, Pardanani A. CALR mutations and a new diagnostic algorithm for MPN. Nat Rev Clin Oncol 2014;11: 125.

[48] Pietra D, Rumi E, Ferretti VV, et al. Differential clinical effects of different mutation subtypes in CALR-mutant myeloproliferative neoplasms. Leukemia 2016;30(2):431.

[49] Levy DE, Lee C-k. What does Stat3 do? J Clin Invest 2002; 109(9):1143–8.

[50] Jerez A, Clemente MJ, Makishima H, et al. STAT3 mutations indicate the presence of subclinical T-cell clones in a subset of aplastic anemia and myelodysplastic syndrome patients. Blood 2013;122(14):2453–9.

[51] Bulavin DV, Demidov ON, Saito Si, et al. Amplification of PPM1D in human tumors abrogates p53 tumor-suppressor activity. Nat Genet 2002;31(2):210.

[52] Montalban-Bravo G, Kanagal-Shamanna R, Sasaki K, et al. NPM1 mutations define a specific subgroup of MDS and MDS/MPN patients with favorable outcomes with intensive chemotherapy. Blood Adv 2019;3(6):922.

[53] Peng J, Zuo Z, Fu B, et al. Chronic myelomonocytic leukemia with nucleophosmin (NPM1) mutation. Eur J Haematol 2016;96(1):65–71.

[54] Makishima H, Yoshida K, Nguyen N, et al. Somatic SETBP1 mutations in myeloid malignancies. Nat Genet 2013;45(8):942.

[55] Meggendorfer M, Bacher U, Alpermann T, et al. SETBP1 mutations occur in 9% of MDS/MPN and in 4% of MPN cases and are strongly associated with atypical CML, monosomy 7, isochromosome i(17)(q10), ASXL1 and CBL mutations. Leukemia 2013;27:1852.

[56] Liu Y-R, Zhu H-H, Ruan G-R, et al. NPM1-mutated acute myeloid leukemia of monocytic or myeloid origin exhibit distinct immunophenotypes. Leuk Res 2013; 37(7):737–41.

[57] Döhner H, Estey E, Grimwade D, et al. Diagnosis and management of AML in adults. 2017 ELN recommendations from an international expert panel. Blood 2017; 129(4):424.

[58] Preudhomme C, Sagot C, Boissel N, et al. Favorable prognostic significance of CEBPA mutations in patients with de novo acute myeloid leukemia: a study from the Acute Leukemia French Association (ALFA). Blood 2002;100(8):2717.

[59] Thiede C, Koch S, Creutzig E, et al. Prevalence and prognostic impact of NPM1 mutations in 1485 adult patients with acute myeloid leukemia (AML). Blood 2006; 107(10):4011.

[60] Thol F, Damm F, Lüdeking A, et al. Incidence and prognostic influence of DNMT3A mutations in acute myeloid leukemia. J Clin Oncol 2011;29:2889–96.

[61] Ley TJ, Ding L, Walter MJ, et al. DNMT3A mutations in acute myeloid leukemia. N Engl J Med 2010;363(25): 2424–33.

[62] Marcucci G, Maharry K, Wu Y-Z, et al. IDH1 and IDH2 gene mutations identify novel molecular subsets within de novo cytogenetically normal acute myeloid leukemia: a Cancer and Leukemia Group B study. J Clin Oncol 2010;28(14):2348.

[63] Paschka P, Schlenk RF, Gaidzik VI, et al. IDH1 and IDH2 mutations are frequent genetic alterations in acute myeloid leukemia and confer adverse prognosis in cytogenetically normal acute myeloid leukemia with NPM1 mutation without FLT3 internal tandem duplication. J Clin Oncol 2010;28(22):3636–43.

[64] Tallman M. Prognostic significance of molecular markers and targeted regimens in the management of acute myeloid leukemia. J Natl Compr Canc Netw 2018;16(5S):656–9.

[65] Larrosa-Garcia M, Baer MR. FLT3 inhibitors in acute myeloid leukemia: current status and future directions. Mol Cancer Ther 2017;16(6):991.

[66] DiNardo CD, Stein EM, de Botton S, et al. Durable remissions with ivosidenib in IDH1-mutated relapsed or refractory AML. N Engl J Med 2018;378(25):2386–98.

[67] Stein EM, DiNardo CD, Pollyea DA, et al. Enasidenib in mutant IDH2 relapsed or refractory acute myeloid leukemia. Blood 2017;130(6):722.

[68] Coleman WB, Tsongalis GJ. Diagnostic molecular pathology: a guide to applied molecular testing. London: Academic Press; 2017.

[69] Noguera NI, Ammatuna E, Zangrilli D, et al. Simultaneous detection of NPM1 and FLT3-ITD mutations by capillary electrophoresis in acute myeloid leukemia. Leukemia 2005;19:1479.

[70] Jones AV, Ward D, Lyon M, et al. Evaluation of methods to detect CALR mutations in myeloproliferative neoplasms. Leuk Res 2015;39(1):82–7.

[71] Behdad A, Weigelin HC, Elenitoba-Johnson KSJ, et al. A clinical grade sequencing-based assay for CEBPA mutation testing: report of a large series of myeloid neoplasms. J Mol Diagn 2015;17(1):76–84.

[72] Fazekas AJ, Steeves R, Newmaster SG. Improving sequencing quality from PCR products containing long mononucleotide repeats. Biotechniques 2010;48(4): 277–85.

[73] Yannakou CK, Jones K, McBean M, et al. ASXL1 c.1934dup;p.Gly646Trpfs*12—a true somatic alteration requiring a new approach. Blood Cancer J 2017;7(12): 656.

[74] Schnittger S, Eder C, Jeromin S, et al. ASXL1 exon 12 mutations are frequent in AML with intermediate risk karyotype and are independently associated with an adverse outcome. Leukemia 2012;27:82.

Infectious Disease

Advances in Molecular Pathology 2 (2019) 77–88
ADVANCES IN MOLECULAR PATHOLOGY

Impact of Molecular Diagnostics on Antimicrobial Stewardship

Sheila M. Johnson, PhD[a], Mackenzie E. Collins, BS[a], Melissa B. Miller, PhD[a,b,*]
[a]Clinical Microbiology Laboratory, University of North Carolina Health Care, Chapel Hill, NC, USA; [b]Department of Pathology and Laboratory Medicine, University of North Carolina School of Medicine, Chapel Hill, NC, USA

KEYWORDS
• Molecular diagnostics • Molecular microbiology • Antimicrobial stewardship • Antibiotic resistance

KEY POINTS

- Molecular diagnostics are useful in cases whereby phenotypic testing may be unreliable or organisms are slow growing or uncultivable.
- Rapid molecular identification and resistance detection are proving to be essential for the timely and accurate diagnosis and treatment of infections.
- Combined with an effective stewardship program, rapid molecular diagnostics can have a beneficial impact on patient outcomes.

INTRODUCTION

Antibiotics revolutionized medicine and are responsible for saving millions of lives from previously lethal diseases [1]. Unfortunately, more than 47 million unnecessary antibiotic prescriptions are written every year in US doctors' offices, emergency departments, and nursing homes [2]. A study by the Centers for Disease Control and Prevention (CDC) and Pew Charitable Trusts revealed that outpatients were often prescribed antibiotics not recommended by current clinical guidelines, even when antibiotic treatment was indicated. For instance, recommended first-line antibiotics were only used 52% of the time for sinus, middle ear infections, and sore throat [3]. This antibiotic misuse perpetuates the worldwide problem of antibiotic resistance, now recognized as a serious threat to public health [4]. Bacteria have developed resistance to nearly every antibiotic produced to date [1].

The CDC estimates that 23,000 deaths and more than 2 million illnesses are caused by antibiotic-resistant bacteria [5]. Development of new antibiotics is subjected to challenging regulatory requirements and can be expensive for pharmaceutical companies, thus rendering the process slow [6–8]. In 2010, the Infectious Diseases Society of America launched the "10 × '20 Initiative," which is a collaboration of global stakeholders committed to support new antimicrobial research and development with a goal of developing 10 new antibacterial drugs by 2020 [9]. A 2019 review of the initiative indicates great progress: 11 new approved antibiotics, 15 more in phase 2 or 3 development, and 9 drugs in phase 1 [10].

Disclosure Statement: S.M. Johnson and M.E. Collins have nothing to disclose. M.B. Miller serves on the scientific advisory boards of Luminex Molecular Diagnostics, Curetis, and BioFire Diagnostics and is a consultant for Shield Diagnostics.

*Corresponding author. Clinical Microbiology Laboratory, University of North Carolina Health Care, Chapel Hill, NC. *E-mail address:* melissa.miller@unchealth.unc.edu
twitter: @shedamarie (S.M.J.); @melmillerphd (M.B.M.)

https://doi.org/10.1016/j.yamp.2019.07.006
2589-4080/19/

SIGNIFICANCE

Antimicrobial Stewardship

The CDC identified risks associated with antibiotic resistance in their publication, "Antibiotic Resistance Threats in the United States, 2013" [1], which also highlighted the benefits of antibiotic stewardship programs. Antibiotic stewardship (now often referred to as antimicrobial stewardship) is a part of the 2015 National Action Plan for Combating Antibiotic-Resistant Bacteria, which set a goal for all hospitals to have antibiotic stewardship programs by 2020 to include 20% reductions of inappropriate antibiotic prescriptions [11].

Antimicrobial stewardship has 3 main goals: treat patients with the most appropriate antimicrobial at the correct dose and duration; prevent antimicrobial overuse, misuse, and abuse; and minimize the development of resistance. Examples of antibiotic misuse include the sustained use of broad-spectrum antibiotics, treatment of colonization and self-limited bacterial infections, and treatment of viral infections and noninfectious processes causing fever. The benefits of stewardship are considerable; patient safety and quality of care are improved by reduced treatment failures and increased infection cure rates [12], appropriate prescriptions for therapy and prophylaxis [13,14], and reduced antibiotic resistance [15,16] and rates of *Clostridium difficile* infections [17–19]. Often, the outcomes of these initiatives also result in cost savings through reduced intensive care unit (ICU) and hospital stays [8,20,21].

Traditional Microbiology

Historically, microorganism identification has relied on microscopy, culture, and biochemical testing. Traditional microscopy provides stain and morphology characteristics that can be useful for early therapeutic decisions. For bacterial identification, clinical specimens are inoculated to a range of selective and differential media and incubated under conditions to support growth. Biochemical testing may then be performed to further identify the organism [22,23].

From the time of specimen collection through organism identification and antimicrobial susceptibility testing (AST), patients often receive broad, empiric antibiotic coverage [24]. Frequently, antimicrobial susceptibilities of the identified organism are required to target therapy. Traditional susceptibility methods include broth microdilution, disc diffusion, and MIC gradient test strip testing. Interpretive criteria known as breakpoints facilitate translation of results into "susceptible," "intermediate," "susceptible dose dependent," or "resistant" categories that typically correlate with pharmacodynamic properties and/or clinical treatment outcome [25].

Challenges

Bacterial growth rate in culture is a limiting factor that delays organism identification and AST. For the most cultivable bacteria, the time from specimen collection to final result can take multiple days [22,26]. In addition, the sensitivity of culture is low for patients treated with antimicrobials or with infections because of slow-growing, fastidious, and intracellular organisms [22,26–28]. This turnaround time can significantly delay any deescalation of antibiotics and consequently hamper stewardship efforts.

Interventions to improve antibiotic use require the identification and resistance profile of the organism causing an infection; thus, successful antimicrobial stewardship programs rely on timely microbiology results. New rapid molecular tests allow the microbiology laboratory to provide diagnostic results much earlier and have a positive impact on antimicrobial stewardship goals owing to faster turnaround time for both identification of organisms and detection of resistance determinants. Current molecular diagnostic strategies include hybridization, nucleic acid amplification, mass spectrometry, and sequencing technologies.

MOLECULAR DIAGNOSTICS

Molecular Identification Panels

Hybridization and nucleic acid amplification approaches are reasonably affordable and easy to use. Assays are often designed as multiplexed panels that identify pathogens associated with a particular clinical syndrome, including bloodstream, respiratory, gastrointestinal (GI), and central nervous system infections [29]. Furthermore, resistance determinants are often integrated into molecular identification panels.

Bloodstream infections

Molecular identification of organisms from blood cultures has been shown to significantly improve patient outcomes by decreasing the time to result over culture, thus allowing targeted therapy to be initiated sooner. Table 1 [30–36] lists Food and Drug Administration (FDA)-approved assays designed to identify organisms causing bloodstream infections (BSIs) and associated performance characteristics. In addition, with proper interpretation, early molecular identification can also identify potentially contaminated blood cultures and consequently decrease overtreatment. A limitation to

TABLE 1
Food and Drug Administration–Cleared Multiplex Assays for Diagnosis of Bloodstream Infections

Technology	Assay name (Manufacturer)	No. of Organism Targets	No. of Resistance Targets	Performance Statistics (Reference)	Run time, h	Time Reduced to Antibiotic Optimization, h (Reference)
DNA microarray	Verigene BC-GP (Luminex Corp, Austin, TX)	8	3	94.6% sensitivity [39] Polymicrobial infections, missed targets in 28% cases [35]	2.5	12.5–27 [35]
	Verigene BC-GN (Luminex Corp)	7	6	98% sensitivity [35] Polymicrobial infections, missed targets in 46% cases [35]	2.5	11–14 [35]
PCR based	ePlex BCID-GP (GenMark Dx, Carlsbad, CA)	20	4	97% sensitivity; 99% PPV [40]	1.5	24–48 [40]
	ePlex BCID-GN (GenMark Dx)	21	6	99% sensitivity; 96% PPV [40]	1.5	24–48 [40]
Probe based	PhenoTest (Accelerate Dx, Tuscon, AZ)	14	20	94.5%/98.9% (PPA/NPA) [37] 96.5% agreement for resistance targets [37]	1.5	24–48 [37]
Nested PCR	FilmArray BCID (BioFire/BMX, Salt Lake City, UT)	24	3	>96% sensitivity [35] 46% false positive, 30% false negative in polymicrobial infections [35]	1.5	33.5 [38]
Rescue PCR	iC-GPC (iCubate, Huntsville, AL)	5	3	>95% sensitivity [35] 14.8% false negative for *Streptococcus pneumoniae* [35]	4–5	ND
Magnetic resonance	T2Bacteria Panel (T2 Biosystems, Lexington, MA)	5	13	89.5% sensitivity, 98.4% specificity [41]	3–5	ND
Nucleic acid amplification	Xpert MRSA/SA (Cepheid, Sunnyvale, CA)	1	1	>98% sensitivity [35]	<1	40.8 [36]

Abbreviations: ND, not determined; PPV, positive predictive value; PPA, positive percent agreement; NPA, negative percent agreement.

this approach is that it still requires incubation of blood culture bottles before initiation of identification methods. However, once blood culture bottles become positive, the turnaround time for molecular identification of organisms and resistance genes is 1 to 3 hours.

The first randomized controlled study to assess clinical outcomes from implementation of a molecular blood culture identification panel examined its impact with and without stewardship intervention. Compared with the control group, both molecular panel groups had decreased broad-spectrum antibiotic use (45 hours vs 56 hours), more narrow-spectrum antibiotic use (71–85 hours vs 42 hours), faster antibiotic escalation (6 hours vs 24 hours), and less treatment of contaminants (8%–11% vs 25%). Only the molecular testing plus stewardship group saw a shorter time to antibiotic deescalation (21 hours) when compared with the control group (34 hours) and molecular testing alone (38 hours). In this study, the groups did not differ in mortality, length of stay (LOS), or cost [37].

Combined with an effective stewardship program, molecular diagnostics and AST can shorten LOS and ICU days plus reduce health care–acquired infections and mortality. To illustrate this point, Bauer and colleagues [31] used the GeneXpert system (Cepheid, Sunnyvale, CA, USA) to identify and differentiate methicillin-resistant and methicillin-susceptible *Staphylococcus aureus* and coagulase-negative *Staphylococcus* species from positive blood cultures. Over the course of 4 months and 82 patients, the average decrease in ICU LOS was 6.2 days; vancomycin treatment was reduced by 1.7 days, and an overall savings of $21,000 was calculated per patient.

It has been shown, however, that antimicrobial stewardship must be in place for rapid diagnostics to have beneficial impact on mortality risk, LOS, and patient outcomes. In a 2017 review, Timbrook and colleagues [38] observed implementation of molecular diagnostics in BSIs only decreased mortality risk when used in conjunction with antimicrobial stewardship. Rapid molecular testing together with antimicrobial stewardship has been shown to enable shorter LOS (6 days vs 11 days) and shorter time to appropriate therapy (39.3 hours vs 64.7 hours) in contrast to molecular testing in the absence of stewardship [39].

Several multiplex systems also offer antimicrobial resistance testing independent of identification (Table 2) [40–47]. In an evaluation of the ELITe MGB system (ELITechGroup Molecular Diagnostics, Torino, Italy), Bianco and colleagues [48] detected resistance genes from 192 positive blood cultures representing both gram-negative bacilli (112) and gram-positive cocci (80) and compared their results to parallel conventional AST. From the time of blood culture positivity, the turnaround time for conventional AST ranged from 1 to 2 days, whereas average ELITe MGB assay test time was 2.5 hours. Antimicrobial therapy was changed in 67 cases following receipt of phenotypic AST results; based on molecular results, 41 patients could have been treated with appropriate therapy 24 hours earlier. Although antimicrobial resistance testing by rapid molecular methods has the potential to improve clinical decision making, it is somewhat limited by the positive and negative predictive values. In order to adjust antimicrobial therapy based on the positive identification of a resistance gene, the diagnostic test should have a high positive predictive value. In addition, the test would need a high negative predictive value to permit any narrowing of therapy if no resistance markers were detected [49].

Although the diagnostic strategies above depend on a positive blood culture, the T2 Magnetic Resonance Assay (T2MR; T2 Biosystems, Lexington, MA, USA) has the ability to detect organisms directly from whole blood. This system offers panels for *Candida* species, Lyme disease, bacteria, and antimicrobial resistance markers. In a multicenter trial, T2MR was used to monitor candidemia clearance in patients on antifungal therapy. The T2MR assay successfully detected candidemia in specimens with corresponding positive blood cultures (7/7) in addition to specimens with negative blood cultures (7/23) [50]. Although the performance of blood cultures can be diminished [51], T2MR is not inhibited by therapeutic levels of antifungal agents and could be a useful tool to determine optional duration of treatment. The T2Bacteria panel detects 5 ESKAPEc organisms responsible for greater than 50% of all BSIs: *Enterococcus faecium*, *S aureus*, *Klebsiella pneumoniae*, *Pseudomonas aeruginosa*, and *Escherichia coli*. When compared with blood culture results of 1427 patients in a prospective multicenter pivotal clinical trial, the T2Bacteria panel detected 127 subjects with evidence of infection, compared with 39 subjects by blood culture for T2Bacteria target organisms, demonstrating a potential positive impact on therapy owing to either change in or confirmation of appropriate therapy [52]. Although more data are needed regarding the routine performance of T2MR and its potential role in antimicrobial stewardship, the decrease in time to result it offers over traditional blood cultures indicates it may have a significant impact in certain patient populations.

TABLE 2
Multiplex Assays for Resistance Determination

Technology	Assay Name (Manufacturer)	FDA Approval	No. of Resistance Targets	Performance Statistics (Reference)	Run Time, h	Specimen
Nucleic acid amplification	Xpert CARBA-R (Cepheid)	Yes	5 carbapenemases	100% sensitivity; 98.1 specificity [45]	<1	Rectal swabs, isolates
Magnetic resonance	T2Resistance Panel (T2 Biosystems)	RUO[a]	5 carbapenemases 2 ESBL 2 AmpC 2 *van* 2 *mec*	TBD	3–5	Whole blood
DNA microarray	Check-MDR CT103XL (Check-Points, Wageningen, Netherlands)	RUO	11 carbapenemases 21 ESBL 7 AmpC	100% sensitivity; 100% specificity [46]	7.5	Isolates
	Check-MDR CT201 (Check-Points)	RUO	5 carbapenemases 12 ESBL	100% sensitivity; 100% specificity [47]	7.5	Isolates
	Check-MDR CT101 (Check-Points)	RUO	2 carbapenemases 12 ESBL 7 AmpC	100% sensitivity; 100% specificity [48]	7.5	Isolates
Ligation-mediated PCR	Check-MDR Carba (Check-Points)	RUO	5 carbapenemases	100% sensitivity; 100% specificity [49]	4.5	Isolates
	Check-MDR ESBL (Check-Points)	RUO	3 ESBL	99% sensitivity; 92.2% specificity [50]	4.5	Isolates
PCR based	Check-Direct CPE (Check-Points)	RUO	4 carbapenemases	100% sensitivity; 100% specificity [51]	2	Rectal swabs, isolates
	CRE ELITe MGB (ELITech Group, Torino, Italy)	Europe only	5 carbapenemases	99.3% sensitivity; 100% specificity [52]	<3	Rectal swabs, blood culture
	ESBL ELITe MGB (ELITech Group)	Europe only	4 CTX-M	99.3% sensitivity; 100% specificity [52]	<3	Rectal swabs, blood culture

Abbreviations: ESBL, extended-spectrum beta-lactamase; *mec*, genes encoding methicillin resistance; RUO, research use only; TBD, to be determined; *van*, genes encoding vancomycin resistance.

[a] Not yet available.

Infections other than bloodstream

Accurate, rapid viral detection in conjunction with education and stewardship efforts also leads to a decrease in unnecessary antibiotic use. Rogers and colleagues [53] found that positive viral results after implementation of the FilmArray Respiratory Panel (BioFire Diagnostics LLC, Salt Lake City, UT, USA) in a children's hospital reduced the time to result (6.5 hours vs 19 hours), the time in isolation (72 hours vs 84 hours), and the duration of antibiotic use (2.7 days vs 3.2 days) when compared with batched polymerase chain reaction (PCR) testing. In adults, another study also showed significantly decreased time to positive viral test results when using the FilmArray Respiratory Panel (1.7 hours vs 7.7 hours). In addition, they found that diagnosis of influenza by multiplex PCR was associated with significantly lower odds ratios for admission, LOS, and duration of antimicrobial use when compared with conventional methods [54]. Additional studies evaluating the recently approved FilmArray Pneumonia panel also detail the potential for timely antibiotic adjustment in 165/243 (68%) [55] and 50/63 (79%) [56] of patients tested.

Compared with stool culture, molecular GI panel studies have demonstrated a positive impact on clinical management. Outcomes include using targeted antimicrobial therapy over empirical and prompt discontinuation of antibiotics in patients with Shiga-like toxin-producing *E coli* [57] in addition to fewer imaging studies, shorter LOS, and decreased health care costs [58]. Coordinated with an effective stewardship program, molecular GI panels have also been shown to reduce inappropriate antibiotic use. For example, Keske and colleagues [59] evaluated the impact of molecular GI panel usage before and after antimicrobial stewardship intervention with an emphasis on the diagnosis and management of diarrhea. Among inpatients, the investigators observed a reduction of inappropriate antibiotic use (25.8% vs 42.9%) after implementation of a stewardship program that included education and training of health care providers.

Although results often offer great positive predictive value, not all pathogens or resistance genes can be covered by multiplex assays, and most molecular panels are limited to common syndrome-causing pathogens [60]. Furthermore, multiplexed panels are able to identify multiple organisms within a specimen, including those that may represent asymptomatic infection, colonization, or contamination. Interpretation of these results is often challenging for clinicians [24]. Hitchcock and colleagues [61] describe such challenges in their study of GI panel use in patients hospitalized greater than 72 hours. In their retrospective review of 481 FilmArray GI panel tests performed over 18 months, 29 were positive (6%), with the majority (23/29) positive for viral targets. Of the 4 cases positive for bacterial targets, none were consistent with acute infectious gastroenteritis, and the results could not be confirmed. After accounting for chronic viral shedding and probable false positives, the yield was only 3% (12/406), indicating limited utility of this assay in this patient population when an infectious gastroenteritis syndrome is not evident. Such results can compromise stewardship efforts because of initiation of unnecessary antimicrobial therapy as well as additional diagnostic testing and hospitalization costs.

Considerable data exist to support the contribution of molecular identification panels to antimicrobial stewardship efforts, and initial evaluations of the FilmArray Meningitis/Encephalitis (ME) panel anticipated improved stewardship and patient outcomes (BioFire Diagnostics, Salt Lake City, UT) [62,63]; however, reports confirming the impact of the ME panel on antimicrobial stewardship are limited. On the contrary, many published studies reveal test overutilization [64], no difference in LOS [65], and no reduction of antimicrobial therapy despite a negative result [65–67]. Due to the potential mortality associated with central nervous system infections, clinicians are unlikely to discontinue therapy until confirmatory culture or other clinical results are available [68].

Mass Spectrometry

Matrix-assisted laser desorption time-of-flight mass spectrometry (MALDI-TOF MS) is a technological advance that has quickly become an essential asset in the clinical microbiology laboratory. Initially used in high-complexity clinical chemistry and hematology applications, MALDI-TOF has been applied to microbial identification using spectral databases and user-friendly software [26]. The average turnaround time for isolate identification by MALDI-TOF is on the order of minutes; automated identification systems can take 5 to 8 hours, whereas traditional biochemical methods may take 24 to 48 hours [69,70].

Microorganism identification by MALDI-TOF MS has clearly made significant contributions to antimicrobial stewardship efforts. Reports indicate that MALDI-TOF MS on isolates from positive blood cultures can reduce time to identification by approximately 28 hours and shorten time to effective antimicrobial therapy resulting in lower rates of ICU LOS, recurrence, and mortality [71,72]. For example, when compared with conventional biochemical testing, organism identification by MALDI-TOF MS shortened the time to appropriate antimicrobial therapy by 1 day (2.5 days vs 3.3 days), but the reduction in mortality was not statistically significant [73]. In combination with antimicrobial stewardship, organism identification by MALDI-TOF also shortens the time to optimal therapy (34.4 hours vs 58.7 hours [74] and 43.1 hours vs 75.2 hours [75]), reduces LOS (9 days vs 15 days) [75], and decreases the duration of unnecessary antibiotic therapy in cases of blood culture contamination (1.31 days vs 3.89 days [74] and 11.8 hours vs 48.2 hours [75]). Additional studies show MALDI-TOF identification plus stewardship review and intervention reduced 30-day mortality (12% vs 21% of patients) and resulted in an annual cost savings of $2.34 million ($2439 per BSI) [76]. These savings calculations included costs related to testing implementation, pharmacy review, and intervention time.

To further reduce time to identification, protocols using MALDI-TOF to identify bacteria from direct patient specimens are ongoing. The most promising reports detail direct identification from positive blood cultures. Currently, the reported accuracy of these methods is greater than 85% for monomicrobial cultures; polymicrobial cultures still remain a challenge [77,78]. To evaluate the impact to clinical management, Clerc and colleagues [79] compared the direct MALDI-TOF from positive blood culture procedure with Gram stain alone. Direct MALDI-TOF identification influenced antimicrobial management in 71/202 (35.1%) gram-negative BSIs, while Gram stain alone influenced 42/202 (20.8%). Frequently, direct MALDI-TOF identification resulted in early appropriate broadening of antimicrobial therapy.

Additional methods are in development to use MALDI-TOF MS beyond microbial identification. Detection of antimicrobial resistance and epidemiologic strain typing are 2 potential applications of interest. Strategies for antimicrobial resistance determination by MALDI-TOF MS include detecting the modifications to antibiotics-caused bacterial enzymatic activity, detecting antimicrobial resistance through bacterial peak pattern or mass peak profile analysis, and detecting resistance by semiquantification of bacterial growth in the presence of a given antibiotic [80]. Several studies report successful resistance detection including *S aureus* methicillin resistance [81,82], vancomycin resistance in *Enterococcus* [83], *Acinetobacter* and *Klebsiella* resistance to carbapenems [84–86], and extended beta-lactamase production among Enterobacteriaceae [87]. Strain typing by MALDI-TOF MS is another promising application that could reduce delays and potentially reduce costs in hospital epidemiology and outbreak investigations [82,83,88].

Sequencing Technologies

More recently, high throughput "next-generation" whole-genome sequencing (WGS) has enabled the examination of entire pathogen genomes. In addition to bacterial identification, strain typing, and resistance gene determination, WGS also supports microbiology, epidemiology, and public health objectives [89]. For example, shortly after the description of *Candida auris* in Japan, the multidrug-resistant yeast was identified from invasive infections in several countries, and it was unknown whether the organism emerged independently or was spread from a single source. WGS analysis determined that isolates were grouped into unique clades by geographic region, suggesting an independent emergence of different clonal populations [90]. WGS is also emerging as the new gold standard method for strain comparison because of its high discriminatory capacity, proving useful in investigations such as carbapenem-resistant *K pneumoniae* transmission among inpatients and between hospitals [91,92] and multidrug-resistant *Mycobacterium abscessus* subspecies massiliense in cystic fibrosis patients [93]. Having institution-specific sequence-based data for multidrug-resistant organisms enhances stewardship efforts by providing the data needed to develop appropriate empiric therapy and treatment algorithms.

One advantage to testing antimicrobial resistance by WGS is the ability to screen an entire genome simultaneously for resistance determinants. In addition, the sequence data are subsequently available for further analyses and purposes [94]. Retrospective analysis identified the emergence of *mcr-1* colistin resistance in Germany; 4 previously unidentified colistin-resistant isolates were detected upon database review and analysis of 577 Enterobacteriaceae genomes [95]. Genotypic versus phenotypic resistance can be a limitation and warrants consideration. Commonly acquired resistance genes like beta-lactamases or aminoglycoside-modifying enzymes can be detected, and the conservative approach is to treat these organisms as resistant. However, complicated regulatory systems, such as vancomycin heteroresistance and AmpC hyperproduction, are difficult to reliably detect by molecular methods [96–98]. Furthermore, it is necessary to recognize new genes or allelic variants of current resistance mechanisms as they arise [99].

WGS methods are also useful in cases whereby phenotypic testing may be unreliable and organisms are slow-growing or uncultivable. For example, WGS of *Mycobacterium tuberculosis* can identify resistance significantly more quickly than culture-based susceptibility methods [89,100] that may not be available for 1 to 2 months. During this time, patients are routinely started on first-line 4-drug therapy. Köser and colleagues [100] reported a case of tuberculosis in a patient on first-line therapy for 3 months before phenotypic susceptibility results determined the patient had multidrug-resistant tuberculosis; extensively drug-resistant tuberculosis was confirmed 3 weeks later. Upon readmission, WGS was performed directly on the first culture-positive broth. In a matter of days, sequence analysis revealed a mixed infection, confirmed the phenotypic susceptibility results, and identified resistance to an additional 5 drugs.

SUMMARY

As a result of inappropriate prescribing practices, many patients are at risk for developing antibiotic-resistant infections. Stewardship programs aim to ensure patients receive the "right antibiotic, at the right time, with the right dose and duration" [5]. A systematic review and meta-analysis of 145 studies revealed abundant evidence that implementation of antimicrobial stewardship objectives do in fact result in positive clinical outcomes with regard to adverse events, resistance rates, and cost [101].

Rapid molecular diagnostics and susceptibility testing are proving to be essential for the timely and accurate diagnosis and treatment of infections, even shifting toward becoming standard of care. More outcome studies comparing molecular versus conventional identification and susceptibility testing are necessary. These studies plus further improvements in prescribing practices are an essential step toward advancing antimicrobial stewardship goals.

REFERENCES

[1] Centers for Disease Control and Prevention. Antibiotic resistance threats in the United States, 2013. US Dep Heal Hum Serv; 2013. Available at: https://www.cdc.gov/drugresistance/pdf/ar-threats-2013-508.pdf.

[2] Fleming-Dutra KE, Hersh AL, Shapiro DJ, et al. Prevalence of inappropriate antibiotic prescriptions among us ambulatory care visits, 2010-2011. JAMA 2016. https://doi.org/10.1001/jama.2016.4151.

[3] Hersh AL, Fleming-Dutra KE, Shapiro DJ, et al. Frequency of first-line antibiotic selection among us ambulatory care visits for otitis media, sinusitis, and pharyngitis. JAMA Intern Med 2016. https://doi.org/10.1001/jamainternmed.2016.6625.

[4] Lapi F, Wilchesky M, Kezouh A, et al. Fluoroquinolones and the risk of serious arrhythmia: a population-based study. Clin Infect Dis 2012. https://doi.org/10.1093/cid/cis664.

[5] Centers for Disease Control and Prevention. Antibiotic use in the United States, 2017: progress and opportunities. US Dep Heal Hum Serv; 2017. https://www.cdc.gov/antibiotic-use/stewardship-report/pdf/stewardship-report.pdf.

[6] Gould IM, Bal AM. New antibiotic agents in the pipeline and how they can help overcome microbial resistance. Virulence 2013. https://doi.org/10.4161/viru.22507.

[7] Piddock LJV. The crisis of no new antibiotics—what is the way forward? Lancet Infect Dis 2012. https://doi.org/10.1016/S1473-3099(11)70316-4.

[8] Doron S, Davidson LE. Antimicrobial stewardship. Mayo Clin Proc 2011. https://doi.org/10.4065/mcp.2011.0358.

[9] Infectious Diseases Society of America. The 10 × '20 Initiative: pursuing a global commitment to develop 10 new antibacterial drugs by 2020. Clin Infect Dis 2010;50(8):1081–3.

[10] Talbot GH, Jezek A, Murray BE, et al. The Infectious Diseases Society of America's 10 × '20 Initiative (Ten New Systemic Antibacterial Agents FDA-approved by 2020): is 20 × '20 a possibility? Clin Infect Dis 2019. https://doi.org/10.1093/cid/ciz089.

[11] The White House Administration. National action plan for combating antibiotic-resistant bacteria. Open Gov Natl Action Plans; 2015. https://www.cdc.gov/drugresistance/pdf/national_action_plan_for_combating_antibotic-resistant_bacteria.pdf.

[12] Malani AN, Richards PG, Kapila S, et al. Clinical and economic outcomes from a community hospital's antimicrobial stewardship program. Am J Infect Control 2013. https://doi.org/10.1016/j.ajic.2012.02.021.

[13] Stach LM, Hedican EB, Herigon JC, et al. Clinicians' attitudes towards an antimicrobial stewardship program at a children's hospital. J Pediatric Infect Dis Soc 2012. https://doi.org/10.1093/jpids/pis045.

[14] Kaki R, Elligsen M, Walker S, et al. Impact of antimicrobial stewardship in critical care: a systematic review. J Antimicrob Chemother 2011. https://doi.org/10.1093/jac/dkr137.

[15] Valiquette L, Cossette B, Garant M-P, et al. Impact of a reduction in the use of high-risk antibiotics on the course of an epidemic of *Clostridium difficile*-associated disease caused by the hypervirulent NAP1/027 strain. Clin Infect Dis 2007. https://doi.org/10.1086/519258.

[16] DiazGranados CA. Prospective audit for antimicrobial stewardship in intensive care: impact on resistance and clinical outcomes. Am J Infect Control 2012. https://doi.org/10.1016/j.ajic.2011.07.011.

[17] Nowak MA, Nelson RE, Breidenbach JL, et al. Clinical and economic outcomes of a prospective antimicrobial

stewardship program. Am J Health Syst Pharm 2012. https://doi.org/10.2146/ajhp110603.

[18] Bishop J, Parry MF, Hall T. Decreasing *Clostridium difficile* infections in surgery: impact of a practice bundle incorporating a resident rounding protocol. Conn Med 2013;77(2):69–75.

[19] Leung V, Gill S, Sauve J, et al. Growing a "positive culture" of antimicrobial stewardship in a community hospital. Can J Hosp Pharm 2011. https://doi.org/10.4212/cjhp.v64i5.1065.

[20] Griffith M, Postelnick M, Scheetz M. Antimicrobial stewardship programs: methods of operation and suggested outcomes. Expert Rev Anti Infect Ther 2012. https://doi.org/10.1586/eri.11.153.

[21] Sick AC, Lehmann CU, Tamma PD, et al. Sustained savings from a longitudinal cost analysis of an internet-based preapproval antimicrobial stewardship program. Infect Control Hosp Epidemiol 2013. https://doi.org/10.1086/670625.

[22] Laupland KB, Valiquette L. The changing culture of the microbiology laboratory. Can J Infect Dis Med Microbiol 2013. https://doi.org/10.1155/2013/101630.

[23] Van Belkum A, Durand G, Peyret M, et al. Rapid clinical bacteriology and its future impact. Ann Lab Med 2013. https://doi.org/10.3343/alm.2013.33.1.14.

[24] Messacar K, Parker SK, Todd JK, et al. Implementation of rapid molecular infectious disease diagnostics: the role of diagnostic and antimicrobial stewardship. J Clin Microbiol 2017. https://doi.org/10.1128/JCM.02264-16.

[25] Turnidge J, Paterson DL. Setting and revising antibacterial susceptibility breakpoints. Clin Microbiol Rev 2007. https://doi.org/10.1128/CMR.00047-06.

[26] Clark AE, Kaleta EJ, Arora A, et al. Matrix-assisted laser desorption ionization-time of flight mass spectrometry: a fundamental shift in the routine practice of clinical microbiology. Clin Microbiol Rev 2013. https://doi.org/10.1128/CMR.00072-12.

[27] Austin B. The value of cultures to modern microbiology. Antonie Van Leeuwenhoek 2017. https://doi.org/10.1007/s10482-017-0840-8.

[28] Fenollar F, Raoult D. Molecular diagnosis of bloodstream infections caused by non-cultivable bacteria. Int J Antimicrob Agents 2007. https://doi.org/10.1016/j.ijantimicag.2007.06.024.

[29] Ramanan P, Bryson AL, Binnicker MJ, et al. Syndromic panel-based testing in clinical microbiology. Clin Microbiol Rev 2018. https://doi.org/10.1128/CMR.00024-17.

[30] She RC, Bender JM. Advances in rapid molecular blood culture diagnostics: healthcare impact, laboratory implications, and multiplex technologies. J Appl Lab Med 2018. https://doi.org/10.1373/jalm.2018.027409.

[31] Bauer KA, West JE, Balada-Llasat J-M, et al. An antimicrobial stewardship program's impact. Clin Infect Dis 2010. https://doi.org/10.1086/656623.

[32] Starr KF, Robinson DC, Hazen KC. Performance of the accelerate diagnostics Pheno™ system with resin-containing BacT/ALERT® Plus blood culture bottles. Diagn Microbiol Infect Dis 2019. https://doi.org/10.1016/j.diagmicrobio.2019.01.002.

[33] Messacar K, Hurst AL, Child J, et al. Clinical impact and provider acceptability of real-time antimicrobial stewardship decision support for rapid diagnostics in children with positive blood culture results. J Pediatric Infect Dis Soc 2017. https://doi.org/10.1093/jpids/piw047.

[34] Wojewoda CM, Sercia L, Navas M, et al. Evaluation of the Verigene gram-positive blood culture nucleic acid test for rapid detection of bacteria and resistance determinants. J Clin Microbiol 2013. https://doi.org/10.1128/JCM.00831-13.

[35] Huang TD, Melnik E, Bogaerts P, et al. Evaluation of the ePlex blood culture identification panels for detection of pathogens in bloodstream infections. J Clin Microbiol 2019;57(2). https://doi.org/10.1128/JCM.01597-18.

[36] De Angelis G, Posteraro B, De Carolis E, et al. T2Bacteria magnetic resonance assay for the rapid detection of ESKAPEc pathogens directly in whole blood. J Antimicrob Chemother 2018. https://doi.org/10.1093/jac/dky049.

[37] Banerjee R, Teng CB, Cunningham SA, et al. Randomized trial of rapid multiplex polymerase chain reaction-based blood culture identification and susceptibility testing. Clin Infect Dis 2015. https://doi.org/10.1093/cid/civ447.

[38] Timbrook TT, Morton JB, Mcconeghy KW, et al. The effect of molecular rapid diagnostic testing on clinical outcomes in bloodstream infections: a systematic review and meta-analysis. Clin Infect Dis 2017. https://doi.org/10.1093/cid/ciw649.

[39] Vardakas KZ, Anifantaki FI, Trigkidis KK, et al. Rapid molecular diagnostic tests in patients with bacteremia: evaluation of their impact on decision making and clinical outcomes. Eur J Clin Microbiol Infect Dis 2015. https://doi.org/10.1007/s10096-015-2466-y.

[40] Cepheid. Xpert Carba-R® [package insert] 2016 Sunnyvale, CA.

[41] Cuzon G, Naas T, Bogaerts P, et al. Evaluation of a DNA microarray for the rapid detection of extended-spectrum β-lactamases (TEM, SHV and CTX-M), plasmid-mediated cephalosporinases (CMY-2-like, DHA, FOX, ACC-1, ACT/MIR and CMY-1-like/MOX) and carbapenemases (KPC, OXA-48, VIM, IMP and NDM). J Antimicrob Chemother 2012. https://doi.org/10.1093/jac/dks156.

[42] Naas T, Cuzon G, Bogaerts P, et al. Evaluation of a DNA microarray (check-MDR CT102) for rapid detection of TEM, SHV, and CTX-M extended-spectrum β-lactamases and of KPC, OXA-48, VIM, IMP, and NDM-1 carbapenemases. J Clin Microbiol 2011. https://doi.org/10.1128/JCM.02607-10.

[43] Bogaerts P, Hujer AM, Naas T, et al. Multicenter evaluation of a new DNA microarray for rapid detection of clinically relevant *bla* genes from β-lactam-resistant

gram-negative bacteria. Antimicrob Agents Chemother 2011. https://doi.org/10.1128/AAC.00353-11.

[44] Cuzon G, Naas T, Bogaerts P, et al. Probe ligation and real-time detection of KPC, OXA-48, VIM, IMP, and NDM carbapenemase genes. Diagn Microbiol Infect Dis 2013. https://doi.org/10.1016/j.diagmicrobio.2013.05.004.

[45] Nijhuis R, van Zwet A, Stuart JC, et al. Rapid molecular detection of extended-spectrum β-lactamase gene variants with a novel ligation-mediated real-time PCR. J Med Microbiol 2012. https://doi.org/10.1099/jmm.0.047910-0.

[46] Check-points. Check-direct CPE user manual Wageningen (Netherlands). http://www.check-points.eu/downloads/manuals/Check-Direct%20CPE_IFU_080-06_EN_1sep2014.pdf.

[47] Girlich D, Bernabeu S, Fortineau N, et al. Evaluation of the CRE and ESBL ELITe MGB® kits for the accurate detection of carbapenemase- or CTX-M–producing bacteria. Diagn Microbiol Infect Dis 2018. https://doi.org/10.1016/j.diagmicrobio.2018.02.001.

[48] Bianco G, Boattini M, Iannaccone M, et al. Detection of antibiotic resistance genes from blood cultures: performance assessment and potential impact on antibiotic therapy management. J Hosp Infect 2019. https://doi.org/10.1016/j.jhin.2019.03.007.

[49] Fleece ME, Pholwat S, Mathers AJ, et al. Molecular diagnosis of antimicrobial resistance in *Escherichia coli*. Expert Rev Mol Diagn 2018. https://doi.org/10.1080/14737159.2018.1439381.

[50] Mylonakis E, Zacharioudakis IM, Clancy CJ, et al. Efficacy of T2 magnetic resonance assay in monitoring candidemia after initiation of antifungal therapy: the serial therapeutic and antifungal monitoring protocol (STAMP) trial. J Clin Microbiol 2018. https://doi.org/10.1128/JCM.01756-17.

[51] Riedel S, Eisinger SW, Dam L, et al. Comparison of BD Bactec Plus Aerobic/F Medium to VersaTREK Redox 1 blood culture medium for detection of *Candida* spp. in seeded blood culture specimens containing therapeutic levels of antifungal agents. J Clin Microbiol 2011. https://doi.org/10.1128/JCM.02260-10.

[52] T2Biosystems. Clinical trial data supporting FDA clearance of the T2bacteria panel versus blood culture for the diagnosis of bacteremia. Available at: https://www.t2biosystems.com/wp-content/uploads/2018/08/T2Bacteria-Pivotal-Trial-White-Paper.pdf. Accessed April 11, 2019.

[53] Rogers BB, Shankar P, Jerris RC, et al. Impact of a rapid respiratory panel test on patient outcomes. Arch Pathol Lab Med 2015. https://doi.org/10.5858/arpa.2014-0257-OA.

[54] Rappo U, Schuetz AN, Jenkins SG, et al. Impact of early detection of respiratory viruses by multiplex PCR assay on clinical outcomes in adult patients. J Clin Microbiol 2016. https://doi.org/10.1128/jcm.00549-16.

[55] Buchan B, Windham S, Faron M, et al. Clinical evaluation and potential impact of a semi-quantitative multiplex molecular assay for the identification of pathogenic bacteria and viruses in lower respiratory specimens. American Thoracic Society 2018 International Conference, San Diego, CA, Poster A107.

[56] Alviset S, Gastli N, Charpentier J, et al. Impact of the FilmArray pneumonia panel on antimicrobial stewardship in pneumonia patients. Presented at 29th European Congress of Clinical Microbiology & Infectious Diseases. Amsterdam (Netherlands), April 13-16, 2019.

[57] Cybulski RJ, Bateman AC, Bourassa L, et al. Clinical impact of a multiplex gastrointestinal polymerase chain reaction panel in patients with acute gastroenteritis. Clin Infect Dis 2018. https://doi.org/10.1093/cid/ciy357.

[58] Beal SG, Tremblay EE, Toffel S, et al. A gastrointestinal PCR panel improves clinical management and lowers health care costs. J Clin Microbiol 2018. https://doi.org/10.1128/JCM.01457-17.

[59] Keske Ş, Zabun B, Aksoy K, et al. Rapid molecular detection of gastrointestinal pathogens and its role in antimicrobial stewardship. J Clin Microbiol 2018. https://doi.org/10.1128/JCM.00148-18.

[60] Uprety P, Mitchell SL, Krock BL, et al. The current state of metagenomics in infectious disease. Adv Mol Pathol 2018;1(1):81–9.

[61] Hitchcock MM, Gomez CA, Banaei N. Low yield of FilmArray GI panel in hospitalized patients with diarrhea: an opportunity for diagnostic stewardship intervention. J Clin Microbiol 2018. https://doi.org/10.1128/JCM.01558-17.

[62] Leber AL, Everhart K, Balada-Llasat J-M, et al. Multicenter evaluation of BioFire FilmArray meningitis/encephalitis panel for detection of bacteria, viruses, and yeast in cerebrospinal fluid specimens. J Clin Microbiol 2016. https://doi.org/10.1128/jcm.00730-16.

[63] Messacar K, Breazeale G, Robinson CC, et al. Potential clinical impact of the film array meningitis encephalitis panel in children with suspected central nervous system infections. Diagn Microbiol Infect Dis 2016. https://doi.org/10.1016/j.diagmicrobio.2016.05.020.

[64] Radmard S, Reid S, Ciryam P, et al. Clinical utilization of the FilmArray meningitis/encephalitis (ME) multiplex polymerase chain reaction (PCR) assay. Front Neurol 2019;10. https://doi.org/10.3389/fneur.2019.00281.

[65] Dack K, Pankow S, Ablah E, et al. Contribution of the BioFire® FilmArray® meningitis/encephalitis panel: assessing antimicrobial duration and length of stay. Kans J Med 2019;12(1):1–3.

[66] Chang D, Okulicz JF, Nielsen LE, et al. A tertiary care center's experience with novel molecular meningitis/encephalitis diagnostics and implementation with antimicrobial stewardship. Mil Med 2018;183(1–2):e24–7.

[67] Eichinger A, Hagen A, Meyer-Bühn M, et al. Clinical benefits of introducing real-time multiplex PCR for cerebrospinal fluid as routine diagnostic at a tertiary care pediatric center. Infection 2019;47(1):51–8.

[68] Dien Bard J, Alby K. Point-counterpoint: meningitis/encephalitis syndromic testing in the clinical laboratory.

Ledeboer NA. J Clin Microbiol 2018;56(4). https://doi.org/10.1128/JCM.00018-18.

[69] Seng P, Drancourt M, Gouriet F, et al. Ongoing revolution in bacteriology: routine identification of bacteria by matrix-assisted laser desorption ionization time-of-flight mass spectrometry. Clin Infect Dis 2009. https://doi.org/10.1086/600885.

[70] Singhal N, Kumar M, Kanaujia PK, et al. MALDI-TOF mass spectrometry: an emerging technology for microbial identification and diagnosis. Front Microbiol 2015. https://doi.org/10.3389/fmicb.2015.00791.

[71] Vlek ALM, Bonten MJM, Boel CHE. Direct matrix-assisted laser desorption ionization time-of-flight mass spectrometry improves appropriateness of antibiotic treatment of bacteremia. PLoS One 2012. https://doi.org/10.1371/journal.pone.0032589.

[72] Huang AM, Newton D, Kunapuli A, et al. Impact of rapid organism identification via matrix-assisted laser desorption/ionization time-of-flight combined with antimicrobial stewardship team intervention in adult patients with bacteremia and candidemia. Clin Infect Dis 2013. https://doi.org/10.1093/cid/cit498.

[73] Ge M-C, Kuo A-J, Liu K-L, et al. Routine identification of microorganisms by matrix-assisted laser desorption ionization time-of-flight mass spectrometry: success rate, economic analysis, and clinical outcome. J Microbiol Immunol Infect 2017;50(5):662–8.

[74] Nagel JL, Huang AM, Kunapuli A, et al. Impact of antimicrobial stewardship intervention on coagulase-negative *Staphylococcus* blood cultures in conjunction with rapid diagnostic testing. J Clin Microbiol 2014. https://doi.org/10.1128/JCM.00682-14.

[75] Beganovic M, Costello M, Wieczorkiewicz SM. Effect of matrix-assisted laser desorption ionization–time of flight mass spectrometry (MALDI-TOF MS) alone versus MALDI-TOF MS combined with real-time antimicrobial stewardship interventions on time to optimal antimicrobial therapy in patients with posit. J Clin Microbiol 2017;55(5):1437–45.

[76] Patel TS, Kaakeh R, Nagel JL, et al. Cost analysis of implementing matrix- assisted laser desorption ionization-time of flight mass spectrometry plus real-time antimicrobial stewardship intervention for bloodstream infections. J Clin Microbiol 2017. https://doi.org/10.1128/JCM.01452-16.

[77] Christner M, Rohde H, Wolters M, et al. Rapid identification of bacteria from positive blood culture bottles by use of matrix-assisted laser desorption-ionization time of flight mass spectrometry fingerprinting. J Clin Microbiol 2010. https://doi.org/10.1128/JCM.01831-09.

[78] Stevenson LG, Drake SK, Murray PR. Rapid identification of bacteria in positive blood culture broths by matrix-assisted laser desorption ionization-time of flight mass spectrometry. J Clin Microbiol 2010;48(2):444–7.

[79] Clerc O, Prod'hom G, Vogne C, et al. Impact of matrix-assisted laser desorption ionization time-of-flight mass spectrometry on the clinical management of patients with gram-negative bacteremia: a prospective observational study. Clin Infect Dis 2013;56(8):1101–7.

[80] Oviaño M, Bou G. Matrix-assisted laser desorption ionization–time of flight mass spectrometry for the rapid detection of antimicrobial resistance mechanisms and beyond. Clin Microbiol Rev 2019;32(1). https://doi.org/10.1128/CMR.00037-18.

[81] Josten M, Reif M, Szekat C, et al. Analysis of the matrix-assisted laser desorption ionization-time of flight mass spectrum of *Staphylococcus aureus* identifies mutations that allow differentiation of the main clonal lineages. J Clin Microbiol 2013. https://doi.org/10.1128/JCM.00518-13.

[82] Wolters M, Rohde H, Maier T, et al. MALDI-TOF MS fingerprinting allows for discrimination of major methicillin-resistant *Staphylococcus aureus* lineages. Int J Med Microbiol 2011. https://doi.org/10.1016/j.ijmm.2010.06.002.

[83] Griffin PM, Price GR, Schooneveldt JM, et al. Use of matrix-assisted laser desorption ionization-time of flight mass spectrometry to identify vancomycin-resistant enterococci and investigate the epidemiology of an outbreak. J Clin Microbiol 2012. https://doi.org/10.1128/JCM.01000-12.

[84] Álvarez-Buylla A, Picazo JJ, Culebras E. Optimized method for *Acinetobacter* species carbapenemase detection and identification by matrix-assisted laser desorption ionization-time of flight mass spectrometry. J Clin Microbiol 2013. https://doi.org/10.1128/JCM.00181-13.

[85] Kempf M, Bakour S, Flaudrops C, et al. Rapid detection of carbapenem resistance in *Acinetobacter baumannii* using matrix-assisted laser desorption ionization-time of flight mass spectrometry. PLoS One 2012. https://doi.org/10.1371/journal.pone.0031676.

[86] Cai JC, Hu YY, Zhang R, et al. Detection of OmpK36 porin loss in *Klebsiella* spp. by matrix-assisted laser desorption ionization-time of flight mass spectrometry. J Clin Microbiol 2012. https://doi.org/10.1128/JCM.00503-12.

[87] Sparbier K, Schubert S, Weller U, et al. Matrix-assisted laser desorption ionization-time of flight mass spectrometry-based functional assay for rapid detection of resistance against β-lactam antibiotics. J Clin Microbiol 2012. https://doi.org/10.1128/JCM.05737-11.

[88] Wolk DM, Clark AE. Matrix-assisted laser desorption time of flight mass spectrometry. Clin Lab Med 2018;38(3):471–86.

[89] Kwong JC, Mccallum N, Sintchenko V, et al. Whole genome sequencing in clinical and public health microbiology. Pathology 2015. https://doi.org/10.1097/PAT.0000000000000235.

[90] Lockhart SR, Etienne KA, Vallabhaneni S, et al. Simultaneous emergence of multidrug-resistant *Candida auris* on 3 continents confirmed by whole-genome sequencing and epidemiological analyses. Clin Infect Dis 2017. https://doi.org/10.1093/cid/ciw691.

[91] Snitkin ES, Zelazny AM, Thomas PJ, et al. Tracking a hospital outbreak of carbapenem-resistant *Klebsiella*

pneumoniae with whole-genome sequencing. Sci Transl Med 2012. https://doi.org/10.1126/scitranslmed.3004129.

[92] Spencer MD, Winglee K, Passaretti C, et al. Whole genome sequencing detects inter-facility transmission of carbapenem-resistant *Klebsiella pneumoniae*. J Infect 2019;78(3):187–99.

[93] Bryant JM, Grogono DM, Greaves D, et al. Whole-genome sequencing to identify transmission of Mycobacterium abscessus *Mycobacterium abscessus* between patients with cystic fibrosis: a retrospective cohort study. Lancet 2013. https://doi.org/10.1016/S0140-6736(13)60632-7.

[94] Su M, Satola SW, Read TD. Genome-based prediction of bacterial antibiotic resistance. J Clin Microbiol 2018. https://doi.org/10.1128/jcm.01405-18.

[95] Falgenhauer L, Waezsada S-E, Yao Y, et al. Colistin resistance gene mcr-1 in extended-spectrum β-lactamase-producing and carbapenemase-producing Gram-negative bacteria in Germany. Lancet Infect Dis 2016; 16(3):282–3.

[96] Zankari E, Hasman H, Cosentino S, et al. Identification of acquired antimicrobial resistance genes. J Antimicrob Chemother 2012. https://doi.org/10.1093/jac/dks261.

[97] Stoesser N, Batty EM, Eyre DW, et al. Predicting antimicrobial susceptibilities for *Escherichia coli* and *Klebsiella pneumoniae* isolates using whole genomic sequence data. J Antimicrob Chemother 2013. https://doi.org/10.1093/jac/dkt180.

[98] Gordon NC, Price JR, Cole K, et al. Prediction of *Staphylococcus aureus* antimicrobial resistance by whole-genome sequencing. J Clin Microbiol 2014. https://doi.org/10.1128/JCM.03117-13.

[99] Anjum MF, Zankari E, Hasman H. Molecular methods for detection of antimicrobial resistance. Microbiol Spectr 2017;5(6). https://doi.org/10.1128/microbiolspec.ARBA-0011-2017.

[100] Köser CU, Bryant JM, Becq J, et al. Whole-genome sequencing for rapid susceptibility testing of *M. tuberculosis*. N Engl J Med 2013. https://doi.org/10.1056/nejmc1215305.

[101] Schuts EC, Hulscher MEJL, Mouton JW, et al. Current evidence on hospital antimicrobial stewardship objectives: a systematic review and meta-analysis. Lancet Infect Dis 2016. https://doi.org/10.1016/S1473-3099(16)00065-7.

Advances in Molecular Pathology 2 (2019) 89–97
ADVANCES IN MOLECULAR PATHOLOGY

Application of Next-Generation Sequencing in Public Health Epidemiology and Outbreak Investigation

Anthony Tran, DrPH, MPH, D(ABMM)[a,*], Marie-Claire Rowlinson, PhD, D(ABMM)[b]
[a]District of Columbia Department of Forensic Sciences, Public Health Laboratory Division, 401 East Street, Southwest, Washington, DC 20024, USA; [b]Florida Department of Health, Bureau of Public Health Laboratories, 1217 North Pearl Street, Jacksonville, FL 32202, USA

KEYWORDS
- Whole-genome sequencing (WGS) • Next-generation sequencing (NGS) • Public health laboratory
- Epidemiology • Outbreaks • Public health

KEY POINTS
- Next-generation sequencing and whole-genome sequencing provide much more discriminatory power than traditional molecular epidemiologic tools for outbreak investigations and surveillance.
- Whole-genome sequencing not only plays a role in outbreak investigations, but also in clinical diagnostic applications that will allow for more rapid identification and drug-susceptibility testing.
- The future of whole-genome sequencing will allow for real-time field sequencing so that key epidemiologic data can to be obtained immediately without the need for a traditional laboratory.

INTRODUCTION

Molecular epidemiology for infectious diseases is an essential part of public health outbreak investigation and subsequent intervention. Molecular techniques have been deployed in public health infectious disease detection and surveillance for over 30 years, with the use of sequence analysis becoming the foundation of molecular surveillance [1]. Molecular typing methods can be used broadly to study the distribution, dynamics, and determinants of disease in human populations, and can be used at a more granular level to identify patterns of infection, sources of transmission, and support outbreak investigations. These methods analyze the relatedness of organisms at a molecular level and can discriminate between strains to varying degrees depending on the methodology, and are considerably better than phenotypic methods at discrimination between clones. The field is rapidly evolving as molecular microbiological techniques continue to advance along with analytical and computational tools. Notably, next-generation sequencing (NGS) has become a powerful tool in this domain [2].

The terms "next-generation sequencing" and "whole-genome sequencing" (WGS) are commonly used interchangeably. However, NGS is appropriate in describing any sequencing technology that performs massively parallel, high-throughput, or deep sequencing; whereas WGS implies that the entire genome of an organism is sequenced. NGS and WGS applications are used in the clinical and public health laboratory. The chemistries of the instruments and sequencing and detection methods differ—NGS systems can generally be

Disclosure: The authors have nothing to disclose.

*Corresponding author, *E-mail address:* anthony.tran@dc.gov

https://doi.org/10.1016/j.yamp.2019.07.007
2589-4080/19/

compared or characterized by looking at the number of reads generated and the length of those reads. Commercial systems for NGS include offerings from Illumina (San Diego, CA), Oxford Nanopore Technologies (Oxford, UK), Pacific Biosciences (Menlo Park, CA), and Thermo Fisher Scientific Ion Torrent (Waltham, MA) [3,4]. Other systems are applicable to research settings or are likely to become commercially available in the future as the technology evolves and is constantly improving (ie, lower cost, better accuracy).

NGS technology only recently became cost-effective, rapid, and sufficiently simplified such that it can be implemented in the clinical and public health laboratory. The application of NGS to date for infectious diseases has been predominantly in surveillance and outbreak investigation; nevertheless its use in clinical diagnostic practice will continue to expand [5–7]. As the technology along with the necessary quality parameters and appropriate analysis become more established and standardized, it is safe to assume that this will become more commonplace in the clinical and public health laboratory. Its current applications have already shown how a higher-resolution and more discriminatory method can positively change public health as well as individual patient care. A seminal paper from the United Kingdom on the application of WGS for outbreak investigation describes how WGS was used to characterize methicillin-resistant *Staphylococcus aureus* (MRSA) isolates suspected in an outbreak at a neonatal intensive care unit [8]. The outbreak was confirmed, along with transmission dynamics and determination of the resistome. This informed infection control to prevent further transmission and supported appropriate treatment of patients. In the United States, WGS was initiated statewide for all *Listeria* isolates in 2013 as a collaborative effort between the Centers for Disease Control and Prevention (CDC), the US Department of Agriculture, the National Institutes of Health, and the Association of Public Health Laboratories (and its member public health laboratories). This technology, used for the investigation of organisms that cause foodborne illness, as part of the national PulseNet program, and in replacement of traditional pulsed-field gel electrophoresis (PFGE), was shown to enhance listeriosis surveillance. During the pilot period described in the paper, more outbreaks were identified, clusters were detected in a timelier manner, and a greater number of cases were linked to food sources [9]. In addition to the use of NGS for epidemiologic purposes, its use in diagnostics continues to be explored. One example is the use of WGS for genotyping of tuberculosis (TB) for epidemiologic surveillance and identification of drug resistance. The use of WGS for TB epidemiology is well-described. In a study by Walker and colleagues [10], researchers compared WGS with current genotyping methods for TB (MIRU-VNTR) on 390 *Mycobacterium tuberculosis* complex (MTBC) isolates and determined that WGS provided greater resolution. This paper prompted continued efforts at Public Health England to perform WGS and implement it routinely, not only in surveillance and cluster detection, but also for diagnostic purposes. Resistance mutations were characterized and matched with resistance phenotype for validation of resistance-causing mutations [11]. At a US public health reference laboratory, a diagnostic assay has been developed and implemented using WGS. The diagnostic use of this assay is to identify the species within the MTBC, and predict drug resistance, in addition to genotyping for surveillance [12].

This paper discusses and explores the use of NGS and WGS for outbreak tracing and surveillance from various perspectives of outbreaks and diseases of public health and clinical importance.

SIGNIFICANCE

Foodborne Illnesses

The CDC estimates that 48 million people get sick, 128,000 are hospitalized, and 3000 die from foodborne illness annually in the United States [13]. CDC's PulseNet program is a national network that collects and analyzes laboratory data, and that compares enteric bacteria with one another to identify clusters of food and waterborne disease that might otherwise go unrecognized. Bacteria in the PulseNet USA program include: *Salmonella* spp, *Listeria* spp, Shiga toxin-producing *Escherichia coli*, *Campylobacter* spp, *Shigella* spp, *Vibrio parahemolyticus* and *V. cholerae*, and *Cronobacter* spp. The PulseNet program turned 20 years old in 2016 and has become an essential program in the United States in the detection and prevention of local and multistate outbreaks [14].

Historically, the PulseNet program used PFGE data for molecular surveillance but has been transitioning to WGS since 2013, with PFGE due to cease completely in Spring 2019. PFGE methodology involves analysis of the bacterial genome by restriction enzyme digestion. Enteric bacteria are digested with a restriction enzyme, DNA fragments are pulsed through an alternating electric field, resulting in a pattern of DNA fragments, or "fingerprint." Fingerprint patterns are compared with those of other isolates using standardized software. This analysis enables the development of a dendrogram to pictorialize how one isolate is related to another. Fingerprints with indistinguishable patterns are considered part of a "cluster." A cluster is considered when there are more cases than expected at a geographic location over a certain period of time (60 days). Fig. 1 shows *Salmonella* PFGE fingerprints and the associated dendrogram. The figure illustrates different *Salmonella* serotypes and highlights how an analysis is made; in this picture the 2 Javiana serotype strains are identical and can be shown to be distinct from the other serotypes. The 2 Typhimurium serotypes are the same serotype but are not identical.

Standardization is crucial between laboratories to assure that fingerprints from 1 laboratory can be accurately compared with those from another laboratory. Public health laboratory scientists must be certified to perform testing, and analysis and data uploading to PulseNet must be performed according standardized CDC protocols.

Although PFGE was the gold standard method of PulseNet over 20 years, WGS has shown to provide more discriminatory data than PFGE [15]. NGS for PulseNet involves the following standard steps: DNA extraction, library preparation (shearing the DNA and adding indexes) and amplification, template preparation and sequencing. However, data analysis is crucial to ensure that bacteria can be compared with one another in a biologically relevant way, that is, also discriminatory. For PulseNet "whole-genome multilocus sequence typing" (wgMLST) methodology is currently the standard protocol since it can be easily standardized and provides stable nomenclature. This sequencing method is based on the classic multilocus sequence typing (MLST) method that has been used for molecular typing of bacteria for several years. Classic MLST schemes look at 7 defined loci in the genome, usually housekeeping genes, with each locus being assigned an allele number so that bacterial strains can be identified by an allelic profile, which is a combination of the 7 allele numbers. Using wgMLST, more loci can be analyzed, between 1500 and 4000, which translates to a higher typing resolution. Looking at allelic variation, as opposed to single-nucleotide polymorphisms (SNPs), means that recombinations, deletions, and insertions at multiple positions can be counted as single evolutionary events [16]. Fig. 2 is a diagram of wgMLST analysis which shows a dendrogram based on WGS data. This dendrogram shows that the 2 Newport serotypes are similar but not identical and are distinct from the other serotypes.

A challenge with the use of wgMLST schemes is that they require allelic curation, which can take some time to establish. Nevertheless, the same standardization, certification, and quality metrics apply to WGS as to PFGE. Since 2013, CDC has used WGS to detect *Listeria* spp. outbreaks. Using WGS has many benefits over PFGE for the following reasons: it replaces several methods in 1 test, detects more *Listeria* spp. clusters; provides more discrimination for determination of outbreaks, even if those outbreaks are small; provides more discrimination for linking infected patients to potential food sources; and has identified new food sources such as caramel apples and packaged salads that were not originally linked to the outbreak [9,17].

Identification of a food source is vital in the timely recall of food to prevent further illness. Similar conclusions are drawn from a PulseNet Canada publication that showed how WGS improved outbreak detection for *E coli* O157:H7 compared with conventional methods, by accurately identifying outbreak and nonoutbreak isolates. WGS offered a higher-resolution analysis and was ultimately determined to provide

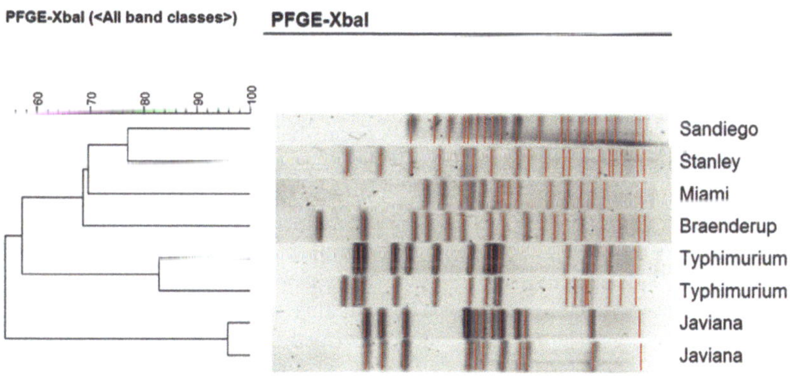

FIG. 1 Salmonella dendrogram and PFGE patterns.

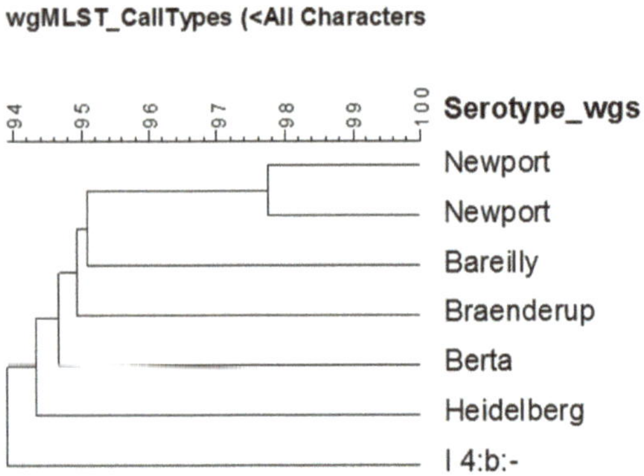

FIG. 2 Salmonella wgMLST dendrogram.

more accurate classification of isolates that were outbreak related and could therefore direct limited epidemiologic resources more effectively [18].

There are many examples in which WGS has provided essential information on which public health action could be taken. For example, CDC identified a *Salmonella enterica* serotype Newport cluster in January 2017, which had indistinguishable PFGE patterns entered into the PulseNet national database. Although PFGE was performed to identify isolates in the cluster, WGS was used to show strain relatedness between patients, dairy cattle, and leftover ground beef, suggesting a common source, most likely the dairy cattle [19]. In August 2017, an outbreak of multidrug-resistant *Campylobacter jejuni* was linked to puppy exposures. The cluster was identified in Florida by wgMLST, which indicated that the *Campylobacter* spp. cluster was drug resistant. This outbreak was ultimately epidemiologically linked to 6 pet store companies, with 118 human cases (29 in pet store employees) from 18 states [20]. Further information about PulseNet can be found on the CDC Web site, www.cdc.gov/pulsenet.

Legionnaires' Disease

Legionnaires' disease (LD) causes severe pneumonia, and often can be fatal if left untreated; however, these infections are infrequently diagnosed [21,22]. This may be because of the fastidious nature of the bacteria, combined with the fact that nearly all clinical diagnoses are made using a urine antigen test (UAT) [22]. Unfortunately, this assay only detects serogroup 1 of *Legionella pneumophila*, which is only 1 of 15 serogroups that cause LD, and does not detect other species of *Legionella* that also cause disease, such as *Legionella micadei* and *Legionella longbeachae* [23]. The lower sensitivity may also lead to falsely negative screening results, thus leading to a missed diagnosis [23]. Although culture remains the gold standard, it is not routinely performed in many hospitals, thus most LD diagnoses are made via the UAT.

Because culture is not routinely performed, outbreak investigations must rely heavily on epidemiologic investigation along with rigorous environmental sampling. If *Legionella* isolates can be obtained from patients, and environmental sampling also yields isolates, then further testing to match clinical isolates to their environmental counterparts should be done. This would allow for definitive linkages to the common source of the outbreak.

WGS has been widely used recently to provide insights into *L pneumophila* populations in water systems in buildings, including potable water sources such as sinks and showers and nonpotable water sources such as cooling towers [24,25]. Previously, it was not feasible to trace back transmission to these artificial water systems without the use of WGS because of the ubiquitous nature of resident *L pneumophila* populations in these buildings. Traditional methods such as PFGE and sequence-based typing (SBT) are often not sufficiently discriminatory to determine true causation of an outbreak [25]. The ability of WGS to provide complete genomic information, thus conferring the highest resolution, has made it the gold standard for these types of investigations. Longitudinal studies of environmental sources of *L pneumophila* have shown that homogenous PFGE profiles have yielded heterogeneous populations by WGS [26]. Similar retrospective studies on archived clinical isolates of *L pneumophila* have yielded comparable conclusions [27–29].

A prime example for the use of WGS to assist in outbreak tracing of LD was a 2015 outbreak in New York City (NYC). This was the largest outbreak of LD in NYC history and the largest in the United States since its discovery in 1976 [30]. In total, 138 cases of LD, including 16 deaths, were linked to a single cooling tower in the South Bronx. Twenty-six patients were diagnosed via culture as having *L pneumophila* serogroup 1 (Lp1). All 26 patients' isolates were indistinguishable by PFGE, SBT, and WGS, thus indicating that the cause of their infection was from a common source. The investigation led to 55 cooling towers from 46 buildings in the "outbreak zone" being sampled and tested. Lp1 DNA was found in 21 of the 55 (38%) of the cooling towers, with 14 (66.7%) yielding successful cultures. WGS of these 14 isolates revealed that only 1 of the cooling towers matched all 26 of the patient isolates. Further analysis by WGS revealed that this clone, named F4469, has been endemic in the Bronx since 2007 causing sporadic outbreaks of LD [31]. It remains unclear why this clone caused such a large outbreak in 2015 despite being resident in NYC for so many years.

Influenza and Other Healthcare-Associated Infections

Influenza virus is a major contributor of influenza-like illness reported to hospitals during the winter months. Seasonal influenza epidemics occur worldwide in both Northern and Southern hemispheres during winter. There are an estimated 500,000 deaths annually due to influenza worldwide [32]. In the United States, the CDC estimated that 48.8 million people contracted influenza during the 2017 to 2018 season, with nearly 1 million hospitalizations and 79,400 deaths [33]. Health care-associated infections (HAIs) with influenza are a major issue because of the severity of the disease, especially in vulnerable hospitalized populations that may be immunocompromised, at extremes of age, or pregnant. This, combined with the high risk of transmission due to cohorting in open areas of emergency department waiting rooms and triage, are of significant concern for hospital infection control professionals [34].

Traditionally, HAIs of influenza virus were commonly identified through molecular diagnostic methods, such as real-time reverse transcription polymerase chain reaction, which provide results of the influenza species along with contact tracing of patient and staff movements within the hospital. Those patients who overlap in time and space and were diagnosed with a specific influenza virus and subtype, if available, were assumed to be have transmitted to each other [34]. Unfortunately, this method is not completely accurate and is mainly based on epidemiologic information gathered during the investigation. During the winter months when influenza virus transmission is high, many infected patients will present with the same influenza subtype (eg, H1N1 or H3N2). Subtyping alone does not provide a sufficient molecular epidemiologic link. Recently, WGS has been used to further characterize the influenza virus detected from patients, and can definitively pinpoint the index patient [34–36].

In 1 outbreak investigation, epidemiologists thought that the cause of a hospital outbreak in a ward was due to 2 index patients. However, after WGS analysis, it was determined that only 1 patient was the cause of the outbreak while the other was not linked [34]. This illustrates how traditional methods of testing and epidemiologic investigation led to the incorrect conclusions, which were later modified because of information gained from WGS. Another example provides insight into a cluster of influenza B subtype B/Yamagata over a 4-week period, when 17 of 20 patients were linked to each other by either a shared room or common ward. WGS was able to provide a rapid detailed analysis of the samples that matched the epidemiologic link supporting these common shared spaces and relationships [35]. Infection control preventionists were able to quickly determine the cause and make critical policy changes to avoid future HAI outbreaks.

In addition to HAI investigations, the usefulness of WGS has been expanded by researchers to analyze the genetic makeup of avian-influenza origin viruses to better understand how these viruses cross between animal species. Studies examining H3N2 in canines, H5N1 in migratory birds, and H7N9 in humans over time have helped us better understand how SNPs may lead to cross-species transmission of influenza [37–39]. This information will help public health authorities to better predict potential reassortant events.

NGS can be applied to investigation of HAI for many other infectious disease organisms as well. One example is the nontuberculous mycobacterium, *Mycobacterium chimaera*, which caused HAIs associated with a heater-cooler device during cardiac surgery [40]. Analysis provided strong evidence for point-source contamination of the heater-cooler devices and global dissemination of this strain of *M chimaera*. NGS will prove particularly useful in outbreaks and determination of source when organisms exhibit drug resistance and/or are hard to identify. *Candida auris* is an organism that is hard to identify in the clinical laboratory and exhibits considerable antimicrobial resistance (AR), making the prevention of the spread of this organism a major public health priority. Sequencing analysis was crucial in elucidating the emergence of this AR threat and will continue to be a valuable tool in tracking and preventing its spread [41]. The use of NGS for determination of AR in a range of organisms goes beyond epidemiology and infection prevention efforts. NGS will play a future role in routine prediction of AR in the clinical laboratory, not just for bacteria but also for mycobacteria, viruses, and fungi. Genotyping efforts for HIV and hepatitis C virus will also benefit from the greater discriminatory power of NGS methods [42–44].

Tuberculosis

TB is one of the top causes of death worldwide. In 2017, the World Health Organization estimated that 10 million people became ill with TB and 1.6 million died, with 0.3 million of those among HIV-positive people, in whom TB is the leading killer. Another challenge with TB is multidrug resistance (MDR). There were 558,000 new cases of TB that were resistant to the most effective first-line drug, rifampin [45]. Although the incidence of TB continues to decline both worldwide and in the United States, the rate of decline is not sufficient to meet the goals of the "End TB Strategy" and, ultimately, TB elimination. In the United States there were 9029 new cases of TB in 2018, a rate of 2.8 cases per 100,000 persons [46]. Globally, and in the United States, the diagnosis and treatment of TB and MDR-TB remains a public health priority. NGS has seen considerable use in the epidemiology of infectious diseases and can be applied to TB epidemiology. There is limited genetic diversity within *Mycobacterium tuberculosis* compared with other microorganisms and, thus, NGS can be used effectively to determine epidemiologic factors where traditional typing methods fall short. NGS can be used to determine transmission dynamics, differentiate between relapse and reinfection, elucidate within-host diversity, and identify drug resistance as being primary versus acquired. Systematic reviews highlight the higher discriminatory power of NGS while also cautioning about the need for more investigation related to the methodologies used for analysis, the setting of thresholds for defining epidemiologic relatedness, and an understanding of genetic diversity in *M tuberculosis* strains [47–49]. Continuing advances are being made with NGS in its use for epidemiologic study and surveillance, and now as a diagnostic tool. NGS can be used for routine diagnostics for TB, particularly for determination of drug resistance. Walker and colleagues [11] characterized mutations across 23 candidate genes to determine whether they were benign or caused resistance, and compared the results with phenotypic information. The WGS data matched closely to phenotype data, although correct characterization of all mutations was not achieved; also, there were some resistance phenotypes for which a mutation could not be attributed. There are a few possible reasons for this, including the fact that phenotypic drug susceptibility testing is an imperfect methodology, and that mutations that cause resistance could arise outside of the candidate genes or regions that were characterized. Nevertheless, this paper suggested that WGS had the potential to be implemented routinely to predict drug resistance in a clinical laboratory, which would significantly decrease turnaround time (TAT) for patient-management decisions. A study across 8 laboratories in Europe and North America assessed the real-time performance and cost implications of implementing WGS for TB diagnostics and concluded that the WGS workflow achieved a faster TAT, reduced overall cost, and that prediction of drug susceptibility was accurate; however, WGS cannot yet completely replace other testing methodologies [50,51]. Subsequently, WGS was routinely implemented in 2017 by Public Health England. In the US public health laboratory system, a large state public health laboratory implemented WGS for TB diagnosis in February 2016 for all new TB cases. In October 2018, after extensive parallel WGS and growth-based drug-susceptibility testing (DST), this state public health laboratory implemented a reduced drug-susceptibility testing algorithm for TB. With this novel algorithm, isolates from new TB cases have WGS performed with a TAT of approximately 1 week. Fig. 3 highlights 2 workflows and the time-saving that WGS affords.

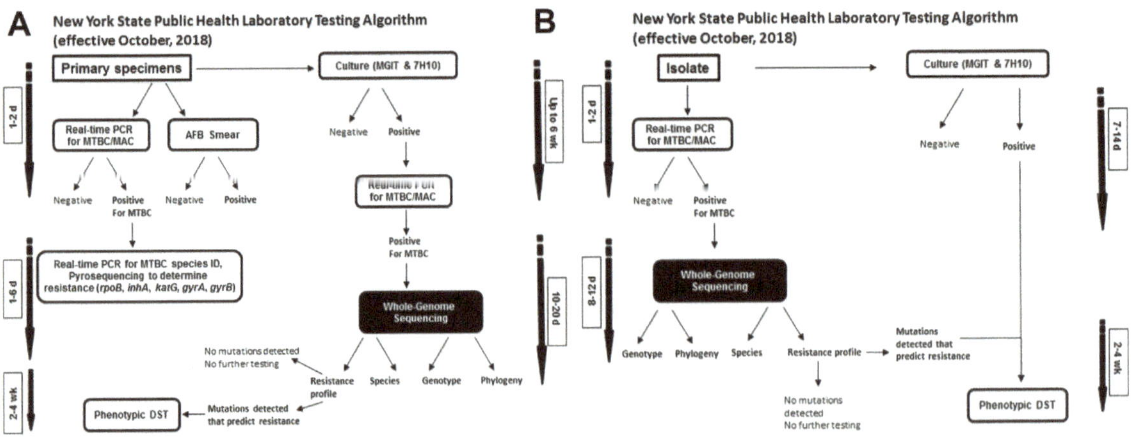

FIG. 3 New York State Department of Health simplified WGS algorithm for tuberculosis testing.

TB strains that are determined by WGS to be pan-susceptible (ie, no predicted mutations in genes known to be associated with resistance) do not have DST performed, which has reduced the need for DST in the laboratory by 80% [12]. This algorithm has provided greater resolution in prediction of drug resistance in a timelier manner than conventional methods. The CDC's Division of TB Elimination is supporting sequencing efforts for the implementation of WGS for TB genotyping in the United States by 2020 to replace the current MIRU-VNTR genotyping method. As NGS/WGS is implemented at the national and global level, efforts to standardize protocols will be essential. The ReSeq TB Database is a worldwide repository of curated sequences and metadata related to mutations associated with drug resistance in *M tuberculosis* [52,53]. The Comprehensive Resistance Prediction for Tuberculosis: an International Consortium is a collaboration whose goal is to diagnose and treat drug-resistant TB more quickly through efforts, such as WGS, to accurately predict genetic resistance [54,55]. Through these efforts, NGS/WGS has the potential to prevent transmission, prevent or shorten outbreaks, and more accurately and quickly identify multidrug-resistant TB and extensively drug-resistant TB.

FUTURE CONSIDERATIONS

Continued advances in WGS technology are making it easier for laboratories to enter into the sequencing arena. The current needs for pure samples (eg, bacterial isolates, amplified viral RNA, fungi) is shifting to a metagenomics approach in which primary source material, such as cerebral spinal fluid, blood, tissue, respiratory secretions, and stool can be sequenced. The challenge of metagenomics sequencing will be how to analyze the massive amount of data generated, because DNA from various sources, including the host and not just the primary pathogen, will be present [56]. The key will be having a sophisticated and curated bioinformatics pipeline that will be able to analyze and sort out the data to make it digestible for the end user. Advances in metagenomics sequencing for outbreak investigations and diagnosis are already underway, with numerous successful examples. The US Food and Drug Administration has sequenced *Cyclospora cayetanensis* from stool samples collected in Nepal and provides the groundwork for SNP analysis for future outbreak tracing [57]. This metagenomics approach is critical for public health as hospital laboratories begin to implement culture-independent diagnostic technologies, thus decreasing the availability of culture for molecular epidemiologic purposes. For example, using shotgun metagenomics for diagnosis of *Brugia malayi* in a 34-year-old who had no clear diagnosis after several visits to hospitals in the United States and China for nearly a year [58], after an eye discharge sample was obtained, WGS performed, and data analyzed, the parasite was determined to be the causative agent of the symptoms.

The landscape of field epidemiology is also evolving in response to advances in WGS. The MinION platform from Oxford Nanopore Technologies has allowed WGS to be conducted outside of a traditional laboratory, requiring only a laptop and a USB cable for power and connectivity. This technology has supported WGS outbreak surveillance in remote areas such as in Liberia during the world's largest Ebola outbreak, and also in Brazil to conduct real-time monitoring of Zika virus [59,60]. In both cases, transporting of samples to the laboratory was not possible, therefore conducting WGS in the field was the only way to obtain real-time outbreak surveillance data critical for public health action.

SUMMARY

WGS is an invaluable tool for definitively identifying and pinpointing sources of outbreaks from numerous diseases and infections. As this technology continues to become more affordable and user-friendly, the use and incorporation of WGS will continue to increase. Although public health laboratories are best situated to provide support for large-scale outbreaks, WGS technology should soon be accessible to all laboratories to support more localized outbreak tracing as well.

ACKNOWLEDGMENTS

Mycobacteriology Laboratory at the Wadsworth Center, New York State Department of Health.

REFERENCES

[1] Robertson BH, Nicholson JK. New microbiology tools for public health and their implications. Annu Rev Public Health 2005;26:281–302.

[2] Riley LW, Blanton RE. Advances in molecular epidemiology of infectious diseases: definitions, approaches, and scope of the field. Microbiol Spectr 2018;6(6). https://doi.org/10.1128/microbiolspec.AME-0001-2018.

[3] Levy SE, Myers RM. Advancements in next-generation sequencing. Annu Rev Genomics Hum Genet 2016;17:95–115.

[4] Reuter JA, Spacek DV, Snyder MP. High-throughput sequencing technologies. Mol Cell 2015;58(4):586–97.

[5] Didelot X, Bowden R, Wilson DJ, et al. Transforming clinical microbiology with bacterial genome sequencing. Nat Rev Genet 2012;13(9):601–12.
[6] Koser CU, Ellington MJ, Cartwright EJ, et al. Routine use of microbial whole genome sequencing in diagnostic and public health microbiology. PLoS Pathog 2012; 8(8):e1002824.
[7] Oakeson KF, Wagner JM, Mendenhall M, et al. Bioinformatic analyses of whole-genome sequence data in a public health laboratory. Emerg Infect Dis 2017; 23(9):1441–5.
[8] Koser CU, Holden MT, Ellington MJ, et al. Rapid whole-genome sequencing for investigation of a neonatal MRSA outbreak. N Engl J Med 2012;366(24):2267–75.
[9] Jackson BR, Tarr C, Strain E, et al. Implementation of nationwide real-time whole-genome sequencing to enhance listeriosis outbreak detection and investigation. Clin Infect Dis 2016;63(3):380–6.
[10] Walker TM, Ip CL, Harrell RH, et al. Whole-genome sequencing to delineate *Mycobacterium tuberculosis* outbreaks: a retrospective observational study. Lancet Infect Dis 2013;13(2):137–46.
[11] Walker TM, Kohl TA, Omar SV, et al. Whole-genome sequencing for prediction of *Mycobacterium tuberculosis* drug susceptibility and resistance: a retrospective cohort study. Lancet Infect Dis 2015;15(10):1193–202.
[12] Shea J, Halse TA, Lapierre P, et al. Comprehensive whole-genome sequencing and reporting of drug resistance profiles on clinical cases of *Mycobacterium tuberculosis* in New York State. J Clin Microbiol 2017;55(6):1871–82.
[13] Centers for Disease and Prevention. Foodborne Illnesses and Germs | Food Safety | CDC. Centers for Disease Control and Prevention. 2019. Available at: https://www.cdc.gov/foodsafety/foodborne-germs.html. Accessed April 4, 2019.
[14] Announcement. 20th Anniversary of PulseNet: the National Molecular Subtyping Network for Foodborne Disease Surveillance — United States, 2016. MMWR Morb Mortal Wkly Rep 2016;65:636.
[15] Ribot EM, Hise KB. Future challenges for tracking foodborne diseases: PulseNet, a 20-year-old US surveillance system for foodborne diseases, is expanding both globally and technologically. EMBO Rep 2016;17(11): 1499–505.
[16] Nadon C, Van Walle I, Gerner-Smidt P, et al. PulseNet International: vision for the implementation of whole genome sequencing (WGS) for global food-borne disease surveillance. Euro Surveill 2017; 22(23) [pii:30544].
[17] Self JL, Conrad A, Stroika S, et al. Notes from the field: outbreak of listeriosis associated with consumption of packaged salad - United States and Canada, 2015-2016. MMWR Morb Mortal Wkly Rep 2016;65(33):879–81.
[18] Rumore J, Tschetter L, Kearney A, et al. Evaluation of whole-genome sequencing for outbreak detection of Verotoxigenic Escherichia coli O157:H7 from the Canadian perspective. BMC Genomics 2018;19(1):870.
[19] Marshall KEH, Tewell M, Tecle S, et al. Protracted outbreak of *Salmonella* Newport infections linked to ground beef: possible role of dairy cows - 21 states, 2016-2017. MMWR Morb Mortal Wkly Rep 2018; 67(15):443–6.
[20] Montgomery MP, Robertson S, Koski L, et al. Multidrug-resistant *Campylobacter jejuni* outbreak linked to puppy exposure - United States, 2016-2018. MMWR Morb Mortal Wkly Rep 2018;67(37):1032–5.
[21] Fields BS, Benson RF, Besser RE. Legionella and Legionnaires' disease: 25 years of investigation. Clin Microbiol Rev 2002;15(3):506–26.
[22] Pierre DM, Baron J, Yu VL, et al. Diagnostic testing for Legionnaires' disease. Ann Clin Microbiol Antimicrob 2017;16:59.
[23] Herwaldt LA, Marra AR. *Legionella*: a reemerging pathogen. Curr Opin Infect Dis 2018;31(4):325–33.
[24] David S, Mentasti M, Lai S, et al. Spatial structuring of a *Legionella pneumophila* population within the water system of a large occupational building. Microb Genom 2018;4(10). https://doi.org/10.1099/mgen.0.000226.
[25] Wuthrich D, Gautsch S, Spieler-Denz R, et al. Air-conditioner cooling towers as complex reservoirs and continuous source of *Legionella pneumophila* infection evidenced by a genomic analysis study in 2017, Switzerland. Euro Surveill 2019;24(4). https://doi.org/10.2807/1560-7917.ES.2019.24.4.1800192.
[26] Wells M, Lasek-Nesselquist E, Schoonmaker-Bopp D, et al. Insights into the long-term persistence of *Legionella* in facilities from whole-genome sequencing. Infect Genet Evol 2018;65:200–9.
[27] Raphael BH, Huynh T, Brown E, et al. Culture of clinical specimens reveals extensive diversity of *Legionella pneumophila* strains in Arizona. mSphere 2019;4(1) [pii: e00649-18].
[28] Mercante JW, Morrison SS, Desai HP, et al. Genomic analysis reveals novel diversity among the 1976 Philadelphia Legionnaires' disease outbreak isolates and additional st36 strains. PLoS One 2016;11(9):e0164074.
[29] Schjorring S, Stegger M, Kjelso C, et al. Genomic investigation of a suspected outbreak of *Legionella pneumophila* ST82 reveals undetected heterogeneity by the present gold-standard methods, Denmark, July to November 2014. Euro Surveill 2017;22(25) [pii:30558].
[30] Fitzhenry R, Weiss D, Cimini D, et al. Legionnaires' disease outbreaks and cooling towers, New York City, New York, USA. Emerg Infect Dis 2017;23(11):1769–76.
[31] Lapierre P, Nazarian E, Zhu Y, et al. Legionnaires' disease outbreak caused by endemic strain of *Legionella pneumophila*, New York, New York, USA, 2015. Emerg Infect Dis 2017;23(11):1784–91.
[32] Fauci AS. Seasonal and pandemic influenza preparedness: science and countermeasures. J Infect Dis 2006; 194(Suppl 2):S73–6.
[33] Centers for Disease and Prevention. Estimated influenza illnesses, medical visits, hospitalizations, and deaths in the United States — 2017–2018 influenza season. 2018.

Available at: https://www.cdc.gov/flu/about/burden/2017-2018.htm. Accessed April 4, 2019.
[34] Houlihan CF, Frampton D, Ferns RB, et al. Use of whole-genome sequencing in the investigation of a nosocomial influenza virus outbreak. J Infect Dis 2018;218(9):1485–9.
[35] Sansone M, Wiman A, Karlberg ML, et al. Molecular characterization of a nosocomial outbreak of influenza B virus in an acute care hospital setting. J Hosp Infect 2019;101(1):30–7.
[36] MacFadden DR, McGeer A, Athey T, et al. Use of genome sequencing to define institutional influenza outbreaks, Toronto, Ontario, Canada, 2014-15. Emerg Infect Dis 2018;24(3):492–7.
[37] Xiao YL, Ren L, Zhang X, et al. Deep sequencing of H7N9 influenza A viruses from 16 infected patients from 2013 to 2015 in shanghai reveals genetic diversity and antigenic drift. mSphere 2018;3(5) [pii:e00462-18].
[38] Voorhees IEH, Dalziel BD, Glaser A, et al. Multiple incursions and recurrent epidemic fade-out of h3n2 canine influenza A virus in the United States. J Virol 2018;92(16) [pii:e00323-18].
[39] Nonthabenjawan N, Cardona C, Amonsin A, et al. Time-space analysis of highly pathogenic avian influenza H5N2 outbreak in the US. Virol J 2016;13(1):147.
[40] Hasan NA, Epperson LE, Lawsin A, et al. Genomic analysis of cardiac surgery-associated *Mycobacterium chimaera* infections, United States. Emerg Infect Dis 2019;25(3):559–63.
[41] Lockhart SR, Etienne KA, Vallabhaneni S, et al. Simultaneous emergence of multidrug-resistant *Candida auris* on 3 continents confirmed by whole-genome sequencing and epidemiological analyses. Clin Infect Dis 2017;64(2):134–40.
[42] Su M, Satola SW, Read TD. Genome-based prediction of bacterial antibiotic resistance. J Clin Microbiol 2019;57(3) [pii:e01405-18].
[43] Tzou PL, Ariyaratne P, Varghese V, et al. Comparison of an in vitro diagnostic next-generation sequencing assay with sanger sequencing for HIV-1 genotypic resistance testing. J Clin Microbiol 2018;56(6) [pii:e00105-18].
[44] Longmire AG, Sims S, Rytsareva I, et al. GHOST: global hepatitis outbreak and surveillance technology. BMC Genomics 2017;18(Suppl 10):916.
[45] World Health Organization. Global tuberculosis report 2018. Geneva (Switzerland): World Health Organization; 2018.
[46] World TB Day — March 24, 2019. MMWR Morb Mortal Wkly Rep 2019;68:257.
[47] Roetzer A, Diel R, Kohl TA, et al. Whole genome sequencing versus traditional genotyping for investigation of a *Mycobacterium tuberculosis* outbreak: a longitudinal molecular epidemiological study. PLoS Med 2013;10(2):e1001387.
[48] Hatherell HA, Colijn C, Stagg HR, et al. Interpreting whole genome sequencing for investigating tuberculosis transmission: a systematic review. BMC Med 2016;14:21.
[49] Nikolayevskyy V, Kranzer K, Niemann S, et al. Whole genome sequencing of *Mycobacterium tuberculosis* for detection of recent transmission and tracing outbreaks: a systematic review. Tuberculosis (Edinb) 2016;98:77–85.
[50] Pankhurst LJ, Del Ojo Elias C, Votintseva AA, et al. Rapid, comprehensive, and affordable mycobacterial diagnosis with whole-genome sequencing: a prospective study. Lancet Respir Med 2016;4(1):49–58.
[51] Satta G, Lipman M, Smith GP, et al. *Mycobacterium tuberculosis* and whole-genome sequencing: how close are we to unleashing its full potential? Clin Microbiol Infect 2018;24(6):604–9.
[52] Cirillo DM, Miotto P, Tagliani E. Reaching consensus on drug resistance conferring mutations. Int J Mycobacteriol 2016;5(Suppl 1):S31–2.
[53] ReSeqTB. Available at: https://platform.reseqtb.org/. Accessed April 4, 2019.
[54] Allix-Beguec C, Arandjelovic I, Bi L, et al. Prediction of susceptibility to first-line tuberculosis drugs by DNA sequencing. N Engl J Med 2018;379(15):1403–15.
[55] Comprehensive resistance prediction for tuberculosis: an International Consortium. Available at: http://www.crypticproject.org/. Accessed April 4, 2019.
[56] Forbes JD, Knox NC, Ronholm J, et al. Metagenomics: the next culture-independent game changer. Front Microbiol 2017;8:1069.
[57] Cinar HN, Gopinath G, Jarvis K, et al. The complete mitochondrial genome of the foodborne parasitic pathogen *Cyclospora cayetanensis*. PLoS One 2015;10:e0128645.
[58] Gao D, Yu Q, Wang G, et al. Diagnosis of a malayan filariasis case using a shotgun diagnostic metagenomics assay. Parasit Vectors 2016;9:86.
[59] Hoenen T, Groseth A, Rosenke K, et al. Nanopore sequencing as a rapidly deployable ebola outbreak tool. Emerg Infect Dis 2016;22(2):331–4.
[60] Faria NR, Sabino EC, Nunes MRT, et al. Mobile real-time surveillance of Zika virus in Brazil. Genome Med 2016;8:97.

Advances in Molecular Pathology 2 (2019) 99–110
ADVANCES IN MOLECULAR PATHOLOGY

Next-Generation Sequencing Approaches to Predicting Antimicrobial Susceptibility Testing Results

Rebecca Yee, PhD, Patricia J. Simner, PhD, D(ABMM)*
Division of Medical Microbiology, Department of Pathology, Johns Hopkins University School of Medicine, Meyer B1-193, 600 North Wolfe Street, Baltimore, MD 21287-7093, USA

KEYWORDS
• Whole genome sequencing (WGS) • Targeted NGS • Metagenomic next-generation sequencing (mNGS)
• Clinical microbiology • Antimicrobial resistance • Predictions

KEY POINTS

- Next-generation sequencing (NGS) methods allow for a comprehensive detection of resistance genes within an organism or microbiome, known as the resistome.
- NGS-based detection of antimicrobial resistance can be further applied to predict phenotypic antimicrobial susceptibility testing (AST) using either a rule-based or a model-based approach.
- Most studies evaluating the accuracy of whole genome sequencing have applied second-generation, short-read sequencing methods, and have demonstrated good (>90%) predicted AST agreement for most antimicrobial agent-organism combinations.
- Newer, third-generation, long-read sequencing methods have increased applicability to patient care due to their real-time analysis capabilities.

INTRODUCTION

One of the largest global public health crises is the increase of antimicrobial-resistant infections. Internationally, more than 700,000 people (~23,000 Americans) die from antimicrobial-resistant infections annually. This number is projected to grow to 10 million deaths per year by 2050 [1]. Collective global action is required to face this threat and the promotion of novel, rapid diagnostics to reduce the unnecessary use of antimicrobials needs to be prioritized [1,2].

Next-generation sequencing (NGS) is gaining momentum as a diagnostic tool in Clinical Microbiology Laboratories. Three different applications of NGS have been developed to study antimicrobial resistance (AMR): (1) whole genome sequencing (WGS) with or without assembly of the genome of the pathogen of interest with detection of AMR genes; (2) targeted NGS with different methods for enrichment (ie, polymerase chain reaction amplification of AMR genes followed by NGS); or (3) metagenomic NGS (mNGS) to allow

Disclosure Statement: P.J. Simner reports grants and personal fees from Accelerate Diagnostics, grants from BD Diagnostics, Inc., grants from bioMerieux, Inc., grants from Check-Points Diagnostics, BV, grants from Hardy Diagnostics, personal fees from Roche Diagnostics, personal fees from Opgen Inc, personal fees from CosmosID, outside the submitted work; travel funds from Oxford Nanopore Technologies.

*Corresponding author, *E-mail address:* psimner1@jhmi.edu

https://doi.org/10.1016/j.yamp.2019.07.008

for pan-nucleic acid detection, including AMR genes, directly from patient specimens. These applications have been used to investigate the role of the resistome in tracking antimicrobial resistant organisms [3,4], to define novel mechanisms of resistance [5,6], to study the evolution of resistance within a patient's bacterial isolates [7], and to study the resistome of various microbiomes [8]. The resistome encompasses all the AMR genes in a given organism or microbiome [9].

An exciting development from NGS applications over the past 5 years is its ability to predict phenotypic antimicrobial susceptibility testing (AST) results among bacteria, which is the focus of this review. The resistome can then be translated based on the presence or absence of genes or single nucleotide polymorphisms (SNPs) to predict susceptibility or resistance to antimicrobial agents, using a rule-based approach. Machine learning and statistical models are other novel tools being developed to predict AST using NGS applications [10]. The authors describe the current state of NGS applications to predict AST using both second-generation short-read sequencing and third-generation long-read sequencing methods.

GENOTYPE VERSUS PHENOTYPE DILEMMA

Phenotypic AST methods ask the question "What concentration of the antimicrobial agent inhibits growth of the organism?" Clinicians have grown confident and reliant on phenotypic AST results to guide treatment of patients through many years of experience. Phenotypic AST methods are well-standardized approaches that can provide a minimum inhibitory concentration (MIC) or disk diffusion zone diameter result that can be set up and interpreted following the Clinical and Laboratory Standards Institute (CLSI) or European Committee on Antimicrobial Susceptibility Testing (EUCAST) guidelines [11,12]. The major drawback to this method is the slow turnaround time because it is a growth-dependent method. For nonfastidious organisms, the standard time to result from specimen receipt is 48 to 72 hours (Fig. 1). This is further delayed if pure or sufficient growth is not obtained on the first day of isolation, if a slower growing organism is isolated, or if an organism is multidrug-resistant (MDR) requiring the testing of additional antimicrobial agents beyond those present in standard panels. Many new methods have been introduced over the past 10 years to provide more rapid resistance detection such as simplex or multiplex nucleic acid amplification tests (NAT) of AMR genes, chromogenic agars, or rapid phenotypic tests (chromogenic or lateral flow assays) but none have yielded comprehensive results to predict the complete phenotypic AST profile. Nonetheless, these methods have introduced resistance mechanism–guided predictions to pave the way for NGS methodologies.

Contrary to most beliefs, phenotypic AST methods are an imperfect standard, as there can be significant variation in results for certain antimicrobial agent-organism combinations (greater than the standard error of AST ± 1 doubling dilution) and subtle testing differences between testers or automated instruments lead to further variability [13]. This variability is not accounted for in the clinical setting, as it is not practical to perform replicate MIC tests for clinical care. Furthermore, the prescribed methods are highly standardized from inoculum density, media, temperature, atmosphere, and incubation period, which do not reflect the variation in the environment and expression of phenotype that can occur during human infections [13]. Interpretation of phenotypic results is independent of the mechanism of resistance and will only detect AMR if expressed in vitro. It is known that expression of resistance can vary based on heteroresistant subpopulations, mixed infections, biofilm formation, further selection, and persistence based on selective pressures, which can all lead to resistance in vivo that were not detected in vitro, leading to the possibility of ineffective antibiotic prescribing [10].

Genotypic methods for detection of resistance answer the following question: "Is there a gene that predicts that a specific antimicrobial agent will not be effective against the pathogen recovered?" Genotypic methods to predict phenotype overcome some major limitations of phenotypic AST, with arguably the most important one being the capability of providing faster results (ie, 1–4 hour TAT). An additional benefit of this approach is that it can be performed directly from the specimen or from cultured growth. Most simplex or multiplex NAT tests introduced for clinical care to date detect a few high-profile acquired resistance genes such as *mecA* in *Staphylococcus aureus*, *vanA/B* in enterococci, and extended-spectrum β-lactamase ($bla_{CTX\text{-}M}$) or carbapenemase genes (bla_{KPC}, bla_{NDM}, bla_{VIM}, bla_{IMP}, and $bla_{OXA\text{-}48}$) among gram-negative organisms. Although clinicians are generally comfortable responding to these tests by broadening therapy when an unanticipated resistance gene is identified, they often display a hesitancy to narrow therapy when a resistance gene has not been identified and prefer to wait till the AST profile becomes available [14]. Furthermore, there is a lack of understanding of the precise function of all the

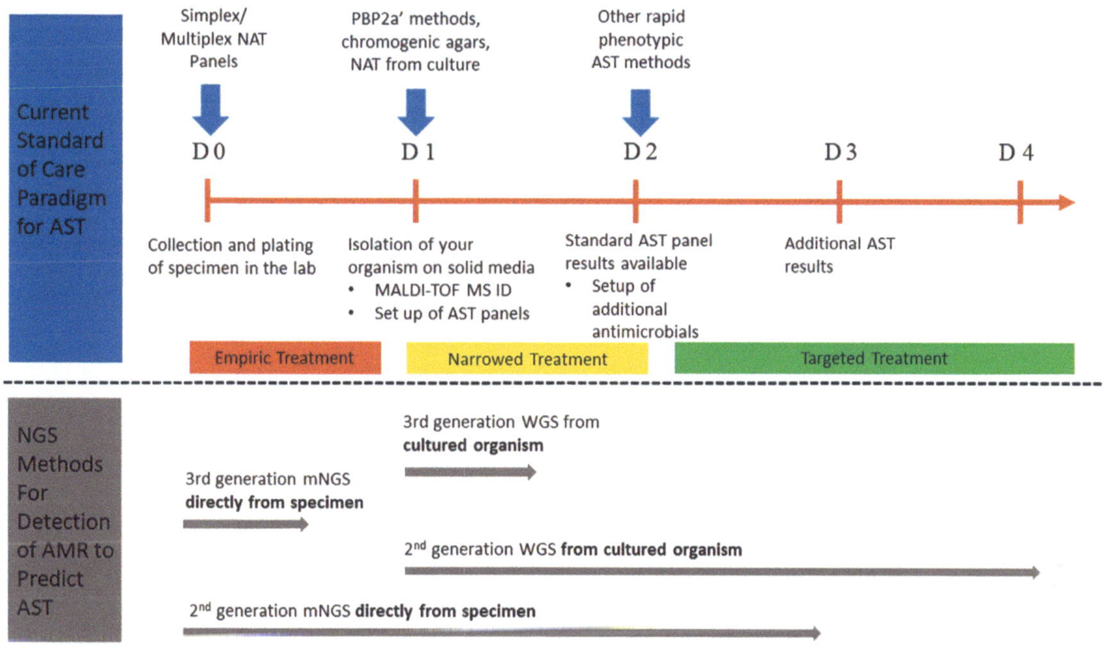

FIG. 1 Summary of current standard of care and NGS methods for antimicrobial susceptibility testing (AST). (*Top half*) The current paradigm for identification and AST in the clinical microbiology laboratory has an average TAT of 2 to 3 days from specimen receipt to finalized AST results. Newer, rapid methods (designated by blue arrows based on TAT) to predict antimicrobial resistance have been introduced for clinical care including nucleic acid amplification tests (NAT), chromogenic agars, and rapid phenotypic tests (eg, chromogenic, lateral flow, and/or agglutination tests). (*Bottom half*) The current TAT based on the literature for second-generation and third-generation next-generation sequencing methods performed directly from specimen using a metagenomic NGS (mNGS) approach or from cultured organism using a whole genome sequencing (WGS) approach.

AMR genes (ie, which antibiotics they inactivate) and so clinical microbiology laboratories need to work closely with their antimicrobial stewardship teams and infectious disease colleagues to convey the results in a way that positively affects patient care. Lastly, the detection of an AMR gene does not always correlate with expression and may lead to discordant genotype/phenotype results. Recent guidance describes using a more conservative approach to genotype/phenotype discrepancies such that when a resistance gene is detected despite susceptibility in vitro the AST should be reported as resistant [12]. The major limitation of the current genotypic methods is that they are limited to the specific targets in the assay, whereas NGS applications have the capability of overcoming this by detecting the entire resistome of organisms or the microbiome and therefore providing a comprehensive prediction of AST.

SHORT-READ VERSUS LONG-READ SEQUENCING TECHNOLOGIES FOR ANTIMICROBIAL SUSCEPTIBILITY TESTING

Sequencing technologies used to detect AMR genes can be divided into short-read (ie, second-generation) and long-read (ie, third-generation) sequencing technologies. The advantages and disadvantages of these technologies as they relate to AMR detection are summarized in Table 1. Most of the initial studies applying NGS for AMR used second-generation sequencing platforms applying methods that required DNA fragmentation, amplification, and sequencing of the genome in a highly paralleled format that generates short reads (50–600 base pairs) with high accuracy (~0.1% error rate) [15]. Despite its lower cost (~$50–100/per genome in large batches), the genome assemblies using short reads often result in fragmented assemblies especially around repetitive regions often

TABLE 1
Advantages and disadvantages of short-read sequencing versus long-read sequencing for detection of antimicrobial resistance

	Definition	Advantages	Disadvantages
Second-generation short-read sequencing	NGS technologies where nucleic acid is fragmented and amplified followed by sequencing of many different clusters of short reads (50–500 bp) taking place in parallel where base detection is monitored by different methods, including pyrophosphate release (454), hydrogen release (Ion Torrent), release of fluorescent reversible-terminator nucleotides (Illumina), or fluorescent ligated probes (SOLiD)	• High accuracy (~0.1% error rate) ○ Strain typing capability ○ SNP level analysis ○ Detection of chromosomal mutations leading to AMR, entire AMR genes, and distinction of allelic variants • Multiplexing capability driving lower costs	• Long TAT • Whole genomes are often difficult to assemble around repetitive regions leading to fragmented assemblies • Unable to link AMR genes to genetic context by mNGS methods
Third-generation long-read sequencing	NGS technologies that allow for long-read (1–100kb) single-molecular sequencing by monitoring incorporation of fluorescently labeled nucleotides (Pacific Biosciences, PacBio) or monitoring an electrical signal as nucleic acid is fed through a nano-sized pore (Oxford Nanopore Technology; ONT)	• Real-time analysis • Shorter TAT • Live streaming capability (ONT) • Easier to assemble WGS due to long reads • Plasmids are easily assembled and typed • AMR genes are easily detected • Provides genetic context directly from clinical specimens	• Lower accuracy (3%–15% error rate) ○ SNP level analysis is not possible ○ Chromosomal mutations leading to AMR or allelic variants are not reliably detected • High concentration of input nucleic acid is required

surrounding AMR genes on the chromosome or mobile genetic elements (ie, plasmids), areas with high sequence homology, or regions with extreme guanine-cytosine content [10,15]. Furthermore, the sequencing run itself generally requires large batches to maintain lower costs and can take 24 to 48 hours depending on the sequencing chemistry resulting in a long TAT, therefore negating any potential benefit as a rapid diagnostic tool to predict AST for clinical care. Illumina has dominated the market with its low-cost sequencing-by-synthesis method driving large-scale projects evaluating WGS to predict AST and evaluating mNGS as an agnostic tool for diagnosing infectious diseases [16].

Newer third-generation sequencing technologies, such as Oxford Nanopore Technologies (ONT) and Pacific Biosciences (PacBio), rely on real-time single-molecule sequencing producing long reads (on average 1–100 kbp) with higher per base error rates (3%–15%) [15]. The lower accuracy of long-read sequencing permits detection of resistance based on the presence or absence of AMR genes but the higher error rate make it difficult to determine a specific allele (eg, *bla*$_{KPC-2}$ vs *bla*$_{KPC-3}$) or identify SNPs in chromosomal genes leading to AMR. On the other hand, the long reads allow for more complete assemblies through repetitive regions, enable complete plasmid assemblies, and provide context to AMR genes detected by mNGS approaches directly from specimens [17].

ONT has perhaps the greatest adaptability compared with other NGS technologies as a diagnostic tool because it allows for real-time base-calling and streaming analysis of results within minutes of starting the sequencing run [18]. Furthermore, it has been demonstrated that a sequencing run of an hour using R9.4 flow cells generates sufficient information to study the entire resistome of an organism to allow for rule-based prediction models [17,19]. The biggest limitation is the high error rate, as chromosomal mutations as small as an SNP can result in drastic changes to prediction models. There are 3 main types of errors produced by ONT sequencing: (1) random errors, (2) homopolymer errors, and (3) methylation errors. Generating sufficient sequencing depth (at least 100x coverage) can overcome most random errors. However, systematic errors in the form of homopolymer indels and methylation errors still result in disagreement compared with Illumina- or hybrid Illumina–corrected assemblies (ie, use of short-reads to correct errors in long-read data) [17,19]. A few different bioinformatics programs have the ability to correct known errors or use lineage-based models to mitigate the low SNP calling accuracy [17,20]. Lastly, the costs of ONT sequencing remain relatively high (~$600–1000). Newer more affordable technologies such as the ONT Flongel disposable flow cells (~$100/flow cell) and more rapid automated protocols will allow more adaptability in the clinical setting.

DIFFERENT PREDICTION MODELS

There are 2 prediction models used to correlate AMR detection with AST phenotype: (1) rule-based approaches using databases of AMR loci and (2) model-based approaches using machine learning and/or statistical models. These approaches are briefly described here to set context. Readers are encouraged to read the more in-depth review by Su and colleagues [10] on this topic. These approaches try to predict AST by correlating the identification of AMR genes to the clinical breakpoints set by CLSI/EUCAST for individual antimicrobial agent/organism combinations or more precisely to the MIC. A report from the EUCAST subcommittee recommended that genotypic-phenotypic concordance from WGS data should primarily be the epidemiologic cut-off value and that a secondary comparator could be the clinical breakpoints to determine clinical impact [21]. However, the US Food and Drug Administration intends to hold molecular-based predictions for phenotypic AST to the same standards as phenotypic qualitative AST devices with broth microdilution as the reference standard where categorical agreement (>89.9%) and error rates would be assessed.

For the rule-based approach, AMR genes or k-mers (small portions of genes, <50 bp) are detected/analyzed using either raw reads or assembled genomes using software that searches databases of AMR loci. For bacteria, common broad AMR pipelines include ResFinder, the Comprehensive Antimicrobial Resistance Database (CARD), Basic Local Alignment Search Tool (BLAST), Antibiotic Resistance Gene-ANNOTation, short read sequencing typing, and National Center for Biotechnology Information's (NCBI) National Database of Antibiotic Resistant Organisms [22,23]. Organism-specific databases have also been generated, such as the *Mycobacterium tuberculosis* (MTB) databases (UVP, Mykrobe, TBDReaMDB, MUBII-TB-DB) [10]. It is important to note that not all databases perform similarly and different results can be obtained using the various databases and bioinformatics pipelines [24].

Detection of AMR genes is the first step; the next step is to correlate the AMR gene or SNP identified to expected phenotypes. Some databases provide correlation to phenotypic results based on genetic studies that link AMR genes to phenotypes. However, caution must be taken as not all predictions have been validated to accurately predict resistance. Moreover, NGS methods may be inadequate in detecting mechanisms of resistance that have not been fully elucidated, such as variations in lipopolysaccharides, alterations of cell membrane permeability, and efflux pump changes, among others [21]. Although detection and acquisition of enzymes known to cleave certain drugs (eg, β-lactamase genes), loss-of-function mutations (eg, porin knockout models), or mutations leading to altered target specificity (eg, *gyrA* and *parC* mutations leading to fluoroquinolone resistance) are relatively easy to interpret, mutations in coding or noncoding regions of the genome that alter the structure, dynamics, and substrate specificity of proteins, enzymes, and cell wall components pose greater challenges [16]. Without a comprehensive understanding of the impact of a mutation or combination of mechanisms on AMR, predicting effects on susceptibility can be difficult and is a noteworthy limitation of WGS [21]. Thus, if considering AMR detection via WGS to forecast AST results for clinical care, specific prediction models need to be further developed and validated. For some mechanisms, prediction is simple such as the presence or absence of *mecA* to predict methicillin susceptibility in *S aureus*. However, for most cases it is far more complex. For example, fluoroquinolone resistance among *Enterobacterales* is predicted based on single-step or 2-step mutations in the quinolone resistance determining region of *gyrA* and/or *parC* and the presence/absence of plasmid-mediated quinolone resistance genes and different combination thereof. Alternatively, Tamma and colleagues [17] have shown that detection of simply harboring aminoglycoside-modifying (eg, aminoglycoside acetyltransferases, aminoglycoside nucleotidyltransferases, aminoglycoside phosphotransferases) enzyme-encoding genes is not sufficient enough to accurately predict phenotypic AST of aminoglycosides in *Klebsiella pneumoniae*. A 90% to 100% agreement is achieved when an isolate harbored

5 or more aminoglycoside-modifying genes, whereas 2 or less predicted an agreement less than 50%. For studies using rule-based prediction models, the software, database, and prediction algorithms should be specified to the reader.

For model-based approaches, using either machine learning approaches and/or statistical models, the classifier is trained based on a set of genomes with known phenotypes without linking individual AMR genes. Similar to rule-based methods, the models can use k-mers, raw reads, contigs, or assemblies to then predict phenotypic results. The classifier is either provided specific sets of prediction rules or is taught what SNPs, indels, AMR genes, or other genetic features are important to predict phenotype [10]. Rule-based approaches to analyzing WGS data include assumptions about the phenotypes they are trying to predict. Machine learning methods allow the end user to perform analyses without making these assumptions and provide a more unbiased and robust approach [10].

ACCURACY OF WHOLE GENOME SEQUENCING TO PREDICT ANTIMICROBIAL SUSCEPTIBILITY TESTING

WGS is a well-studied and well-adapted method to predict phenotypic AST. A pure culture of an organism of interest is obtained and the genome is sequenced with or without assembly yielding a wealth of information about the epidemiology, virulence, and AMR determinants of the organism. WGS for AST offers the potential to provide rapid, consistent, and accurate predictions of known resistance phenotypes. Studies evaluating both short- and long-read sequencing have been completed and are summarized in the following sections.

SUMMARY OF SHORT-READ WHOLE GENOME SEQUENCING TO PREDICT ANTIMICROBIAL SUSCEPTIBILITY TESTING

Most initial studies applying WGS to predict AST were performed using second-generation sequencing, mostly completed on the Illumina platforms. Performance characteristics of WGS for detection of phenotypic resistance against different mechanisms of action or various antimicrobial agents (cell wall inhibitors, quinolones, protein synthesis inhibitors, antifolate agents, aminoglycosides, and in some cases, RNA synthesis inhibitors) are summarized in Fig. 2. Most studies used rule-based approaches but a few groups have used model-based approaches.

For gram-negative organisms, sensitivities greater than 90% among all the agents tested were achieved in *Escherichia coli*, *Campylobacter* species, *Salmonella* spp., *K pneumoniae*, and *Shigella sonnei* [25–29]. The specificities of all the respective agents tested were greater than 95% with the exception of trimethoprim and streptomycin that had a specificity of 80% and 75%, respectively, in isolates of *S sonnei*. Despite having a specificity of greater than 90% for the agents tested, variations in the sensitivities suggest that AMR mechanisms are complex and can be specific to a particular agent and organism.

Most studies have focused on the accuracy of AMR gene detection to phenotypic AST without describing the potential impact on patient care. One study by Shelburne and colleagues [30] attempt to address this by performing a proof-of-concept study using WGS to predict empirical therapy with β-lactam agents among patients with febrile neutropenia. They demonstrated that more than 60% of the evaluated *Pseudomonas aeruginosa* and *Enterobacter cloacae* bloodstream isolates had β-lactam resistance due to chromosomal mutations, which traditional β-lactamase NAT methodologies cannot detect. Using the context of their patient population, they demonstrate the feasibility of using WGS as a more comprehensive approach to guide antimicrobial treatment decisions (sensitivity of 87% and specificity of 98%) for patients with life-threatening infections with *E coli*, *K pneumoniae*, *E cloacae*, and *P aeruginosa*.

For gram-positive organisms such as *S aureus* and *Enterococcus* spp., the detection of resistance against cell wall inhibitors and fluoroquinolones can be achieved with a sensitivity of greater than 90% and 80%, respectively [31–33]. The sensitivities for detection of resistance to protein synthesis inhibitors were less reliable for both organisms at 82% for clindamycin against *S aureus* and 73% for quinupristin-dalfopristin against *Enterococcus* spp. However, greater than 92% sensitivity was achieved for all other protein synthesis inhibitors. Such discrepancies demonstrate the need for a more comprehensive database of resistance mechanisms. The Mykrobe predictor database show low concordance in strains with constitutive clindamycin resistance [31,32]; 8 out of 30 resistant *Enterococcus faecium* lacked known genes [33]. Despite variable sensitivities, all drug classes tested in gram-positive organisms resulted to close to greater than 90% specificity.

Overall, the sensitivities for detection of resistance using WGS is the highest for agents acting on the cell wall and most variable for antifolate agents and protein synthesis inhibitors for both gram-negative and gram-positive bacteria. Based on our literature search, the

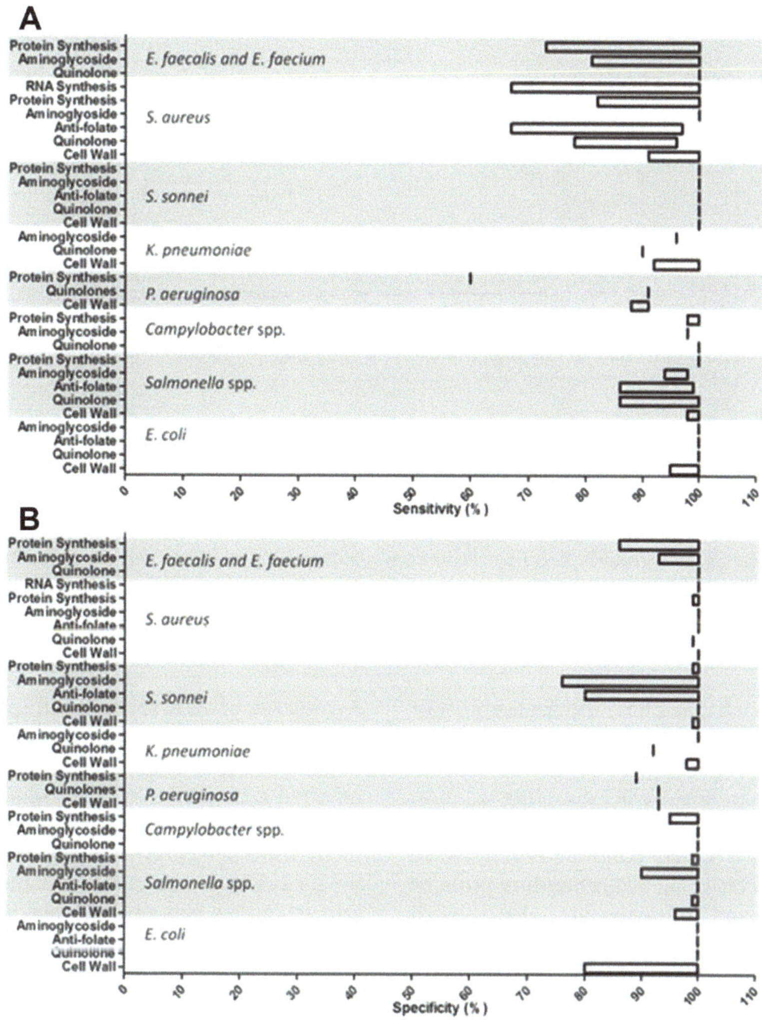

FIG. 2 Performance characteristics of second-generation WGS methods in predicting AST in gram-negative and gram-positive bacteria. (**A**) The sensitivity and (**B**) specificity of rule-based approaches in predicting phenotypic resistance of various antimicrobial agents. Data are grouped by indicated organism, and the specific antimicrobial agents based on mechanisms of action can be found in Supplementary Table 1. (*Data from* Refs [25–29,31–34,59].)

lowest sensitivity (60%) was achieved in detection for amikacin resistance in *P. aeruginosa* where only 63 of 105 isolates contained a genetic element that predicts resistance and analyses were further complicated when protein expression of these genetic elements varied among the isolates [34]. Although aminoglycoside resistance, in particular gentamicin, can be detected with a sensitivity approaching 100%, the ability to predict kanamycin resistance is lower, in the range of 81% to 100% [25,33]. The limitations in a rule-based approach may help explain why we see variations among different agents in the same antimicrobial class and using a model-based approach may adjust for these variations. Only a few studies using model-based approaches have been performed and they demonstrate comparable accuracy to rule-based approaches (Supplementary Table 1) [35–39].

Although the limited model-based studies only showed equivalent accuracy compared with rule-based approaches, it is worthy to note the advantage of using

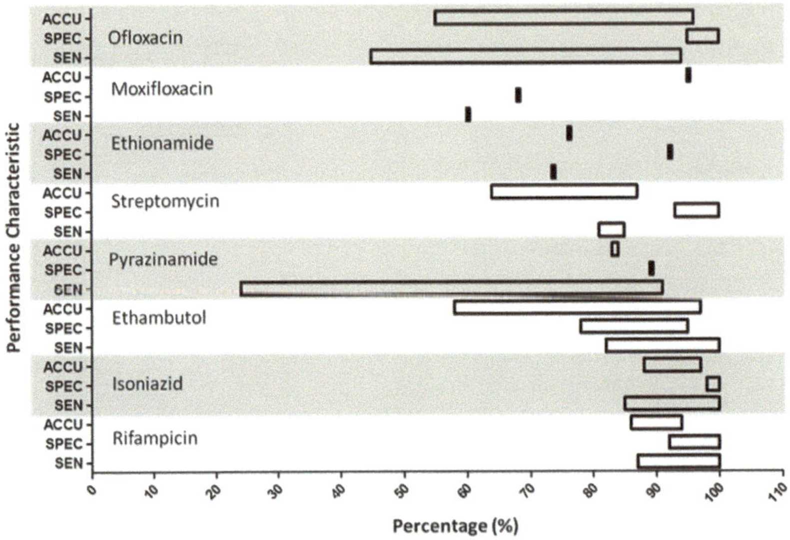

FIG. 3 Comparison of sensitivity and specificity from rule-based approaches and accuracy from model-based approaches in prediction of antimicrobial resistance in *Mycobacterium tuberculosis.* Data are grouped by indicated antimicrobial agent. ACCU, accuracy; SEN, sensitivity; SPEC, specificity. (*Data from* Refs [35,36,42,44–47,60].)

a model-based approach that allows the applicability of WGS to predict MICs of antimicrobial agents. It has been shown that with greater than 97% accuracy, the MIC of beta-lactams to +/−1 MIC doubling dilution can be determined for *Streptococcus pneumoniae* using a model-based approach called Random Forest where input data are sequences of penicillin-binding proteins [40]. Similarly, Eyre and colleagues [41] also showed that an overall accuracy of 99% and 95% was achieved when using their linear regression algorithm to determine the MIC for azithromycin and ciprofloxacin, respectively, in *Neisseria gonorrhoeae.* Furthermore, the same group demonstrated an average accuracy of 95% for nontyphoidal *Salmonella* [37] and 92% for *K pneumoniae* [38] agreement within +/−1 doubling dilution of the MIC.

Using WGS to predict AMR for MTB is extremely useful because WGS data can be generated weeks before phenotypic AST results are available and inform better clinical decision-making processes. This can be particularly helpful for patients infected with MDR or extensively drug-resistant MTB. The overall sensitivity and specificity of WGS to predict first-line MTB agents (rifampicin, isoniazid, and ethambutol) ranges from 80% to 100% (Fig. 3; see Supplementary Table 1) [42–47]. Studies evaluating the performance characteristics of detecting resistance of pyrazinamide, another first-line TB agent, have reported more variable sensitivities of 70% to 91% and specificities of 89% to 99%. One study that only included 24 isolates with detectable pyrazinamide resistance by traditional AST reported a sensitivity of 24% when WGS was used to detect resistance [43,44]. The poor sensitivity of WGS methods to detect AMR for the drug pyrazinamide can be attributed to the complex nature of the drug, unknown mechanism of resistance of the drug, and the plethora of genes currently shown to be associated, which would then entail the development of a sophisticated and routinely updated database due to impending research into AMR genes. For similar reasons, when model-based approaches are used to detect for AMR resistance in *M tuberculosis,* the accuracy is either equivalent or higher than the sensitivities detected by rule-based methods for all antituberculosis agents tested. In the case of pyrazinamide, an accuracy with a range of 89% to 99% has been reported [35,36]. WGS to predict AST for MTB has been widely studied and is likely to be the first WGS-based assay to be available for clinical care.

SUMMARY OF SHORT-READ METAGENOMIC NEXT-GENERATION SEQUENCING TO PREDICT ANTIMICROBIAL SUSCEPTIBILITY TESTING

Most initial efforts applying mNGS directly from specimens as a diagnostic tool for infectious diseases have focused on pathogen detection. However, results from short-read mNGS may also be used to query AMR genes to provide insight into therapeutic management of patients. A proof-of-concept study, evaluating 24 bone and joint infections by mNGS-correlated AMR detection using a mapping approach with the ResFinder database compared with phenotypic AST, found that correct susceptibilities could be inferred in 94.1% of cases [48]. Of note, they only included culture-positive samples that may have overestimated the predictive power of mNGS in this study. Yan and colleagues [49] recently applied the CosmosID bioinformatics platform to query mNGS results positive for staphylococci for the presence of AMR genes to predict AST to methicillin, clindamycin, trimethoprim-sulfamethoxazole, and vancomycin. They found sensitivities ranging from 65.7% (clindamycin) to 85.0% (trimethoprim-sulfamethoxazole) for predicting resistance with a 77.4% sensitivity for predicting methicillin resistance based on detection of the *mecA* gene. Specificity ranged from 65.7% (TMP-SMX) to 100% for methicillin and vancomycin. The same limitations apply to mNGS for AMR detection as they do for pathogen detection [16,50]. However, the focus to identify specific AMR genes to predict phenotype adds further complexity as the entire genome of the organisms may not be represented in the sequenced reads leading to the possibility of very major errors in prediction models. Thus, the data may only be helpful when detecting an AMR gene rather than the absence for patient care. Also, the presence of the gene in the absence of genetic context may lead to false resistance due to the presence of similar loci occurring in commensal organisms. Further studies are required to assess the ability of mNGS to accurately predict AST and its applicability to patient care.

LONG-READ SEQUENCING TO PREDICT ANTIMICROBIAL SUSCEPTIBILITY TESTING

The use of long-read sequencing to detect AMR for prediction of AST is relatively early in development. Although studies evaluating PacBio sequencing have evolved around AMR detection [51–53], none have specifically tackled the issue of predicting AST and thus the focus here will be on ONT sequencing technologies.

Early studies evaluating ONT for detection of AMR were small proof-of concept and feasibility studies limiting evaluations to acquired resistance genes due to the high per base error rate. These studies demonstrated the potential to live-stream data to detect AMR. They illustrated how short sequencing times (1–2 hours depending of version of flow cell) could generate sufficient information to study the entire resistome, highlighting their potential role as a diagnostic tool [18,19,54,55]. Only a few studies to date have systematically evaluated the correlation of AMR to phenotypic AST results to draw conclusions on accuracy.

One such study evaluating MinION WGS reads of 14 *N gonorrhoeae* isolates demonstrated that open access databases were not sufficient to detect AMR in this pathogen and that an in-house developed pipeline with *de novo* assembly and optimized BLAST algorithms were required for accurate prediction of decreased susceptibility in gonococcal isolates. They demonstrated 100% sensitivity of detection to cefixime, ceftriaxone, and ciprofloxacin and 33% sensitivity of azithromycin with 100% specificity for all agents [56]. The investigators concluded that although these results are promising, a larger study with more diverse mechanisms of AMR and strains are required to validate their findings.

A second study evaluated the accuracy of AMR identified by ONT WGS in predicting AST results among carbapenem-resistant *K pneumoniae* clinical isolates and further assessed the potential impact on patient care [17]. This study evaluated 2 different approaches to analysis using hybrid Illumina and Nanopore assemblies as the reference standard. The 2 approaches included (1) a real-time ONT-only approach without correction or assembly identifying acquired/chromosomal AMR genes using Metrichor's Antimicrobial Resistance Mapping Application (ARMA) and (2) an assembly with correction-based Nanopore-only approach. The real-time approach allowed for full annotation of acquired/chromosomal AMR genes within 8 hours from cultured isolates with 77% (range 30%–100% for various antimicrobial agents) agreement to AST. The assembly with correction-based ONT-only approach allowed for both acquired/chromosomal AMR gene detection and chromosomal SNP analysis of select AMR genes within 14 hours with 92% (range 80%–100% for different antimicrobial agents) agreement (same as the reference hybrid approach). The investigators demonstrated that the correction-based assembly approach, compared with a Nanopore-only real-time approach, enhances the ability to identify chromosomal mutations and allelic variants, increasing the accuracy of predictions for fluoroquinolones, aminoglycosides, and tetracyclines. Moreover, they demonstrated the potential to reduce time to effective antimicrobial therapy by a minimum of 20 hours compared with traditional phenotypic AST [17]. This study highlighted the ability of ONT to accurately predict AST for carbapenem-resistant *K pneumoniae* clinical isolates ultimately to beneficially affect patient's care, with the use of a bioinformatics approach to overcome the known inaccuracies with this approach. Bioinformatics improvements enabling real-time alignment (without assembly) coupled with rapid extraction, library preparation, and new types of flow cells (ie, Flongel [Oxford Nanopore Technologies]) and automated technologies will further enhance the accuracy and workflow of the Nanopore real-time approach for clinical use.

Two studies evaluated ONT to predict AST directly from specimens using mNGS. A study by Schmidt and colleagues [55] applied ONT sequencing directly from high-burden (>10^7 CFU/mL) urinary tract infections/spiked urines to detect the pathogen and predict AST of the predominant pathogen directly from urine using ONT "What's In My Pot?" and ARMA [57] real-time analysis approach [58]. They were able to detect the pathogen and 51 of 55 acquired resistance genes by MinION ONT sequencing but were unable to detect resistance-conferring mutations or allelic variants. The optimized protocol allowed for a 4-hour TAT from sample to results demonstrating the potential to optimize therapy before a second dose of a typical antimicrobial agent (ie, within 8 hours).

A most recent study developed a lineage-based approach to predict AST phenotypes using *S pneumoniae* and 5 antimicrobials (penicillin, ceftriaxone, trim ethoprim-sulfamethoxazole, erythromycin, and tetracycline) as the prototype. To predict resistance in isolates and sputum samples the researchers built a database and generated a K-mer-based (18 bp length) representation of lineages to associate to phenotype. Few samples were tested to draw general limiting confidence in the accuracy of their findings. However, this study does suggest an alternative method to overcome ONT sequencing inaccuracies by associating phylogroup to expected AST phenotype. Caution must be taken although, as some resistance has weak association between lineage and resistance phenotype such as plasmid-mediated resistance genes [20]. Thus, further additions to such an algorithm such as association of plasmids with specific phenotypes could be beneficial.

PROMISES AND HURDLES AHEAD

As we continue to use NGS, we are gaining a better understanding of the correlations between AMR detection and phenotypic AST correlations. However, considerable investigations are still needed to provide a foundation for an accurate alternative for phenotypic AST profiles that are heavily relied on clinically. Model-based approaches seem promising providing an accurate alternative to rule-based prediction models and have the capability to predict an MIC $\pm$ 1 doubling dilution. The use of WGS to predict AST is the most advanced with *M tuberculosis* complex. Furthermore, although this review focus on bacteria, there has been significant progress for viruses, fungi, and parasites [16].

SUPPLEMENTARY DATA

Supplementary data related to this article can be found online at https://doi.org/10.1016/j.yamp.2019.07.008.

REFERENCES

[1] O'Neil J. Tackling drug-resistant infections globally: final report and recommendations, the review on antimicrobial resistance 2016 . Available at: https://amr-review.org/sites/default/files/160518_Final%20paper_with%20cover.pdf.

[2] Ardal C, Outterson K, Hoffman SJ, et al. International cooperation to improve access to and sustain effectiveness of antimicrobials. Lancet 2016;387(10015):296–307.

[3] Peacock SJ, Parkhill J, Brown NM. Changing the paradigm for hospital outbreak detection by leading with genomic surveillance of nosocomial pathogens. Microbiology 2018;164(10):1213–9.

[4] Schurch AC, van Schaik W. Challenges and opportunities for whole-genome sequencing-based surveillance of antibiotic resistance. Ann N Y Acad Sci 2017;1388(1): 108–20.

[5] Haidar G, Philips NJ, Shields RK, et al. Ceftolozane-tazobactam for the treatment of multidrug-resistant pseudomonas aeruginosa infections: clinical effectiveness and evolution of resistance. Clin Infect Dis 2017;65(1): 110–20.

[6] Shields RK, Chen L, Cheng S, et al. Emergence of ceftazidime-avibactam resistance due to plasmid-borne blaKPC-3 mutations during treatment of carbapenem-resistant klebsiella pneumoniae infections. Antimicrob Agents Chemother 2017;61(3) [pii:e02097-16].

[7] Simner PJ, Antar AAR, Hao S, et al. Antibiotic pressure on the acquisition and loss of antibiotic resistance genes in Klebsiella pneumoniae. J Antimicrob Chemother 2018; 73(7):1796–803.

[8] Li J, Rettedal EA, van der Helm E, et al. Antibiotic treatment drives the diversification of the human gut resistome. Genomics Proteomics Bioinformatics 2019; 17(1):39–51.

[9] Lanza VF, Baquero F, Martinez JL, et al. In-depth resistome analysis by targeted metagenomics. Microbiome 2018;6(1):11.

[10] Su M, Satola SW, Read TD. Genome-based prediction of bacterial antibiotic resistance. J Clin Microbiol 2019; 57(3) [pii:e01405-18].

[11] EUCAST. Breakpoints tables for interpretation MICs and zone diameter, version 9 2019. Available at: http://www.eucast.org/clinical_breakpoints/.

[12] Clinical and Laboratory Standards Institute. Methods for dilution antimicrobial susceptibility tests for bacteria that grow Aerobically, S29. Wayne (PA): Clinical and Laboratory Standards Institute; 2019.

[13] Clinical and Laboratory Standards Institute. Methods for dilution antimicrobial susceptibility tests for bacteria that grow aerobically. 11th edition. Wayne (PA): Clinical and Laboratory Standards Institute; 2018.

[14] Banerjee R, Teng CB, Cunningham SA, et al. Randomized trial of rapid multiplex polymerase chain reaction-based blood culture identification and susceptibility testing. Clin Infect Dis 2015;61(7):1071–80.

[15] Ameur A, Kloosterman WP, Hestand MS. Single-molecule sequencing: towards clinical applications. Trends Biotechnol 2019;37(1):72–85.

[16] Mitchell SL, Simner PJ. Next-Generation Sequencing in Clinical Microbiology: Are We There Yet? Clin Lab Med 2019;39(3):405–18.

[17] Tamma PD, Fan Y, Bergman Y, et al. Applying rapid whole-genome sequencing to predict phenotypic antimicrobial susceptibility testing results among carbapenem-resistant klebsiella pneumoniae clinical isolates. Antimicrob Agents Chemother 2019;63(1) [pii:e01923-18].

[18] Cao MD, Ganesamoorthy D, Elliott AG, et al. Streaming algorithms for identification of pathogens and antibiotic resistance potential from real-time MinION(TM) sequencing. Gigascience 2016;5(1):32.

[19] Lemon JK, Khil PP, Frank KM, et al. Rapid nanopore sequencing of plasmids and resistance gene detection in clinical isolates. J Clin Microbiol 2017;55(12): 3530–43.

[20] Břinda K, Callendrello A, Cowley L, et al. Lineage calling can identify antibiotic resistance clones within minutes. Pathog Dis 2018;76(2).

[21] Ellington MJ, Ekelund O, Aarestrup FM, et al. The role of whole genome sequencing in antimicrobial susceptibility testing of bacteria: report from the EUCAST Subcommittee. Clin Microbiol Infect 2017;23(1):2–22.

[22] Jia B, Raphenya AR, Alcock B, et al. CARD 2017: expansion and model-centric curation of the comprehensive antibiotic resistance database. Nucleic Acids Res 2017; 45(D1):D566–73.

[23] Zankari E, Hasman H, Cosentino S, et al. Identification of acquired antimicrobial resistance genes. J Antimicrob Chemother 2012;67(11):2640–4.

[24] Mason A, Foster D, Bradley P, et al. Accuracy of different bioinformatics methods in detecting antibiotic resistance and virulence factors from staphylococcus aureus whole-genome sequences. J Clin Microbiol 2018;56(9) [pii: e01815-17].

[25] Stoesser N, Batty EM, Eyre DW, et al. Predicting antimicrobial susceptibilities for Escherichia coli and Klebsiella pneumoniae isolates using whole genomic sequence data. J Antimicrob Chemother 2013;68(10):2234–44.

[26] Zhao S, Tyson GH, Chen Y, et al. Whole-genome sequencing analysis accurately predicts antimicrobial resistance phenotypes in campylobacter spp. Appl Environ Microbiol 2016;82(2):459–66.

[27] Sadouki Z, Day MR, Doumith M, et al. Comparison of phenotypic and WGS-derived antimicrobial resistance profiles of Shigella sonnei isolated from cases of diarrhoeal disease in England and Wales, 2015. J Antimicrob Chemother 2017;72(9):2496–502.

[28] McDermott PF, Tyson GH, Kabera C, et al. Whole-genome sequencing for detecting antimicrobial resistance in nontyphoidal salmonella. Antimicrob Agents Chemother 2016;60(9):5515–20.

[29] Day MR, Doumith M, Do Nascimento V, et al. Comparison of phenotypic and WGS-derived antimicrobial resistance profiles of Salmonella enterica serovars Typhi and Paratyphi. J Antimicrob Chemother 2018;73(2):365–72.

[30] Shelburne SA 3rd, Lasky RE, Sahasrabhojane P, et al. Development and validation of a clinical model to predict the presence of beta-lactam resistance in viridans group streptococci causing bacteremia in neutropenic cancer patients. Clin Infect Dis 2014;59(2):223–30.

[31] Phaku P, Lebughe M, Strauss L, et al. Unveiling the molecular basis of antimicrobial resistance in Staphylococcus aureus from the Democratic Republic of the Congo using whole genome sequencing. Clin Microbiol Infect 2016;22(7):644.e1-5.

[32] Gordon NC, Price JR, Cole K, et al. Prediction of Staphylococcus aureus antimicrobial resistance by whole-genome sequencing. J Clin Microbiol 2014;52(4): 1182–91.

[33] Tyson GH, Sabo JL, Rice-Trujillo C, et al. Whole-genome sequencing based characterization of antimicrobial resistance in Enterococcus. Pathog Dis 2018;76(2).

[34] Kos VN, Deraspe M, McLaughlin RE, et al. The resistome of Pseudomonas aeruginosa in relationship to phenotypic susceptibility. Antimicrob Agents Chemother 2015;59(1):427–36.

[35] Mahe P, Tournoud M. Predicting bacterial resistance from whole-genome sequences using k-mers and stability selection. BMC Bioinformatics 2018;19(1):383.

[36] Davis JJ, Boisvert S, Brettin T, et al. Antimicrobial resistance prediction in PATRIC and RAST. Sci Rep 2016;6: 27930.

[37] Nguyen M, Long SW, McDermott PF, et al. Using machine learning to predict antimicrobial mics and associated genomic features for nontyphoidal salmonella. J Clin Microbiol 2019;57(2) [pii:e01260-18].

[38] Nguyen M, Brettin T, Long SW, et al. Developing an in silico minimum inhibitory concentration panel test for Klebsiella pneumoniae. Sci Rep 2018;8(1):421.

[39] Moradigaravand D, Palm M, Farewell A, et al. Prediction of antibiotic resistance in Escherichia coli from large-scale pan-genome data. PLoS Comput Biol 2018; 14(12):e1006258.

[40] Li Y, Metcalf BJ, Chochua S, et al. Validation of beta-lactam minimum inhibitory concentration predictions for pneumococcal isolates with newly encountered penicillin binding protein (PBP) sequences. BMC Genomics 2017;18(1):621.

[41] Eyre DW, De Silva D, Cole K, et al. WGS to predict antibiotic MICs for Neisseria gonorrhoeae. J Antimicrob Chemother 2017;72(7):1937–47.

[42] Feliciano CS, Namburete EI, Rodrigues Placa J, et al. Accuracy of whole genome sequencing versus phenotypic (MGIT) and commercial molecular tests for detection of drug-resistant Mycobacterium tuberculosis isolated from patients in Brazil and Mozambique. Tuberculosis (Edinb) 2018;110:59–67.

[43] Coll F, McNerney R, Preston MD, et al. Rapid determination of anti-tuberculosis drug resistance from whole-genome sequences. Genome Med 2015;7(1):51.

[44] Walker TM, Kohl TA, Omar SV, et al. Whole-genome sequencing for prediction of Mycobacterium tuberculosis drug susceptibility and resistance: a retrospective cohort study. Lancet Infect Dis 2015;15(10):1193–202.

[45] Chatterjee A, Nilgiriwala K, Saranath D, et al. Whole genome sequencing of clinical strains of Mycobacterium tuberculosis from Mumbai, India: a potential tool for determining drug-resistance and strain lineage. Tuberculosis (Edinb) 2017;107:63–72.

[46] Ezewudo M, Borens A, Chiner-Oms A, et al. Integrating standardized whole genome sequence analysis with a global Mycobacterium tuberculosis antibiotic resistance knowledgebase. Sci Rep 2018;8(1):15382.

[47] Quan TP, Bawa Z, Foster D, et al. Evaluation of whole-genome sequencing for mycobacterial species identification and drug susceptibility testing in a clinical setting: a large-scale prospective assessment of performance against line probe assays and phenotyping. J Clin Microbiol 2018;56(2) [pii:e01480-17].

[48] Ruppe E, Lazarevic V, Girard M, et al. Clinical metagenomics of bone and joint infections: a proof of concept study. Sci Rep 2017;7(1):7718.

[49] Yan Q, Wi YM, Thoendel MJ, et al. Evaluation of the CosmosID bioinformatics platform for prosthetic joint-associated sonicate fluid shotgun metagenomic data analysis. J Clin Microbiol 2019;57(2) [pii:e01182-18].

[50] Simner PJ, Miller S, Carroll KC. Understanding the promises and hurdles of metagenomic next-generation sequencing as a diagnostic tool for infectious diseases. Clin Infect Dis 2018;66(5):778–88.

[51] Carter GP, Schultz MB, Baines SL, et al. Topical antibiotic use coselects for the carriage of mobile genetic elements conferring resistance to unrelated antimicrobials in staphylococcus aureus. Antimicrob Agents Chemother 2018;62(2) [pii:e02000-17].

[52] Hoffmann M, Pettengill JB, Gonzalez-Escalona N, et al. Comparative sequence analysis of multidrug-resistant IncA/C plasmids from salmonella enterica. Front Microbiol 2017;8:1459.

[53] Hujer AM, Higgins PG, Rudin SD, et al. Nosocomial outbreak of extensively drug-resistant acinetobacter baumannii isolates containing blaOXA-237 carried on a plasmid. Antimicrob Agents Chemother 2017;61(11) [pii:e00797-17].

[54] Judge K, Hunt M, Reuter S, et al. Comparison of bacterial genome assembly software for MinION data and their applicability to medical microbiology. Microb Genom 2016;2(9):e000085.

[55] Schmidt K, Mwaigwisya S, Crossman LC, et al. Identification of bacterial pathogens and antimicrobial resistance directly from clinical urines by nanopore-based metagenomic sequencing. J Antimicrob Chemother 2017; 72(1):104–14.

[56] Golparian D, Dona V, Sanchez-Buso L, et al. Antimicrobial resistance prediction and phylogenetic analysis of Neisseria gonorrhoeae isolates using the Oxford Nanopore MinION sequencer. Sci Rep 2018;8(1):17596.

[57] Gire SK, Goba A, Andersen KG, et al. Genomic surveillance elucidates Ebola virus origin and transmission during the 2014 outbreak. Science 2014;345(6202):1369–72.

[58] de Oliveira WK, Carmo EH, Henriques CM, et al. Zika virus infection and associated neurologic disorders in Brazil. N Engl J Med 2017;376(16):1591–3.

[59] Kos VN, McLaughlin RE, Gardner HA. Elucidation of mechanisms of ceftazidime resistance among clinical isolates of pseudomonas aeruginosa by using genomic data. Antimicrob Agents Chemother 2016;60(6):3856–61.

[60] Allix-Beguec C, Arandjelovic I, Bi L, et al. Prediction of susceptibility to first-line tuberculosis drugs by DNA sequencing. N Engl J Med 2018;379(15):1403–15.

Pharmacogenomics

Advances in Molecular Pathology 2 (2019) 111–118
ADVANCES IN MOLECULAR PATHOLOGY

Artificial Intelligence and Pharmacogenomics

A Timely Synergy for Individualizing Medicine

Ravishankar K. Iyer, PhD[a,*], Arjun P. Athreya, MS, PhD[b], Liewei Wang, MD, PhD[b], Richard M. Weinshilboum, MD[b]

[a]Department of Electrical and Computer Engineering, University of Illinois at Urbana-Champaign, 255 Coordinated Science Lab MC 228, 1308 West Main Street, Urbana, IL 61801, USA; [b]Department of Molecular Pharmacology and Experimental Therapeutics, Mayo Clinic, 200 First St SW, Rochester, MN 55905, USA

KEYWORDS

- Pharmacogenomics
- Machine learning
- Artificial intelligence

KEY POINTS

- Use of artificial intelligence to analyze large clinical and biological data sets to address key aspects of individualized medicine using pharmacogenomics is timely.
- Inferring novel mechanisms of drug response and achieving high degrees of accuracy in predicting response to drug therapy are becoming a reality.
- Prospective validation of insights gained from the synergy of artificial intelligence and pharmacogenomics is needed for adoption in routine clinical practice.

INTRODUCTION

Individualized medicine tailors diagnoses and treatment options on an individual patient basis [1–4]. This is a paradigm shift from choosing a treatment based on aggregate therapeutic efficacy (ie, percentage of patients achieving the desired therapeutic benefit in clinical trials). Individualized treatment is greatly needed because not all patients respond to a particular drug, and drug response varies among patients [4].

Reduction of costs in assaying patients' genetic makeup (genome), among other biological measures (eg, hormone levels), has accelerated advances in individualized medicine [5]. There are only a few well-characterized systemic diseases, however, for which dramatically improved treatment outcomes have been achieved by using genomics data in routine clinical settings (eg, targeted therapies in breast cancer) [4,6]. To expand the benefits of individualized medicine to include other widely prevalent complex diseases (mental health disorders, migraines, and so forth), a key question to address is, Can a clinician's assessment of disease severity, augmented with patient-specific

Disclosure Statement: This material is based on work partially supported by the National Science Foundation (NSF) under grant CNS 13-37732; the National Institutes of Health (NIH) under grants U19 GM61388, R01 GM28157, RC2 GM092729, R24 GM078233, RC2 GM092729, and T32 GM072474; and the Mayo Clinic Center for Individualized Medicine. Any opinions, findings, and conclusions or recommendations expressed in this material are those of the author(s) and do not necessarily reflect the views of the NSF or the NIH. L. Wang and R. M. Weinshilboum are cofounders and stockholders in OneOme LLC; other authors have no disclosures to make.

*Corresponding author, *E-mail address:* rkiyer@illinois.edu

https://doi.org/10.1016/j.yamp.2019.08.003
2589-4080/19/

biological measures, help identify a therapeutic agent (eg, drug) and dose with the highest likelihood of achieving the desired therapeutic benefit?

The answer to that question requires intelligence from high-quality data, rich clinical insights/annotations from domain experience (eg, physicians and biologists), and analytical approaches (methods/models) to combine heterogeneous patient-specific measures to generate actionable intelligence. Actionable intelligence is a small set of patient-derived biological/clinical measures that provide clinicians with novel insights on (1) treatment prognoses, (2) prediction of therapeutic efficacy, and (3) disease pathophysiology or drug mechanisms. Analytical approaches for generating actionable intelligence have to augment a clinician's treatment selection criteria prior to the initiation of treatment and/or during follow-up visits that span the entire duration of the treatment. Therefore, methods have to account for static measures (eg, genomics) and time-varying measures with conditional properties (eg, symptom improvement in response to treatment intervention). Given the widely varying differences in disease manifestations and treatment practices, there are no universal theoretic foundations for generating relevant actionable intelligence [7].

Methods embodying artificial intelligence play a crucial role in the generation of actionable intelligence. Artificial intelligence methodologies ranging from machine learning to deep learning and probabilistic graphs extend beyond traditional single-variable and phenotype associations with the capability of finding patterns of multivariate associations that are predictive of complex response phenotypes in high-dimensional data sets (more variables than samples). Innovations in artificial intelligence methodologies capable of harnessing the power of clinical and genome-wide genomic data have shown early success in fulfilling pharmacogenomic promises of individualized medicine, which are to (1) identify variations in biological mechanisms of response to therapy and (2) aid in development of genomics-guided treatment selection for a given patient to maximize his or her chances of achieving the desired therapeutic benefit.

This article reviews recent advances in capabilities to establish patient stratification and associated predictability in treatment outcomes using pharmacogenomics data. The authors base the review in the context of addressing a set of focused treatment-relevant questions that become the basis for designing analytical workflows to achieve the promise of individualized medicine using pharmacogenomic approaches. These questions were defined based on aspects of current clinical practices and the additional degrees of specificity needed in order to achieve individualized treatment management. For each of these questions, the value of the augmented actionable intelligence is summarized from the perspective of pharmacogenomic research, current treatment practices, or future clinical research.

SIGNIFICANCE

Definitions

Artificial intelligence is the field of computing science that uses algorithms in computing systems to conduct tasks otherwise performed by humans [8]. Machine learning (supervised and unsupervised), deep learning, and probabilistic graphs are some example subsets of artificial intelligence that are increasingly being used in medicine and life sciences research. Machine learning is a study of algorithms or statistical models that can perform a task based on inferring patterns in a given data set. Data samples are characterized using features (variables, such as demographics, genes, and metabolites) and sometimes labels (eg, predefined groups of patients, such as responders or nonresponders, in the context of studying drug response). In the context of drug response, supervised machine learning approaches involve building methods/models to predict outcomes defined by categorical labels (eg, Will a patient be a responder or nonresponder to treatment?) or continuous measures (eg, What will the blood pressure be of a patient after treatment?). Supervised machine learning models are developed using training data, where the labels associated with features of data samples are supplied. Then, using features in test data that were not used in training the prediction model, labels are predicted for the test data. True labels are also known for the test data. Accuracies of the predictive models are reported based on how correct the predicted labels were in comparison with the true labels of the test data. Unsupervised machine learning approaches identify structure in the data, that is, subgroups of patients based on many clinical and/or genomic features. Deep learning methods involve developing artificial neural networks (ANNs) that learn to represent data so as to perform tasks based on examples. ANNs are inspired by the neural structure of the human brain and its activation while learning to perform tasks. Probabilistic graphs are commonly used to model dependencies between variables of interest in a given study [9]. Probabilistic graphs are useful in modeling longitudinal variations in variables relating to disease severity in response to drug treatment. By construct, probabilistic graphs offer the mathematical ability to reason with uncertainty, which is important considering that response to drug therapy varies among patients.

Finding the Right Patient Through Patient Stratification

Stratification is at the heart of individualizing medicine because it begins to help reduce the observed variability in drug response among patients. A compelling justification for placing patient stratification at the heart of individualizing medicine can be made on the basis of the therapeutic success in treating breast cancer. That success is based on testing the expression of molecular markers rather than variants, but it makes the point in a powerful fashion. Today, treatment strategies for each breast cancer patient are tailored to a tumor's specific molecular characteristics. That approach involves the association of the phenotype (which is the molecular characteristics of the tumor, such as whether it is estrogen receptor positive, human epidermal growth factor receptor 2 amplified, and/or triple negative), with a set of biomarkers that are prognostic of treatment outcomes [10,11]. After that success, the goal has been to begin reducing variability in treatment response with an attempt to subdivide patient populations based on sex, molecular characteristics, and/or disease symptom severity.

- Stratification by sex: Are there sex differences in biological profiles of patients with major depressive disorder (MDD) pre–antidepressant treatment and post–antidepressant treatment? Many complex diseases often occur predominantly in one sex versus the other, and sex as a variable could be overlooked as a factor in treatment selection. For example, in MDD, lifetime risk is twice as great in women as in men [12]. Sex is often overlooked, however, as a factor in antidepressant selection. Furthermore, many prior machine learning approaches predicting remission from MDD symptoms in response to antidepressant medication using sociodemographic factors did not find sex among the top 10 important predictors [13–15]. When plasma metabolomics was performed on patients prior to, during, and after antidepressant treatment, however, in a large Mayo Clinic study, significant sex differences in metabolome profile were identified at all time points using multivariate analysis of variance [16]. The augmented actionable intelligence is that sex-dependent biological factors could drive response to the same treatment differently in men and women.
- Stratification by molecular characteristics: Can patients be stratified by the molecular characteristics of their disease status? Stratification by molecular characteristics builds on the success of treatment for diseases like breast cancer in which treatment selection is guided by the molecular characterization of the tumor. Unsupervised machine learning methods using distance metrics (eg, k-means clustering and hierarchical clustering) or distributions (eg, Gaussian mixture model–based clustering) are used to identify cell/patient subpopulations based on genomic profiles (eg, transcriptome variations in single cells and messenger RNA expression levels of helper T cell–related transcription factors). Once the subpopulations are inferred, key factors differentiating the subpopulations are identified, such as fold change in the expression of genes, and often are visualized using dimensionality reduction techniques, such as principal component analyses or t-Stochastic Neighbor Embedding. These approaches have not only identified novel signatures of patient subpopulations [17–22] but also provided novel insights into (1) mechanisms of drug response [23–43] and (2) dosing/treatment strategies specific to the inferred subpopulations [44–47]. The augmented actionable intelligence here is that: specific biological factors (eg, genes and transcription factors) can be inferred that could drive response to therapeutics differently among patients. Such factors could serve as candidates that can be taken into the laboratory to experimentally establish mechanisms contributing to individual variation in drug response. In particular, moving beyond single-gene and phenotype associations, these approaches allow simultaneous evalutation of more biomarkers that potentially could lead to improved predictive accuracies while also explaining novel biology of underlying pathophysiology of disease or drug response, or both. This vision is consistent with recent comments on opportunities and challenges relating to the pharmacogenomics of catechol O-methyltransferase [48].
- Stratification by symptom severity: Can patients be stratified by their disease severity? Treatment decisions for many diseases, such as hypertension, are based on quantified severity levels of disease signs or symptoms [49,50]. Many diseases, however, such as MDD, do not have objective parameters that can be measured and are characterized by complex, subjective drug response phenotypes. Severity of depression symptoms is measured using clinician-rated or patient-rated scales, such as the Hamilton Depression Rating Scale (HDRS) or the

Quick Inventory of Depressive Symptomatology (QIDS). Although we have such subjective measures of depression severity, there are no ways to stratify MDD severity that are based on ranges of total depression severity scores at any intermediate time points of treatment. Definitions of antidepressant treatment outcomes, such as remission (the HDRS or QIDS falls below a fixed numerical value) or response (a 50% decrease in HDRS or QIDS, but not falling below that fixed value), are empirically defined based on whether a patient's total depression severity dropped below a threshold or quantum after 4 weeks or 8 weeks of antidepressant treatment [51]. The lack of stratification in diseases, such as MDD, has often limited the ability to understand pathologic mechanisms of variation in disease manifestation or mechanisms of response to drug treatment. One study addressed the need for such stratification and used Gaussian mixture models to algorithmically identify the minimum number of Gaussians or clusters, that best approximated the actual distribution of depressive symptom severity at each time point [16,52,53]. It is of clinical significance that this work inferred 3 clusters after 8 weeks of antidepressant treatment in multiple clinical trials that comprised patients who were labeled as remitters, responders without remission, and nonresponders based on clinical definitions that use empirically defined thresholds of total depression severity [16,52,53]. From the perspective of pharmacogenomics, inferring patient clusters using data-driven approaches that also have clinical significance is important because the associations of multiple biological measures (eg, metabolomics and genomics) now can be investigated, with patients stratified by disease severity and associated drug response. Such associations could lead to improved understanding of the underlying biology of disease pathophysiology, drug response, or both. The augmented human intelligence here is that the identification of patient clusters increases the potential for studying and understanding the underlying pathologic mechanisms that contribute to variation in disease severity as well as trajectories of patient movement between clusters.

Identifying the right drug at the right dose by predicting its efficacy via pharmacogenomic measures: Can a clinician's pretreatment assessment of disease severity, augmented with a patient's pharmacogenomic measures, predict eventual remission of disease symptoms after treatment? Given that high-throughput genomic data are becoming increasingly affordable, it is timely to think that treatment selection among available drugs could potentially be guided based on genomic biomarkers with the potential to accurately predict treatment outcomes. In addressing this possibility, supervised machine learning techniques are being used to develop prediction models that take a set of patient-specific measures (eg, clinical assessments and pharmacogenomic variants) as input data and predict clinical outcomes. The outcomes related to drug response phenotypes could be either categorical (classifiers will be developed) or continuous (regression methods will be developed). The challenge in building predictive models with genome-wide genomics data is that the number of predictor variables far exceeds the number of samples available to train the methods. Hence, different approaches to reducing the number of predictor variables, ranging from using *P* value thresholds of a genome-wide association study (GWAS) to using functionally validated measures as predictor variables, are used.

Instead of using GWAS as the approach to selecting genes, elastic net regression with variable selection was used to prioritize genomic predictors from approximately 500,000 genes in the Genome-based Therapeutic Drugs for Depression study [14]. The area under the receiver operator curve [54] in that work was 0.77 and agreed with prior work, which found that higher scores of interest and activity symptoms on the QIDS or HDRS scale at baseline correlated with lower chances of achieving remission after the acute phase of antidepressant treatment [55]. In a Taiwanese study, remission to antidepressant treatment was predicted using top-hit single-nucleotide polymorphisms (SNPs) (P value $<7.5*10^{-5}$) from GWAS and baseline clinical variables as predictor variables [56]. In that work, multilayer feedforward neural networks that were to predict the remission status achieved an area under the curve of 0.83, whereas specificity was less than 58%. In all these predictive approaches, the predictive performances using genomic predictors were better than those using sociodemographic factors alone as predictors, which is encouraging. None of the identified genes had SNPs, however, that were identified in pharmacogenomic studies of antidepressant response. In addressing this limitation, recent work demonstrated that when clinical assessments are augmented with pharmacogenomic variants inferred using a metabolomics-informed genomics approach to predict response to selective serotonin reuptake inhibitor treatment in patients with MDD, sex-specific predictive accuracies greater than 69% can be achieved, and this predictive performance can be replicated across multiple trials. It is of clinical significance that predictive accuracies when using pharmacogenomic variants were at least 14% higher than when using only sociodemographic measures as predictors [53]. Deep learning approaches using ANNs have been used to identify common variants of cytochrome P450 enzymes that are thought to contribute to adverse drug reactions [57]. Many approaches to identifying genomic profiles predictive of response to treatment or predictive of the correct dose of a given treatment have been developed [58–60]. Finally, in order to minimize errors in predictions, hybrid approaches combining predictive capabilities of deep learning and traditional machine learning approaches were recently shown to be effective in improving predictability of response to anticancer drug therapy by using omics data [58–61]. The augmented human intelligence here is that a few patient-derived pharmacogenomic biomarkers can augment a clinician's disease severity assessments to help predict treatment outcomes prior to the initiation of drug therapy.

Identifying prognostic changes in symptoms at the "right time": Is there a small set of disease symptoms whose early change in severity is prognostic of long-term treatment outcomes? The premise for asking this question lies in the fact that no approaches provide 100% accuracy in prediction. Thus, even when a patient is started on a specific drug treatment guided by biomarkers that predict a better response among other treatment options, 2 additional questions need to be addressed. First, what mechanisms differentiate this variation in response to treatment from a longitudinal perspective? Second, what changes in symptom severity are needed early in the treatment timeline to determine whether the patient is on the right trajectory of achieving the desired therapeutic benefit? Differentiation-guided pharmacogenomics is an approach that stratifies disease states using unsupervised machine learning methods and then identifies genetic/genomic differences in their response to treatment. Differentiation-guided pharmacogenomics has been used to study differential response to therapies in several diseases, such as melanoma, Parkinson's disease, hypertension, bipolar disorder, and autism [62–65]. Trajectory analyses using growth mixture models are another approach that can be used to identify longitudinal change in a variable of interest in unobserved subpopulations [66]. Growth mixture models have been used to infer trajectories of improvement in total depression severity scores leading to any of a group of categorical treatment outcomes [67–70]. A unique feature of the work of Kelley and colleagues [69] was their ability to associate genomic markers with trajectories of remission and nonresponse. Gueorguieva and colleagues [67,68] showed that when trajectories of response were modeled, a third of the patients who were responders at the end of the acute-phase treatment experienced worsening in their depression symptom severity during the extended phase of the treatment. Finally, probabilistic graphs in the form of factor graphs and hidden Markov models have been proposed to identify trajectories of antidepressant response in patients stratified by depression severity [16]. The benefit of this approach was its ability to encode domain-guided knowledge of clinical assessments after 4 weeks of the treatment, which in turn allowed for deriving easily interpretable quantified prognoses for treatment outcomes that are likely to be observed at 8 weeks [16]. The augmented human intelligence here is that the clinical implications of deriving accurate prognoses of eventual treatment outcomes is significant. Current pharmacogenomic approaches often predict initial treatment outcomes and are less able to predict long-term outcomes. With the long-term predictive capabilities of graphical models, if the prognosis forecasts a poor treatment outcome, the clinician could make a change in the treatment to avoid extended weeks of disease burden from a lack of response. In this way, predictive methods using pharmacogenomics biomarkers could first aid in selecting a drug that among others has the highest predicted likelihood of the patient achieving therapeutic benefit, and then, innovations using probabilistic graphs that use symptom assessment data would help ascertain if early response to treatment is prognostic of a long-term therapeutic benefit.

RELEVANCE AND OPPORTUNITIES FOR FUTURE INVESTIGATIONS

Given the rapid aggregation of omics data collected in routine clinical settings, computing innovations in the form of artificial intelligence methodologies serve as an ideal vehicle to accelerate pharmacogenomic research. The reason is that the volume of data far exceeds human capabilities to analyze such data in a timely manner. In the context of pharmacogenomics, this review highlights the use of analytical approaches to generate novel insights with regard to patient stratification, drug mechanisms, or prediction of treatment outcomes that are timely and relevant in the context of individualizing medicine. These promising results highlight opportunities for future studies and for the successful adoption of these approaches in routine clinical practice.

The information outlined above is exciting but preliminary. Today even academic medical centers and health systems that are implementing pharmacogenomic testing are still primarily using one gene at a time, and only a few SNPs in that gene. Testing is typically performed using simple targeted genotyping-based approaches. What has been envisioned in this article is a future world in which many genes, as well as clinical and demographic information, will be combined, and a highly validated and replicated algorithm will be used to provide health care teams with an estimate of the probability that individual patients will or will not achieve the desired therapeutic response—requiring that a health care team respond in an appropriate and agile fashion. This new paradigm will also require different approaches to testing, in that information on many additional variants beyond those traditionally used in pharmacogenomics may have importance. Finally, the same analyses also offer the possibility of providing novel insight into and understanding of mechanisms responsible for the variation that occurs in virtually all drug response phenotypes. We envision a world much different from the one that existed at the beginning of this century, prior to the conclusion of the Human Genome Project and the broad application of artificial intelligence and machine learning to medical data.

SUMMARY

The synergy of innovations in artificial intelligence and pharmacogenomics is timely and much-needed if the promise of individualized medicine is to be achieved. Achieving high degrees of predictability for drug treatment outcomes while also providing novel insight into mechanisms of variation in drug response phenotypes is at the heart of the problem of matching a patient with the best treatment for that individual patient. At this time, the majority of studies demonstrating the synergy of artificial intelligence and pharmacogenomics are retrospective in nature. As a result, clinical trials that use artificial intelligence approaches and are focused on validating insights gained from retrospective analyses are needed in order to enable adoption of artificial intelligence–guided therapeutic management in routine clinical practice.

REFERENCES

[1] Collins FS, Varmus H. A new initiative on precision medicine. N Engl J Med 2015;372(9):793–5.

[2] Evans WE, Relling MV. Moving towards individualized medicine with pharmacogenomics. Nature 2004; 429(6990):464–8.

[3] Lazaridis KN, McAllister TM, Babovic-Vuksanovic D, et al. Implementing individualized medicine into the medical practice. Am J Med Genet C Semin Med Genet 2014;166C(1):15–23.

[4] Weinshilboum R, Wang L. Pharmacogenomics: bench to bedside. Discov Med 2005;5(25):30–6.

[5] Topol EJ. Individualized medicine from prewomb to tomb. Cell 2014;157(1):241–53.

[6] Ritchie MD. The success of pharmacogenomics in moving genetic association studies from bench to bedside: study design and implementation of precision medicine in the post-GWAS era. Hum Genet 2012;131(10): 1615–26.

[7] Palsson B, Zengler K. The challenges of integrating multi-omic data sets. Nat Chem Biol 2010;6(11):787–9.

[8] Russell SJ, Norvig P. Artificial intelligence: a modern approach. Pearson Education Limited; 2016.

[9] Koller D, Friedman N. Probabilistic graphical models: principles and techniques. MIT press; 2009.

[10] Onitilo AA, Engel JM, Greenlee RT, et al. Breast cancer subtypes based on ER/PR and Her2 expression: comparison of clinicopathologic features and survival. Clin Med Res 2009;7(1–2):4–13.

[11] Wang L, Ingle J, Weinshilboum R. Pharmacogenomic discovery to function and mechanism: breast cancer as a case study. Clin Pharmacol Ther 2018;103(2):243–52.

[12] Piccinelli M, Wilkinson G. Gender differences in depression. Critical review. Br J Psychiatry 2000;177:486–92.

[13] Chekroud AM, Zotti RJ, Shehzad Z, et al. Cross-trial prediction of treatment outcome in depression: a machine learning approach. Lancet Psychiatry 2016;3(3):243–50.

[14] Iniesta R, Hodgson K, Stahl D, et al. Antidepressant drug-specific prediction of depression treatment outcomes from genetic and clinical variables. Sci Rep 2018;8(1): 5530.

[15] Iniesta R, Malki K, Maier W, et al. Combining clinical variables to optimize prediction of antidepressant treatment outcomes. J Psychiatr Res 2016;78:94–102.

[16] Athreya A, Iyer R, Neavin D, et al. Augmentation of physician assessments with multi-omics enhances predictability of drug response: a case study of major depressive disorder. IEEE Comput Intell Mag 2018;13(3): 20–31.

[17] Auman JT, McLeod HL. Colorectal cancer cell lines lack the molecular heterogeneity of clinical colorectal tumors. Clin Colorectal Cancer 2010;9(1):40–7.

[18] Jansen R, Moehlendick B, Bartenhagen C, et al. ACGH detects distinct genomic alterations of primary intrahepatic cholangiocarcinomas and matched lymph node metastases and identifies a poor prognosis subclass. Sci Rep 2018;8(1):10637.

[19] Martinez-Cardus A, Martinez-Balibrea E, Bandres E, et al. Pharmacogenomic approach for the identification of novel determinants of acquired resistance to oxaliplatin

in colorectal cancer. Mol Cancer Ther 2009;8(1):194–202.
[20] Stopa EG, Tanis KQ, Miller MC, et al. Comparative transcriptomics of choroid plexus in Alzheimer's disease, frontotemporal dementia and Huntington's disease: implications for CSF homeostasis. Fluids Barriers CNS 2018;15(1):18.
[21] Wang L, Ren Y, Shi X, et al. The population genetics of pharmacogenomics VIP variants in the Sherpa population. Drug Metab Pharmacokinet 2016;31(1):82–9.
[22] Yang X, Bian J, Gong Y, et al. MADEx: a system for detecting medications, adverse drug events, and their relations from clinical notes. Drug Saf 2019;42(1):123–33.
[23] Abdelfatah SA, Efferth T. Cytotoxicity of the indole alkaloid reserpine from Rauwolfia serpentina against drug-resistant tumor cells. Phytomedicine 2015;22(2):308–18.
[24] Anfosso L, Efferth T, Albini A, et al. Microarray expression profiles of angiogenesis-related genes predict tumor cell response to artemisinins. Pharmacogenomics J 2006;6(4):269–78.
[25] Brown CC, Havener TM, Medina MW, et al. Genome-wide association and pharmacological profiling of 29 anticancer agents using lymphoblastoid cell lines. Pharmacogenomics 2014;15(2):137–46.
[26] Chalabi N, Delort L, Le Corre L, et al. Gene signature of breast cancer cell lines treated with lycopene. Pharmacogenomics 2006;7(5):663–72.
[27] Dawood M, Hamdoun S, Efferth T. Multifactorial modes of action of arsenic trioxide in cancer cells as analyzed by classical and network pharmacology. Front Pharmacol 2018;9:143.
[28] Egana-Gorrono L, Escriba T, Boulanger N, et al. Differential microRNA expression profile between stimulated PBMCs from HIV-1 infected elite controllers and viremic progressors. PLoS One 2014;9(9):e106360.
[29] Galvan A, Fladvad T, Skorpen F, et al. Genetic clustering of European cancer patients indicates that opioid-mediated pain relief is independent of ancestry. Pharmacogenomics J 2012;12(5):412–6.
[30] Ghosheh N, Olsson B, Edsbagge J, et al. Highly synchronized expression of lineage-specific genes during in vitro hepatic differentiation of human pluripotent stem cell lines. Stem Cells Int 2016;2016:8648356.
[31] Kadioglu O, Kermani NS, Kelter G, et al. Pharmacogenomics of cantharidin in tumor cells. Biochem Pharmacol 2014;87(3):399–409.
[32] Kamisoglu K, Sukumaran S, Nouri-Nigjeh E, et al. Tandem analysis of transcriptome and proteome changes after a single dose of corticosteroid: a systems approach to liver function in pharmacogenomics. OMICS 2015;19(2):80–91.
[33] Kuete V, Efferth T. Pharmacogenomics of Cameroonian traditional herbal medicine for cancer therapy. J Ethnopharmacol 2011;137(1):752–66.
[34] Liew PL, Huang RL, Weng YC, et al. Distinct methylation profile of mucinous ovarian carcinoma reveals susceptibility to proteasome inhibitors. Int J Cancer 2018;143(2):355–67.
[35] Ooko E, Kadioglu O, Greten HJ, et al. Pharmacogenomic characterization and isobologram analysis of the combination of ascorbic acid and curcumin-two main metabolites of curcuma longa-in cancer cells. Front Pharmacol 2017;8:38.
[36] Park HW, Dahlin A, Qiu W, et al. Gene expression changes in lymphoblastoid cell lines and primary B cells by dexamethasone. Pharmacogenet Genomics 2019;29(3):58–64.
[37] Peng H, Zeng X, Zhou Y, et al. A component overlapping attribute clustering (COAC) algorithm for single-cell RNA sequencing data analysis and potential pathobiological implications. PLoS Comput Biol 2019;15(2):e1006772.
[38] Reikvam H, Tamburini J, Skrede S, et al. Antileukaemic effect of PI3K-mTOR inhibitors in acute myeloid leukaemia-gene expression profiles reveal CDC25B expression as determinate of pharmacological effect. Br J Haematol 2014;164(2):200–11.
[39] Saeed M, Kadioglu O, Khalid H, et al. Activity of the dietary flavonoid, apigenin, against multidrug-resistant tumor cells as determined by pharmacogenomics and molecular docking. J Nutr Biochem 2015;26(1):44–56.
[40] Saeed ME, Abdelgadir H, Sugimoto Y, et al. Cytotoxicity of 35 medicinal plants from Sudan towards sensitive and multidrug-resistant cancer cells. J Ethnopharmacol 2015;174:644–58.
[41] Saeed MEM, Mahmoud N, Sugimoto Y, et al. Molecular determinants of sensitivity or resistance of cancer cells toward sanguinarine. Front Pharmacol 2018;9:136.
[42] Seo EJ, Saeed M, Law BY, et al. Pharmacogenomics of scopoletin in tumor cells. Molecules 2016;21(4):496.
[43] Shah K, Patel S, Mirza S, et al. A multi-gene expression profile panel for predicting liver metastasis: an algorithmic approach. PLoS One 2018;13(11):e0206400.
[44] Ciavarella S, Vegliante MC, Fabbri M, et al. Dissection of DLBCL microenvironment provides a gene expression-based predictor of survival applicable to formalin-fixed paraffin-embedded tissue. Ann Oncol 2018;29(12):2363–70.
[45] Hamdoun S, Jung P, Efferth T. Drug repurposing of the anthelmintic niclosamide to treat multidrug-resistant leukemia. Front Pharmacol 2017;8:110.
[46] Martin R, Rose D, Yu K, et al. Toxicogenomics strategies for predicting drug toxicity. Pharmacogenomics 2006;7(7):1003–16.
[47] Zhang X, Cha IH, Kim KY. Use of a combined gene expression profile in implementing a drug sensitivity predictive model for breast cancer. Cancer Res Treat 2017;49(1):116–28.
[48] Ho MF, Weinshilboum RM. Catechol O-Methyltransferase pharmacogenomics: challenges and opportunities. Clin Pharmacol Ther 2019;106(2):281–3.
[49] Manunta P, Ferrandi M, Cusi D, et al. Personalized therapy of hypertension: the past and the future. Curr Hypertens Rep 2016;18(3):24.

[50] Marik PE, Varon J. Hypertensive crises: challenges and management. Chest 2007;131(6):1949–62.
[51] Rush AJ, Kraemer HC, Sackeim HA, et al. Report by the ACNP Task Force on response and remission in major depressive disorder. Neuropsychopharmacology 2006; 31(9):1841–53.
[52] Athreya AP, Banerjee SS, Neavin D, et al. Data-driven longitudinal modeling and prediction of symptom dynamics in major depressive disorder: integrating factor graphs and learning methods. Paper presented at: IEEE International Conference on Computational Intelligence in Bioinformatics and Computational Biology. 2017.
[53] Athreya AP, Neavin D, Carrillo-Roa T, et al. Pharmacogenomics-driven prediction of antidepressant treatment outcomes: a machine learning approach with multi-trial replication. Clin Pharmacol Ther 2019. [Epub ahead of print].
[54] Krumsiek J, Mittelstrass K, Do KT, et al. Gender-specific pathway differences in the human serum metabolome. Metabolomics 2015;11(6):1815–33.
[55] Uher R, Perlis RH, Henigsberg N, et al. Depression symptom dimensions as predictors of antidepressant treatment outcome: replicable evidence for interest-activity symptoms. Psychol Med 2012;42(5):967–80.
[56] Lin E, Kuo PH, Liu YL, et al. A deep learning approach for predicting antidepressant response in major depression using clinical and genetic biomarkers. Front Psychiatry 2018;9:290.
[57] Liang Z, Huang JX, Zeng X, et al. DL-ADR: a novel deep learning model for classifying genomic variants into adverse drug reactions. BMC Med Genomics 2016; 9(Suppl 2):48.
[58] Kringel D, Ultsch A, Zimmermann M, et al. Emergent biomarker derived from next-generation sequencing to identify pain patients requiring uncommonly high opioid doses. Pharmacogenomics J 2017;17(5):419–26.
[59] Lin WJ, Chen JJ. Biomarker classifiers for identifying susceptible subpopulations for treatment decisions. Pharmacogenomics 2012;13(2):147–57.
[60] Tao Y, Chen YJ, Fu X, et al. Evolutionary ensemble learning algorithm to modeling of warfarin dose prediction for chinese. IEEE J Biomed Health Inform 2019;23(1):395–406.
[61] Su R, Liu X, Wei L, et al. Deep-resp-forest: a deep forest model to predict anti-cancer drug response. Methods 2019. [Epub ahead of print].
[62] Tropea TF, Chen-Plotkin AS. Unlocking the mystery of biomarkers: a brief introduction, challenges and opportunities in Parkinson Disease. Parkinsonism Relat Disord 2018;46(Suppl 1):S15–8.
[63] Anwar MA, Saleh AI, Al Olabi R, et al. Glucocorticoid-induced fetal origins of adult hypertension: association with epigenetic events. Vascul Pharmacol 2016;82: 41–50.
[64] Najjar F, Owley T, Mosconi MW, et al. Pharmacogenetic study of serotonin transporter and 5HT2A genotypes in autism. J Child Adolesc Psychopharmacol 2015;25(6): 467–74.
[65] Severino G, Squassina A, Costa M, et al. Pharmacogenomics of bipolar disorder. Pharmacogenomics 2013; 14(6):655–74.
[66] Ram N, Grimm KJ. Growth mixture modeling: a method for identifying differences in longitudinal change among unobserved groups. Int J Behav Dev 2009;33(6):565–76.
[67] Gueorguieva R, Chekroud AM, Krystal JH. Trajectories of relapse in randomised, placebo-controlled trials of treatment discontinuation in major depressive disorder: an individual patient-level data meta-analysis. Lancet Psychiatry 2017;4(3):230–7.
[68] Gueorguieva R, Mallinckrodt C, Krystal JH. Trajectories of depression severity in clinical trials of duloxetine: insights into antidepressant and placebo responses. Arch Gen Psychiatry 2011;68(12):1227–37.
[69] Kelley ME, Dunlop BW, Nemeroff CB, et al. Response rate profiles for major depressive disorder: characterizing early response and longitudinal nonresponse. Depress Anxiety 2018;35(10):992–1000.
[70] Tokuoka H, Takahashi H, Ozeki A, et al. Trajectories of depression symptom improvement and associated predictor analysis: an analysis of duloxetine in double-blind placebo-controlled trials. J Affect Disord 2016; 196:171–80.

Advances in Molecular Pathology 2 (2019) 119–131
ADVANCES IN MOLECULAR PATHOLOGY

The Evolution of DNA Sequencing in Pharmacogenomics

Steven E. Scherer, PhD

Department of Molecular and Human Genetics, Baylor College of Medicine, Human Genome Sequencing Center, One Baylor Plaza, MS: BCM226, Houston, TX 77030, USA

KEYWORDS

- Pharmacogenetics • Pharmacogenomics • Genotyping • Sequencing • Technological advancements
- Cytochrome P450

KEY POINTS

- The term pharmacogenetics was introduced by 1959, and the Human Genome Project was completed in 2003; since then, advances toward genetically informed prescribing have been made, but it is not yet common.
- Genetic testing in pharmacogenomics has rapidly advanced from genotyping approaches to high-throughput sequencing, which has led to greater accuracy in genotype assignment and revealed the presence of rare variants.
- As of 2019, most pharmacogenomics implementation efforts are the result of research grants or philanthropic endeavors; however, the field is on the cusp of promising breakthroughs in delivering truly personalized drug therapies.

HISTORY AND BACKGROUND

In an article published at the self-declared end of the Human Genome Project [1], the leaders of the public effort, headed by Francis Collins, posited that "genomics holds the promise of individualized medicine, tailoring prescribing practices and management of patients to each person's genetic profile." It might have been guessed at the time that genetically informed prescribing practices would be common some 15 years or more later. Although adoption of pharmacogenomics in clinical practice has perhaps not shown the arc envisioned in 2003, enormous progress has been realized and many of the hurdles yet to be overcome are well elucidated.

Driven by previous observations of association between the symptoms of hemolytic anemia and antimalarial medications, in 1956 the genetic basis of both favism and toxic reaction to primaquine were linked to mutations in *G6PD* [2]. By 1959, the term pharmacogenetics was introduced and defined as the study of the role of inheritance in drug response [3] incorporating both pharmacokinetic and pharmacodynamic effects. The Human Genome Project and its comprehensive breadth pushed the term toward pharmacogenomics (PGx), defined as the examination of genomic variants involved in the targeting, transport, metabolism, and excretion of drugs and the interaction of these variables influencing the efficacy and toxicity of therapeutic agents. The goal of individualized medicine is to move away from trial and error or one-size-fits-all prescribing practices and instead use a combination of genotype and phenotype to enhance drug response while avoiding adverse events.

GENOTYPING

As pharmacogenetics moved from gene cloning to polymerase chain reaction (PCR) of individual gene exons to

Disclosure: The author has nothing to disclose.
E-mail address: sscherer@bcm.edu

https://doi.org/10.1016/j.yamp.2019.08.002
2589-4080/19/

multiplex PCR designed to characterize multiple genes in 1 experiment, the Human Genome Project and its first byproduct, the Human HapMap project [4], accelerated high-throughput genotyping and transformed pharmacogenetics toward pharmacogenomics [5]. As these techniques progressed in enabling a view of the entire human genome, so too did the push to create custom genotyping reagents designed to characterize common variants already linked to variation in drug response [6] and proposals to begin using these results in clinical settings [7]. In addition to targeted genotyping approaches focused on testing 1 gene at a time for a limited number of single nucleotide polymorphisms (SNPs), other genotyping platforms emerged to interrogate multiple genes simultaneously. One of the first custom PGx commercial offerings was from Roche, the AmpliChip cytochrome P (CYP) 450, targeting 23 SNPs across *CYP2C19* and *CYP2D6* to guide psychiatric drug treatment and approved for clinical use in 2005 by the US Food and Drug Administration (FDA). Others included the CodeLink P450, targeting 110 SNPs across 9 genes, and the Illumina ADME (absorption, distribution, metabolism, and excretion) VeraCode, targeting 184 SNPs in 34 genes. The most comprehensive of these offerings in terms of target breadth was the Affymetrix Drug Metabolizing Enzymes and Transporters (DMET) Plus chip, which assayed 1936 SNPs in 231 genes comprising 47 phase I CYP genes, 70 phase II modifier genes, 62 transporter genes, 46 other genes, and capability to detect deletions in 5 genes with targets suggested by several experts, including academics, pharmaceutical company representatives, and others from the PharmaADME Consortium [8]. After validation of the original design [9], modifications were introduced and the product was released in 2008 as the DMET Plus. For a more thorough description, see Ref. [10]. Although sequencing has largely replaced targeted genotyping for clinical diagnosis of hereditary diseases, clinical testing in pharmacogenomics still relies predominantly on targeted genotyping. This reliance is in part caused by the requirements of a quick turnaround time and low cost for pharmacogenomic testing. A major limitation of targeted genotyping is that only variants included in assay design can be identified and reported; therefore, rare variants are undetected.

In conjunction with PGx targeted genotyping for both clinical and research purposes, which confers a statistical power advantage over genome-wide association studies (GWAS) [11], numerous investigators embraced GWAS to expand the pool of potential genetic contributions [12], particularly in hopes of identifying new drug targets. As with GWAS in common disease, a large number of studies failed to show genome-wide significance, failed to replicate, or failed to account for a large percentage of heritability (see rare variant discussion later). In addition, GWAS for PGx were bedeviled by extra challenges. These challenges included small sample sizes caused by the difficult task of identifying nonresponders in a large pool of responders; additionally, adverse events, although both challenging and expensive to treat, are still rare. Furthermore, phenotypes may be difficult to measure and effect size may get lost in the noise unless a single predominant gene, or a very limited number of genes, is involved. In addition, replication studies may also be impaired by low numbers or, in the case of adverse events, potential ethical considerations. However, there have been some limited successes. For example, Takeuchi and colleagues [13] showed genome-wide significance for *VKORC1*, *CYP2C9*, and *CYP4F2* in warfarin dosing. Shuldiner and colleagues [14] showed that the most significant SNP associated with poor clopidogrel response was in linkage disequilibrium (LD) with the *2 allele. However, these two studies confirmed associations already identified by candidate gene studies, and a further example linking adverse myopathy reaction to simvastatin [15] probably could have been shown had a candidate gene analysis been undertaken [16]. For more detailed analyses, particularly concerning adverse drug reaction and GWAS, see Ref. [17].

In an example of an effective strategy, consortia studies sought to identify novel genes associated with differential diastolic blood pressure response to hydrochlorothiazide treatment using the Genetic Epidemiology of Responses to Antihypertensives cohort as the discovery set. They identified a region on chromosome 12q15 with slightly less than genome-wide significance in African Americans [18]. After replication was shown in a cohort from the Pharmacogenomic Evaluation of Antihypertensive Responses clinical trial [19], a custom DNA capture probe set covering the region of interest was designed and used to sequence the response tails of the two cohorts, identifying a novel missense variant in the gene *BEST3* [20]. This gene encodes a calcium-sensitive smooth muscle chloride channel and shows the utility of DNA sequencing follow up to identify specific variation in regions identified by GWAS.

RESOURCES AND IMPLEMENTATION

With the flood of gene variants found to effect drug metabolism since the 1990s, several research consortia (the Pharmacogenomics Research Network [PGRN], https://www.pgrn.org/) and databases were established to catalog and categorize gene-drug relationships. The 2 primary database examples are PharmGKB (https://www.pharmgkb.org/about), established in 2000, and the CYP database, established about a year later and recently translated to PharmVar (www.PharmVar.org). In addition, recognition that translation of drug-gene relationships to clinical implementation required evidence-based and peer-reviewed translation of diplotypes to predicted metabolizer status prompted the establishment of the Clinical Pharmacogenetics Implementation Consortium (CPIC; https://cpicpgx.org/). In Europe, the primary resources are the Dutch Pharmacogenetics Working Group (DPWG) and, more broadly, the European Pharmacogenetics Implementation Consortium (Eu-PIC; http://www.eu-pic.net/), and, in Canada, the Canadian Pharmacogenomics Network for Drug Safety (http://cpnds.ubc.ca/). CPIC rates gene-drug pairs for levels of evidence supporting clinical actionability and publishes guidelines translating genetic test results to drug dosage adjustments or recommendations for alternative therapies [21], using a uniform guideline development process [22]. CPIC coordinates with DPWG and Eu-PIC and is working on coordination with both ClinVar and ClinGen, as well as developing an application programming interface to more easily incorporate guidelines into electronic health records (EHRs). There are currently 23 guidelines available covering 47 drugs and 19 genes, with both reviews and new guidelines issued regularly. In addition, the FDA maintains a table of pharmacogenomic biomarkers in drug labeling currently covering 305 medications categorized as informative PGx, actionable PGx, or testing required (https://www.fda.gov/Drugs).

SEQUENCING

Starting with the Maxam-Gilbert chemical modification/cleavage protocols [23] and the Sanger chain termination, first with radioactively and then fluorescently tagged dideoxy nucleotides [24,25], DNA sequencing progressed rapidly. The introduction of fluorescent dye terminators, the combination of thermostable polymerases and thermal-cycling reactions, and the move from slab gels to refillable multichannel capillary electrophoresis instrumentation all served to establish modern-day Sanger sequencing as the clinical standard and enabled the Human Genome Project. Although several competing manufacturers attempted to break through using variations of this protocol, all but the Applied Biosystems (now part of ThermoFisher Scientific) instruments have disappeared. These capillary instruments are still used to validate clinical variants identified on next-generation platforms and can also be used to perform fragment size analysis.

The need for the much higher throughput and less costly sequencing necessary to generate and annotate the genomes of both other species and large groups of humans drove the sequencing field to introduce multiple versions of so-called next-generation sequencing (NGS). Most of these efforts were broadly based on Sanger sequencing inasmuch as they followed the sequencing by synthesis (SBS) paradigm (as reviewed by Metzker [26] and others). The first platform to come on the market was the 454 sequencer, which was based on pyrosequencing [27] and the detection of a chemically driven light emission in conjunction with the timing of sequentially flowed nucleotides. DNA templates were prepared by nebulizer shearing, adaptor ligation, binding to beads, and emulsion PCR amplification before deposition on glass slides containing millions of reaction microchambers. The resulting read lengths eventually grew to 450 to 600 bases with throughput that totaled at 125 times that offered by Sanger capillary instruments. The Baylor College of Medicine's Human Genome Sequencing Center (BCM-HGSC) collaboratively sequenced and publicly released the genome of James Watson using this platform [28]. Several competing technologies were offered including the SOLiD, Helicos, and Polinator, but they, like 454, are no longer available.

Following quickly on the heels of 454 and using similar, but refined, sequencing library preparation techniques, Rothberg and colleagues [29] introduced the IonTorrent. The sequencing technology was similar except that, instead of tracking pyrophosphate release on nucleotide addition, this technique tracked the other released molecule, a hydrogen ion detected by changes in reaction chamber pH using a semiconductor chip and thus avoiding any use of light detection, lasers, or cameras. The technology is still marketed by ThermoFisher Scientific and, like most current sequencing platforms, comes in various combinations of instrument and accompanying chip capacities.

Based on studies performed at both the Pasteur Institute and Cambridge University in the mid-1990s, Solexa was formed in 1998 and, after further development and acquisition, introduced its first sequencing instrument in 2006. Soon after releasing their follow-up instrument, the Genome Analyzer II (GAII), Solexa was acquired by Illumina and their instrument platform has dominated the market ever since. Using DNA sheared to around 300 base pairs (bp) in length, sequencing libraries are constructed by adaptor ligation followed by hybridization to a solid support known as a flow cell. Bridge amplification results in millions of clustered templates that undergo an SBS reaction cycle using 4 color fluorescently labeled reversible dye-labeled nucleotides. After imaging, the dye-labeled blocker is cleaved and the next round of labeled nucleotides is exposed to the flow cell for a total of up to 300 cycles. Most of the sequencing on this platform has been 100-cycle or 150-cycle reactions and the more recent versions are now using 2 color chemistries. Although capable of enormous automated throughput, the short reads produced, compared with Sanger sequencing, are (1) more error prone, requiring multiple read depth of coverage to arrive at an accurate consensus sequence; (ii) more prone to sequence context bias [30]; and (3) very difficult to assemble, with most projects relying on read mapping to an established reference. As with most current sequencing platforms, most Illumina platforms are also capable of RNA sequencing, chromatin immunoprecipitation sequencing, and to a degree, methylome sequencing.

One of the primary motivations behind transitioning from targeted genotyping to DNA sequencing approaches in pharmacogenomics is to find rare variants. Taken together, rare variation has been shown to generally be associated with an enhanced effect size [31]. Although Sanger sequencing has been useful for single genes, sequencing of multiple genes simultaneously is both desirable and necessary in pharmacogenomics.

Pharmacogenomics Capture Sequencing

As the technologies behind both genotyping and NGS continued to progress, a middle ground of demand was answered by the development of targeted enrichment or capture sequencing [32]. Originally performed using solid-phase oligonucleotide probes attached to a silica matrix, protocols were soon developed using liquid-phase hybridization paired with posthybridization recovery and elution to construct target-enriched sequencing libraries. Such a technology served to both expand the breadth of the genome being interrogated beyond known common variants while keeping costs and complexities at a reasonable level. NimbleGen was soon joined by Agilent and Illumina in commercial offerings in this arena, with a primary focus on whole-exome sequencing (WES). After much work designed to optimize the technology, development of interpretation protocols, and debates over the ethics surrounding which results should be returned to ordering physicians and patients, the BCM-HGSC and Baylor's Department of Molecular and Human Genetics announced the introduction of clinical WES in 2011 and detailed its preliminary findings in diagnosing mendelian disease in 2013 [33].

One of the defining advantages of capture sequencing is the ability to create custom probe sets designed for the investigator's challenge of choice. To this end, the PGRN's Deep Sequencing Resource (DSR) initiated the design of a capture probe set in 2010 that was meant to show the granularity of sequencing results across clinically important pharmacogenomic loci while remaining close in cost with the genotyping array resources the community had relied on to that point. After multiple rounds of polling and discussion, the network settled on 84 genes with capture hybridization probes designed for all known exons within those genes, regions 2 kb upstream and 1 kb downstream of each gene to capture potential regulatory elements and probes designed for all of the SNP loci present on the 2 most-used genotyping arrays, the Affymetrix DMET plus array covered earlier and the Illumina ADME array, thus making the capture reagent backward compatible with most of the previously generated genotyping datasets [34]. Because of the rigorous design, this reagent includes both coding and noncoding variants, which are often important in pharmacogenomics but not included in a routine exome. As with any new technology rollout, it is critical that it be compared with prevailing data generated by orthogonal technologies. In the development of PGRNseq, the PGRN DSR tested the platform for accuracy by comparing the results obtained with genotyping results from the 1000 Genomes Project in 32 Coriell Repository trios samples representing a broad population ancestry together with genotyping results generated from 2 clinical cohorts. With the exception of the human leukocyte antigen (HLA) gene targets, *CYP2D6* and *CYP2A6*, concordance with genotyping results was 99.8%. The resulting PGRNseq reagent yielded 2 primary advantages: the ability to capture rare variants in a targeted, high-throughput manner without resorting to costly WES or whole-genome sequencing (WGS) necessary for statistically powered association studies in the research realm and the opportunity to identify and develop the necessary tools for eventual clinical application of the results.

The National Institutes of Health (NIH) eMERGE (Electronic Medical Records and Genomics) Network (Phase II) took advantage of both of these points in adopting the PGRNseq reagent for the network's PGx project [35]. One quality control test assessed the research sequencing results versus several clinical genotyping results produced using a spectrum of assays [36]. Results were considered for 4077 participants that had a least 1 pharmacogenomic variant called by PGRNseq that was also genotyped using an orthogonal assay across 6 genes in a clinical laboratory. Results determined concordance on a per-sample basis as 0.972 and on a per-variant basis as 0.997. Repeat analyses to resolve discrepancies were performed for a subset of 1792 samples. All of the sequencing discrepancies were found to be caused by sample swaps and almost all the clinical genotyping discrepancies were caused by allele dropouts due to rare variants interfering with genotyping array primer hybridization. The overall conclusion was that this capture sequencing reagent proved highly concordant with established clinical assays and suggested that routine orthogonal validation at loci shown to be amenable to sequencing may be unnecessary in clinical laboratory settings. The second aim of the PGx project was to establish a searchable database of variants and the SPHINX (Sequence and Phenotype Integration Exchange) is the resulting Web tool (https://www.emergesphinx.org/). In addition, an overview of results based on the analysis of more than 5000 participants [37] noted that, after stringent filtering, about half of the observed variants were novel compared with the dbSNP (Single Nucleotide Polymorphism Database) (https://www.ncbi.nlm.nih.gov/snp/), the 1000 Genomes Project Phase III [38], and Exome Aggregation Consortium (ExAC) databases [39]. Furthermore, more than 96% of the participants carried at least 1 high-impact pharmacogenomic gene variant. Several of the participating network members also published findings covering topics such as cost [40], education [41], patient acceptance [42], clinical decision support [43], and site-specific implementation [44–46]. Based on these results, Mayo Clinic's Center for Individualized Medicine and the BCM-HGSC have collaborated on extending Mayo's Right Drug, Right Dose, Right Time: Using Genomic Data to Individualize Treatment (RIGHT) Protocol [47] to 10,000 subjects using a new variant of the PGRNseq capture sequencing reagent and entering results of 13 genes, including genotype and predicted drug metabolizer phenotypes, into subject EHRs (manuscript in preparation).

Whole-Exome Sequencing

At present, the capture sequencing reagent with the greatest clinical utility is WES. Although its primary use is in genetic disease diagnostics, reportable secondary findings may include variants affecting drug toxicities and efficacy. Because WES is limited to the coding regions of human genes, important noncoding variants are not assayed and PGx targets are confined to genes that are easily sequenced using short read technologies. Baylor Genetics offers secondary findings covering several alleles in 3 genes of pharmacologic importance: *CYP2C9*, *CYP2C19*, and *VKORC1*. There is a paucity of reports covering this application, but Cousin and colleagues [48] studied secondary PGx findings in 94 patient samples referred for clinical WES to diagnose genetic disease. These patients were primarily young individuals with neurologic disease, 90% of whom were taking medications, such as anticonvulsants and proton pump inhibitors; 91% of these individuals were found to harbor a variant PGx allele and 20% were deemed immediately actionable. This study pointed out several important and related caveats that may be broadly applicable to clinical PGx testing. First, assays can only point out what is queried; the return of results for limited targets, both within and between genes, can miss important variants or alleles and therefore represent a false-negative. For example, initial warfarin dosing can be derived from these data because of reporting for both *CYP2C9* and *VKORC1*. In contrast, diazepam is metabolized by both the CYP2C19 enzyme, which is tested and reported, and CYP3A4, which is not tested or reported. Second, the Baylor Genetics test does not return a *1/*1 diplotype (absence of genetic variants) for genes found to be wild-type at the reported sites because inference of such a result can lead to error, particularly in US minority populations [49]. For example, the investigators compared the allele frequencies for *CYP2C9* alleles that were tested for (*2 –*6) with frequencies across the range of untested alleles using the ExAC database. The investigators found that the unreported actionable alleles in non-Finnish Europeans have a frequency of 0.58%, but the frequency in African unreported actionable alleles is 15.4%, starkly illustrating the issue.

Whole-Genome Sequencing

In general, directed, capture, or target-enriched sequencing as a means of more broadly covering specific genes or the coding genome in general have been driven, at least in part, by cost considerations. The view has generally been that the field will eventually adopt WGS as the ultimate genotyping tool once the cost comes down to reasonable levels. This view is amplified for PGx in that most investigators agree that a prospective approach is strongly linked with clinical implementation success [50,51]. On the one hand, WGS should offer the most comprehensive assay of variants affecting drug efficacy and toxicity, but, on the other, many of the same concerns and challenges raised using the technologies outlined earlier remain.

However, there are several advantages provided by WGS, including enhanced gene copy number detection, and several investigators are laying the groundwork for this eventual transition. Early examples of the potential for clinical application in disease genes [52,53] have spawned studies designed to assess the quality of various sequencing platform outputs and the breadth of variation present at known PGx gene loci.

In an early demonstration of how WGS might eventually be combined with family history and other biomarker assay results to predict both disease risk and drug response, Ashley and colleagues [54] used the Helicos sequencing platform (no longer available) to generate very short reads to approximately 24-fold coverage and found 2.6 million SNPs and 752 copy number variants, including many of unknown significance. Analyses limited primarily to monogenic traits revealed a potential explanation for the subject's family history of coronary artery disease based on a rare and potentially deleterious variant in the *LPA* gene that was correlated with a high blood lipoprotein (a) laboratory result as well as other variants associated with further disease risk. Pharmacogenomics results predicted resistance to clopidogrel therapy based on the presence of a known inactivating heterozygous variant in *CYP2C19*, a lower than average suggested initial warfarin dosing based on a known variant in *VKORC1* (a novel nonsynonymous SNP of unknown significance was also found in this gene) and a known homozygous variant in *CYP4F2*, and likely successful response to lipid level–lowering medication caused by a lack of known variants affecting drug response in *SLCO1B1*, *CYP2D6*, *CYP2C9*, and *CYP3A4*; these results might inform future therapeutic intervention for this individual. Most of this author group then expanded on this approach by sequencing a family quartet with a known family history of thrombophilia and, by using a combination of an ethnic-specific synthetic reference genome and haplotype phasing, showed the ability to identify multigenic risk for thrombophilia and predict appropriate drug therapy [55].

In a more recent study and based on promising results reported by others [56,57], Cohn and colleagues [58] studied the concordance of WGS results with both WES and directed genotyping in a cohort of 98 pediatric patients. Specifically, a combination of 2 genotyping assays (mass spectrometer–based assays from Agena Biosciences comprising an iPlex *CYP2D6* panel interrogating 29 SNP and indel sites, together with a custom iPlex panel directed at 38 sites across the remaining 18 genes of interest) was used as both a benchmark for variant calling and to assess copy number at the *CYP2D6* locus. Overall concordance observed between genotyping and WGS was greater than 99%. However, several *CYP2D6* alleles proved troublesome, suggesting that supplementary assays may be necessary to accurately assess this locus in a clinical setting. Comparison of previously generated WES results for 12 of the subjects showed outstanding concordance with the 67 genotyping sites but lacked data for 2 of the noncoding sites, and copy number comparisons were not possible with any degree of accuracy. Further findings include that 17 of the 98 subjects had deletions or duplications of *CYP2D6* and that 95 subjects had at least 1 clinically actionable variant, with 72 having variants informing efficacy or dose adjustment and 23 possessing variants linked to high risk of adverse events. In 2014, Mizzi and colleagues [59] used WGS of 482 unrelated individuals performed on the Complete Genomics platform to characterize and annotate variants defined by the DMET Plus genotyping platform. Analyses of the results suggested at least 1012 novel variants that may result in protein inactivation.

A large number of studies have been undertaken to show the frequency of rare variation in genes of pharmacogenomic significance. Examples include analyses targeting the data generated by the National Heart, Lung, and Blood Institute Exome Sequencing Project Consortium, wherein Gordon and colleagues [60] examined approximately 6500 exomes derived from a combination of white and African American individuals at 12 CYP gene loci known to be involved in a large percentage of oxidative drug metabolism pathways. They discovered 730 nonsynonymous alleles and, as might be expected, African Americans had 3 times the variant burden that was present in white people. Caucasians although individually rare, these newly identified, potentially deleterious CYP gene variants were found in approximately 10% of the individuals assayed.

A further example is provided by Wright and colleagues [38], who screened the 1000 Genomes Phase III WGS data (2504 individuals from 26 human populations) for rare variation in 120 PGx genes of interest [61]. After stringent filtering and with focus on only SNPs in protein coding regions, more than 12,000 variants were discovered with more than 90% of them classified as rare (defined as having a minor allele frequency of <0.5%) and greater than 50% were singletons. More than 50% of the genes surveyed contained what the investigators characterized as high-confidence loss-of-function (LOF) variants. Not surprisingly, *CYP2D6* contained the most LOF variants, with the known *4 allele being the most common and one of just 12 LOF variants not classified as rare. Importantly, 97% of the samples contained at least 1 clinically actionable variant and, if just a couple of known variants that are found outside of coding sequence are included, the figure moves to 100%. These analyses also point out some cautions. First, variants tend to segregate by geographic superpopulation and, because of database bias, the European superpopulation had the highest average number of clinical variants; this drives home the need for far more PGx research targeting diverse populations, as pointed out here and by others [62]. Second, short read sequencing technologies and their associated read-mapping software utilities have limitations in accurately assessing several important PGx loci, including the *UGT* and *HLA* genes, as well as critical copy number assessment of *CYP2D6*. Nonetheless, this thorough appraisal of the 1000 Genomes sequencing dataset serves to further drive home the point that, even when confined to protein coding sequences, individual rare variants in aggregate account for almost all of the observed variation, and sequencing represents the best way of finding them.

CYP2D6

No comprehensive assay designed to define pharmacogenomics variants for individualized prescribing practices can avoid the enzyme CYP450, family 2, subfamily D, polypeptide 6, or more commonly, CYP2D6. Involved in the metabolism or activation of approximately 25% of all currently prescribed drugs, it is probably the most studied of the CYP450 enzymes for multiple reasons. Originally identified in 1969 as the enzyme associated with variable response to the tricyclic antidepressant nortriptyline [63], studies by Maghoub and colleagues [64] in 1977 associated an inherited single allele with an observed variable response to the antihypertensive, debrisoquine. In 1979, Eichelbaum and colleagues [65] found that 5% of subjects passed unmodified sparteine, an antiarrhythmic, in their urine because of a single homozygous recessive allele. The gene was cloned in 1988 [66], assigned to the long arm of chromosome 22 [67], and, importantly, found to reside in close proximity to 2 highly homologous pseudogenes, *CYP2D7* and *CYP2D8* [68]. Based on the rapid discovery and characterization of numerous allelic variants in the 1990s, the P450 Nomenclature Committee [69] and its associated database were established. For a more detailed accounting, see Meyer [70].

The gene encoding *CYP2D6* is defined by 9 exons along the minus strand and is situated alongside the 2 pseudogenes and surrounded by DNA repeat regions distributed over approximately 45 kb of chromosome 22q, leading to both genomic instability and extreme challenges to DNA characterization that meets clinical reporting standards [71,72]. As shown by analysis of both the 1000 Genomes Project Phase III [38] and the ExAC [39] databases, the gene is highly polymorphic and not conducive to short read sequencing techniques on their own [73,74]. Substantially more than 100 allelic variants are defined in PharmVar, with the understanding that many of the world's populations are underrepresented in studies used to populate these databases and therefore clinical testing of individuals from underrepresented populations may reveal alleles that are not previously described or characterized. Most alleles at the locus are defined by 1 or more SNPs and complicated by some SNPs being shared between multiple alleles, which makes this gene difficult for clinical testing laboratories and highlights the need for phasing. The resulting phenotypes can vary from no enzyme activity, to reduced/variable activity, to variable response based on the drug in question, to having no effect. Other alleles are defined by structural variation, including gene deletion, copy number variation (as many as 13 copies have been observed), gene hybrids formed between *CYP2D6* and *CYP2D7* [75], partial gene conversion events, and tandem duplications [76]. In contrast with most allelic phenotypes, increased copy number may result in overexpression of the enzyme and a predicted ultrarapid metabolizer phenotype. For a more detailed review of the locus, its variants, and the resulting phenotypes, see the review by Gaedigk [77].

Longer Read Technologies

Inspired by the need to bridge repeats and provide a scaffold for organism sequencing projects lacking a reference sequence, as well as the need to accurately phase human genomes (see earlier), the market for longer reads spawned the development and introduction of 2 primary players using markedly different technologies. The first, Pacific Biosciences (PacBio), starting with the RSII, and then the Sequel, and now Sequel II, uses a unique single molecule system called SMRT (Single Molecule Real Time), which entails the binding of a single double-stranded molecule in conjunction with an engineered polymerase at the bottom of a zeptoliter well designed as a zero mode waveguide (ZMW) [78]. The ZMW well capacities are 150k, 1M and 8M for the models listed respectively. Imaging of phosphor-linked, fluorescently incorporated nucleotides is recorded in real time and although error rates are high, error is stochastic and the circular template allows for multiple reads from the same template, thus generating a circular consensus sequence. Further consensus is generated by there being millions of ZMWs per flow cell and sequence is generated from both template strands. The current Sequel instrument is capable of read lengths approaching 30 to 50 kb, although 7.5 to 12 kb is more typical. One underlying advantage of this method is that single molecule sequencing requires no amplification, thus obviating a potential source of error.

The second platform, produced and marketed by Oxford Nanopore Technologies (ONT), uses a preattached polymerase to "ratchet" a DNA molecule through a charged polymer membrane with imbedded biological pores and an attached detector that measures the differentiating current of each nucleotide as it passes through the pore (for historical and technical reviews, see Refs. [79,80]). There is at least 1 competing technology that uses solid-state nanopores, but it is not yet available. Great progress has recently been made in both throughput and accuracy and, like the PacBio platforms, single molecule sensitivity, long reads (perhaps even longer), and modified base detection present new and exciting possibilities. However, because read length can only be as long as the individual molecules presented, care must be exercised in DNA isolation and sequencing library preparation to prevent shearing. Two major advantages are realized with the compact version of this platform, known as the MinION: very small size coupled with modest power requirements (about the size and same voltage as a USB [universal serial bus] thumb drive) and an affordable startup cost. These advantages result in being able to take sequencing to the field instead of having to bring DNA to the laboratory, as shown in 2 recent publications [81,82].

Together with technology pioneered by 10x Genomics in which a vast collection of DNA barcode tags are attached to short read templates in the library construction process and then used to link subsequent Illumina reads into assemblies of longer haplotypes (for recent applications see Refs. [83,84]), these single molecule/extended read or linked read approaches can effectively counter some of the pitfalls of short read sequencing [85], especially with several clinically actionable PGx targets, including the *HLA* locus [86]; *CYP2A6*; and, most critically, *CYP2D6*. Both of the long read platforms, when applied to *CYP2D6* genotyping, used well-known long-range PCR amplicons [87] as starting material. The PacBio experiments used a combination of genotyping assays, copy number assays, and PacBio sequencing of long-range PCR amplicons produced from both well-characterized controls and recruited subjects [88,89]. In both cases, variant and allele calls were consistent with both prior knowledge in control samples and with the genotyping and copy number results across all samples, with the caveat that each used a different postprocessing tool to correct the PacBio reads and both studies used a limited number of samples. Nonetheless, they both were able to resolve results to the suballele level, correct diplotypes in some cases, and define new variants. Although an earlier ONT study of the CYP2D6 locus using the MinION was successful in variant phasing, it proved disappointing in error rate and thus resolution [90]; a more recent study using 7 control samples and 25 unrelated clinical samples on a GridION instrument with validation by Sanger sequencing produced far more promising results [91]. The ONT results were also able to differentiate and define copy number variation, with questions remaining whether this can be extended to samples having more than 2 copies of the gene on 1 allele and whether this technology can continue making progress in accurately sequencing homopolymer nucleotide runs.

SUMMARY AND WAY FORWARD

As outlined earlier, ideal incorporation of pharmacogenomics in personalized medicine would entail prospective, phased WGS to accurately define all of the relevant alleles affecting drug efficacy while avoiding adverse events and accounting for rare variants and private mutations. Such information could then become one more tool in the caregiver's hands to optimize patient outcomes while simultaneously acknowledging potentially confounding factors to consider, such as drug-drug interactions and environmental impact, including diet. However, there are a multitude of challenges to overcome as clinicians strive for these goals.

All clinical tests in the United States must meet Centers for Medicare & Medicaid Services, Clinical Laboratory Improvement Amendments, and College of American Pathologists requirements while simultaneously maintaining the flexibility to respond to new technologies and information guiding the annotation and interpretation of DNA sequencing results. Further government regulation in this arena is currently adding uncertainty (see Ref. [92] for more detail). Although clinical implementation is still rare, there are now multiple clinical settings in which PGx implementation is established in clinical care, in some cases for years [93–95]. There are also several NIH research initiatives designed to further the field and translate discoveries into clinical practice, such as PGRN, eMERGE, and IGNITE (Implementing Genomics in Practice; https://ignite-genomics.org). There are several reasons why clinical implementation has been slow to date. Until recently, there was a need to more thoroughly standardize what predicted phenotypes can be gleaned from these data. CPIC recently made great progress, both generally [96,97] and more recently in defining a points system for *CYP2D6* predicted phenotypes [98]. The challenges of difficult regions in the genome, such as the HLA and *CYP2D6*, currently demand supplementary tools and platforms to augment short read sequencing, such as amplicons, genotyping, long read technologies, and/or algorithms that recognize complex structure in a subset of samples for reflex to one these techniques [99]. There is an enormous need to better educate providers at all levels as well as the public on what PGx sequencing data are, what they mean, and what their current limits and shortcomings are [41,100,101]. Relatedly, clinical decision support (CDS) software development and integration into EHR systems and between systems represents another hurdle to successful implementation because providers rarely have time to drill down into the details of genomic variants and instead must rely on automated systems to suggest dose adjustments or alternative therapies while avoiding so-called alert fatigue. Several software tools have been developed to extract diplotypes and translate these results to star alleles and metabolizer status, but they represent just the first step in building a workable pipeline [102–106]. For more on CDS, see Refs. [107–112]. In addition, there remains the hurdle, at least in the United States, of reimbursement for these tests [113]. As outlined earlier, PGx testing is most effective if done prospectively and thus represents an investment that must prove its cost-benefit impact, although classic randomized controlled trials may not be the best way to accomplish this. For multiple viewpoints on this topic, see Refs. [114–117]. To date, most implementation is the result of research grants or philanthropic endeavors meant to jump-start implementation. That said, the field is currently on the cusp of promising breakthroughs in delivering truly personalized drug therapies, much as the Human Genome Project was during its conceptual phase not so many years ago [118,119].

ACKNOWLEDGMENTS

The author wishes to acknowledge the following BCM-HGSC colleagues for their contributions to this work: Richard Gibbs, Eric Boerwinkle, Donna Muzny, Eric Venner, Christie Kovar, Viktoriya Korchina, Jianhong Hu, Xiang Qin and Tsung-Jung Wu as well as the Mayo-Baylor RIGHT 10K Pharmacogenomics Consortium. The author's work cited here was supported by National Institutes of Health grants U19 GM61388 and 1UM1HG008898 as well as the Mayo Clinic Center for Individualized Medicine.

REFERENCES

[1] Collins FS, Morgan M, Patrinos A. The Human Genome Project: lessons from large-scale biology. Science 2003;300(5617):286–90.
[2] Alving AS, Carson PE, Flanagan CL, et al. Enzymatic deficiency in primaquine-sensitive erythrocytes. Science 1956;124(3220):484–5.
[3] Vogel F. Moderne problem der humangenetik. Ergeb Inn Med Kinderheilkd 1959;12:52–125.
[4] International HapMap Consortium. A haplotype map of the human genome. Nature 2005;437(7063):1299–320.
[5] Weinshilboum R. Inheritance and drug response [review]. N Engl J Med 2003;348(6):529–37.
[6] Lin M, Aquilante C, Johnson JA, et al. Sequencing drug response with HapMap. Pharmacogenomics J 2005;5(3):149–56.
[7] Evans WE, Relling MV. Moving towards individualized medicine with pharmacogenomics [review]. Nature 2004;429(6990):464–8.
[8] PharmaADME Consortium. Available at: http://www.pharmaadme.org/.
[9] Daly TM, Dumaual CM, Miao X, et al. Multiplex assay for comprehensive genotyping of genes involved in drug metabolism, excretion, and transport. Clin Chem 2007;53(7):1222–30.
[10] Deeken J. The Affymetrix DMET platform and pharmacogenetics in drug development [review]. Curr Opin Mol Ther 2009;11(3):260–8.
[11] Sissung TM, English BC, Venzon D, et al. Clinical pharmacology and pharmacogenetics in a genomics era: the DMET platform [review]. Pharmacogenomics 2010;11(1):89–103.
[12] Potamias G, Lakiotaki K, Katsila T, et al. Deciphering next-generation pharmacogenomics: an information technology perspective. Open Biol 2014;4(7) [pii: 140071].
[13] Takeuchi F, McGinnis R, Bourgeois S, et al. A genome-wide association study confirms VKORC1, CYP2C9, and CYP4F2 as principal genetic determinants of warfarin dose. PLoS Genet 2009;5(3):e1000433.
[14] Shuldiner AR, O'Connell JR, Bliden KP, et al. Association of cytochrome P450 2C19 genotype with the antiplatelet effect and clinical efficacy of clopidogrel therapy. JAMA 2009;302(8):849–57.
[15] SEARCH Collaborative Group, Link E, Parish S, Armitage J, et al. SLCO1B1 variants and statin-

induced myopathy–a genomewide study. N Engl J Med 2008;359(8):789–99.
[16] Daly AK. Genome-wide association studies in pharmacogenomics [review]. Nat Rev Genet 2010;11(4): 241–6.
[17] Daly AK. Using genome-wide association studies to identify genes important in serious adverse drug reactions [review]. Annu Rev Pharmacol Toxicol 2012;52: 21–35.
[18] Turner ST, Bailey KR, Fridley BL, et al. Genomic association analysis suggests chromosome 12 locus influencing antihypertensive response to thiazide diuretic. Hypertension 2008;52(2):359–65.
[19] Duarte JD, Turner ST, Tran B, et al. Association of chromosome 12 locus with antihypertensive response to hydrochlorothiazide may involve differential YEATS4 expression. Pharmacogenomics J 2013;13(3):257–63.
[20] Singh S, Wang Z, Shahin MH, et al. Targeted sequencing identifies a missense variant in the BEST3 gene associated with antihypertensive response to hydrochlorothiazide. Pharmacogenet Genomics 2018; 28(11):251–5.
[21] Relling MV, Klein TE. CPIC: clinical pharmacogenetics implementation consortium of the pharmacogenomics research network. Clin Pharmacol Ther 2011;89(3): 464–7.
[22] Caudle KE, Klein TE, Hoffman JM, et al. Incorporation of pharmacogenomics into routine clinical practice: the Clinical Pharmacogenetics Implementation Consortium (CPIC) guideline development process. Curr Drug Metab 2014;15(2):209–17.
[23] Maxam AM, Gilbert W. Sequencing end-labeled DNA with base-specific chemical cleavages. Methods Enzymol 1980;65(1):499–560.
[24] Sanger F, Coulson AR. A rapid method for determining sequences in DNA by primed synthesis with DNA polymerase. J Mol Biol 1975;94(3):441–8.
[25] Sanger F, Nicklen S, Coulson AR. DNA sequencing with chain-terminating inhibitors. Proc Natl Acad Sci U S A 1977;74(12):5463–7.
[26] Metzker ML. Sequencing technologies - the next generation [review]. Nat Rev Genet 2010;11(1):31–46.
[27] Ronaghi M, Karamohamed S, Pettersson B, et al. Real-time DNA sequencing using detection of pyrophosphate release. Anal Biochem 1996;242(1):84–9.
[28] Wheeler DA, Srinivasan M, Egholm M, et al. The complete genome of an individual by massively parallel DNA sequencing. Nature 2008;452(7189):872–6.
[29] Rothberg JM, Hinz W, Rearick TM, et al. An integrated semiconductor device enabling non-optical genome sequencing. Nature 2011;475(7356):348–52.
[30] Dohm JC, Lottaz C, Borodina T, et al. Substantial biases in ultra-short read data sets from high-throughput DNA sequencing. Nucleic Acids Res 2008;36(16):e105.
[31] Lupski JR, Belmont JW, Boerwinkle E, et al. Clan genomics and the complex architecture of human disease. Cell 2011;147(1):32–43.
[32] Albert TJ, Molla MN, Muzny DM, et al. Direct selection of human genomic loci by microarray hybridization. Nat Methods 2007;4(11):903–5.
[33] Yang Y, Muzny DM, Reid JG, et al. Clinical whole-exome sequencing for the diagnosis of mendelian disorders. N Engl J Med 2013;369(16):1502–11.
[34] Gordon AS, Fulton RS, Qin X, et al. PGRNseq: a targeted capture sequencing panel for pharmacogenetic research and implementation. Pharmacogenet Genomics 2016;26(4):161–8.
[35] Rasmussen-Torvik LJ, Stallings SC, Gordon AS, et al. Design and anticipated outcomes of the eMERGE-PGx project: a multicenter pilot for preemptive pharmacogenomics in electronic health record systems. Clin Pharmacol Ther 2014;96(4):482–9.
[36] Rasmussen-Torvik LJ, Almoguera B, Doheny KF, et al. Concordance between research sequencing and clinical pharmacogenetic genotyping in the eMERGE-PGx Study. J Mol Diagn 2017;19(4):561–6.
[37] Bush WS, Crosslin DR, Owusu-Obeng A, et al. Genetic variation among 82 pharmacogenes: The PGRNseq data from the eMERGE network. Clin Pharmacol Ther 2016;100(2):160–9.
[38] 1000 Genomes Project Consortium, Auton A, Brooks LD, Durbin RM, et al. A global reference for human genetic variation. Nature 2015;526(7571):68–74.
[39] Lek M, Karczewski KJ, Minikel EV, et al, Exome Aggregation Consortium. Analysis of protein-coding genetic variation in 60,706 humans. Nature 2016;536(7616): 285–91.
[40] Bielinski SJ, St Sauver JL, Olson JE, et al. Are patients willing to incur out-of-pocket costs for pharmacogenomic testing? Pharmacogenomics J 2017; 17(1):1–3.
[41] Rohrer Vitek CR, Abul-Husn NS, Connolly JJ, et al. Healthcare provider education to support integration of pharmacogenomics in practice: the eMERGE Network experience. Pharmacogenomics 2017;18(10): 1013–25.
[42] Olson JE, Rohrer Vitek CR, Bell EJ, et al. Participant-perceived understanding and perspectives on pharmacogenomics: the Mayo Clinic RIGHT protocol (Right Drug, Right Dose, Right Time). Genet Med 2017; 19(7):819–25.
[43] Freimuth RR, Formea CM, Hoffman JM, et al. Implementing genomic clinical decision support for drug-based precision medicine [review]. CPT Pharmacometrics Syst Pharmacol 2017;6(3):153–5.
[44] Caraballo PJ, Hodge LS, Bielinski SJ, et al. Multidisciplinary model to implement pharmacogenomics at the point of care. Genet Med 2017;19(4):421–9.
[45] Obeng AO, Kaszemacher T, Abul-Husn NS, et al. Implementing algorithm-guided warfarin dosing in an ethnically diverse patient population using electronic health records and preemptive CYP2C9 and VKORC1 genetic testing. Clin Pharmacol Ther 2016;100(5): 427–30.

[46] Ji Y, Skierka JM, Blommel JH, et al. Preemptive pharmacogenomic testing for precision medicine: a comprehensive analysis of five actionable pharmacogenomic genes using next-generation DNA sequencing and a customized CYP2D6 genotyping cascade. J Mol Diagn 2016;18(3):438–45.

[47] Available at: https://www.genomeweb.com/sequencing-technology/mayo-baylor-collaborate-pharmacogenomics-sequencing-study#.XSeyClB7klI.

[48] Cousin MA, Matey ET, Blackburn PR, et al. Pharmacogenomic findings from clinical whole exome sequencing of diagnostic odyssey patients. Mol Genet Genomic Med 2017;5(3):269–79.

[49] Samwald M, Blagec K, Hofer S, et al. Analyzing the potential for incorrect haplotype calls with different pharmacogenomic assays in different populations: a simulation based on 1000 Genomes data. Pharmacogenomics 2015;16(15):1713–21.

[50] Schildcrout JS, Denny JC, Bowton E, et al. Optimizing drug outcomes through pharmacogenetics: a case for preemptive genotyping. Clin Pharmacol Ther 2012; 92(2):235–42.

[51] Van Driest SL, Shi Y, Bowton EA, et al. Clinically actionable genotypes among 10,000 patients with preemptive pharmacogenomic testing. Clin Pharmacol Ther 2014; 95(4):423–31.

[52] Lupski JR, Reid JG, Gonzaga-Jauregui C, et al. Whole-genome sequencing in a patient with Charcot-Marie-Tooth neuropathy. N Engl J Med 2010;362(13):1181–91.

[53] Bainbridge MN, Wiszniewski W, Murdock DR, et al. Whole-genome sequencing for optimized patient management. Sci Transl Med 2011;3(87):87re3.

[54] Ashley EA, Butte AJ, Wheeler MT, et al. Clinical assessment incorporating a personal genome. Lancet 2010; 375(9725):1525–35.

[55] Dewey FE, Chen R, Cordero SP, et al. Phased whole-genome genetic risk in a family quartet using a major allele reference sequence. PLoS Genet 2011;7(9): e1002280.

[56] Chua EW, Cree SL, Ton KN, et al. Cross-comparison of exome analysis, next-generation sequencing of amplicons, and the iPLEX(®) ADME PGx panel for pharmacogenomic profiling. Front Pharmacol 2016;7:1.

[57] Yang W, Wu G, Broeckel U, et al. Comparison of genome sequencing and clinical genotyping for pharmacogenes. Clin Pharmacol Ther 2016;100(4):380–8.

[58] Cohn I, Paton TA, Marshall CR, et al. Genome sequencing as a platform for pharmacogenetic genotyping: a pediatric cohort study. NPJ Genom Med 2017;2:19.

[59] Mizzi C, Peters B, Mitropoulou C, et al. Personalized pharmacogenomics profiling using whole-genome sequencing. Pharmacogenomics 2014;15(9):1223–34.

[60] Gordon AS, Tabor HK, Johnson AD, et al, Exome Sequencing Project. Quantifying rare, deleterious variation in 12 human cytochrome P450 drug-metabolism genes in a large-scale exome dataset. Hum Mol Genet 2014;23(8):1957–63.

[61] Wright GEB, Carleton B, Hayden MR, et al. The global spectrum of protein-coding pharmacogenomic diversity. Pharmacogenomics J 2018;18(1):187–95.

[62] Drögemöller BI, Wright GE, Niehaus DJ, et al. Whole-genome resequencing in pharmacogenomics: moving away from past disparities to globally representative applications. Pharmacogenomics 2011;12(12):1717–28.

[63] Alexanderson B, Evans DA, Sjöqvist F. Steady-state plasma levels of nortriptyline in twins: influence of genetic factors and drug therapy. Br Med J 1969;4(5686):764–8.

[64] Mahgoub A, Idle JR, Dring LG, et al. Polymorphic hydroxylation of Debrisoquine in man. Lancet 1977; 2(8038):584–6.

[65] Eichelbaum M, Spannbrucker N, Steincke B, et al. Defective N-oxidation of sparteine in man: a new pharmacogenetic defect. Eur J Clin Pharmacol 1979;16(3):183–7.

[66] Gonzalez FJ, Skoda RC, Kimura S, et al. Characterization of the common genetic defect in humans deficient in debrisoquine metabolism. Nature 1988;331(6155):442–6.

[67] Eichelbaum M, Baur MP, Dengler HJ, et al. Chromosomal assignment of human cytochrome P-450 (debrisoquine/sparteine type) to chromosome 22. Br J Clin Pharmacol 1987;23(4):455–8.

[68] Kimura S, Umeno M, Skoda RC, et al. The human debrisoquine 4-hydroxylase (CYP2D) locus: sequence and identification of the polymorphic CYP2D6 gene, a related gene, and a pseudogene. Am J Hum Genet 1989;45(6):889–904.

[69] Daly AK, Brockmöller J, Broly F, et al. Nomenclature for human CYP2D6 alleles. Pharmacogenetics 1996;6(3): 193–201.

[70] Meyer UA. Pharmacogenetics - five decades of therapeutic lessons from genetic diversity [review]. Nat Rev Genet 2004;5(9):669–76.

[71] Yang Y, Botton MR, Scott ER, et al. Sequencing the CYP2D6 gene: from variant allele discovery to clinical pharmacogenetic testing [review]. Pharmacogenomics 2017;18(7):673–85.

[72] Drögemöller BI, Wright GE, Niehaus DJ, et al. Next-generation sequencing of pharmacogenes: a critical analysis focusing on schizophrenia treatment. Pharmacogenet Genomics 2013;23(12):666–74.

[73] Genome accessibility masks for 1000 Genomes data. Available at: http://www.internationalgenome.org/announcements/genome-accessibility-masks/.

[74] Popitsch N, WGS500 Consortium, Schuh A, Taylor JC. ReliableGenome: annotation of genomic regions with high/low variant calling concordance. Bioinformatics 2017;33(2):155–60.

[75] Black JL 3rd, Walker DL, O'Kane DJ, et al. Frequency of undetected CYP2D6 hybrid genes in clinical samples: impact on phenotype prediction. Drug Metab Dispos 2012;40(1):111–9 [Erratum in: Drug Metab Dispos 2012;40(6):1238].

[76] Kramer WE, Walker DL, O'Kane DJ, et al. CYP2D6: novel genomic structures and alleles. Pharmacogenet Genomics 2009;19(10):813–22.

[77] Gaedigk A. Complexities of CYP2D6 gene analysis and interpretation [review]. Int Rev Psychiatry 2013;25(5): 534–53.
[78] Levene MJ, Korlach J, Turner SW, et al. Zero-mode waveguides for single-molecule analysis at high concentrations. Science 2003;299(5607):682–6.
[79] Deamer D, Akeson M, Branton D. Three decades of nanopore sequencing [review]. Nat Biotechnol 2016; 34(5):518–24.
[80] Leggett RM, Clark MD. A world of opportunities with nanopore sequencing [review]. J Exp Bot 2017;68(20): 5419–29.
[81] Castro-Wallace SL, Chiu CY, John KK, et al. Nanopore DNA sequencing and genome assembly on the international space station. Sci Rep 2017;7(1):18022.
[82] Greninger AL, Naccache SN, Federman S, et al. Rapid metagenomic identification of viral pathogens in clinical samples by real-time nanopore sequencing analysis. Genome Med 2015;7:99.
[83] Marks P, Garcia S, Barrio AM, et al. Resolving the full spectrum of human genome variation using Linked-Reads. Genome Res 2019;29(4):635–45.
[84] Chaisson MJP, Sanders AD, Zhao X, et al. Multi-platform discovery of haplotype-resolved structural variation in human genomes. Nat Commun 2019;10(1):1784.
[85] Ameur A, Kloosterman WP, Hestand MS. Single-molecule sequencing: towards clinical applications [review]. Trends Biotechnol 2019;37(1):72–85.
[86] Mimori T, Yasuda J, Kuroki Y, et al. Construction of full-length Japanese reference panel of class I HLA genes with single-molecule, real-time sequencing. Pharmacogenomics J 2019;19(2):136–46.
[87] Gaedigk A, Ndjountché L, Divakaran K, et al. Cytochrome P4502D6 (CYP2D6) gene locus heterogeneity: characterization of gene duplication events. Clin Pharmacol Ther 2007;81(2):242–51.
[88] Qiao W, Yang Y, Sebra R, et al. Long-read single molecule real-time full gene sequencing of cytochrome P450-2D6. Hum Mutat 2016;37(3):315–23.
[89] Buermans HP, Vossen RH, Anvar SY, et al. Flexible and scalable full-length CYP2D6 long amplicon PacBio sequencing. Hum Mutat 2017;38(3):310–6.
[90] Ammar R, Paton TA, Torti D, et al. Long read nanopore sequencing for detection of HLA and CYP2D6 variants and haplotypes. Version 2. F1000Res 2015;4:17.
[91] Liau Y, Maggo S, Miller A, et al. Nanopore sequencing of the pharmacogene CYP2D6 allows simultaneous haplotyping and detection of duplications. BioRchiv 2019. https://doi.org/10.1101/576280.
[92] Ray T. GenomeWeb. FDA Actions on PGx Testing Confuse Genetic Industry Players. 2018. Available at: https://www.genomeweb.com/regulatory-news/fda-actions-pgx-testing-confuse-genetic-industry-players#.XSTWD3t7kmI.
[93] Dunnenberger HM, Crews KR, Hoffman JM, et al. Preemptive clinical pharmacogenetics implementation: current programs in five US medical centers [review]. Annu Rev Pharmacol Toxicol 2015;55:89–106.
[94] Bank PCD, Swen JJ, Guchelaar HJ. Implementation of pharmacogenomics in everyday clinical settings. Adv Pharmacol 2018;83:219–46.
[95] Volpi S, Bult CJ, Chisholm RL, et al. Research directions in the clinical implementation of pharmacogenomics: an overview of US programs and projects [review]. Clin Pharmacol Ther 2018;103(5):778–86.
[96] Caudle KE, Dunnenberger HM, Freimuth RR, et al. Standardizing terms for clinical pharmacogenetic test results: consensus terms from the Clinical Pharmacogenetics Implementation Consortium (CPIC). Genet Med 2017; 19(2):215–23.
[97] Caudle KE, Keeling NJ, Klein TE, et al. Standardization can accelerate the adoption of pharmacogenomics: current status and the path forward [review]. Pharmacogenomics 2018;19(10):847–60.
[98] CPIC Final Consensus CYP2D6genotype to phenotype table-March 2019. Available at: https://cpicpgx.org/wp-content/uploads/2019/03/Final-Consensus-CYP2D6-genotype-to-phenotype-table_-final_Mar2019.pdf.
[99] Black JL III, Sicotte H, Peterson SE, et al. CNVAR: a software tool for genotyping CYP2D6 using short read next generation sequencing technology, 2019. Pacific Symposium on Biocomputing Hawaii, January 3–7, 2019.
[100] McCullough KB, Formea CM, Berg KD, et al. Assessment of the pharmacogenomics educational needs of pharmacists. Am J Pharm Educ 2011;75(3):51.
[101] Stanek EJ, Sanders CL, Taber KA, et al. Adoption of pharmacogenomic testing by US physicians: results of a nationwide survey. Clin Pharmacol Ther 2012; 91(3):450–8.
[102] Numanagić I, Malikić S, Pratt VM, et al. Cypiripi: exact genotyping of CYP2D6 using high-throughput sequencing data. Bioinformatics 2015;31(12): i27–34.
[103] Numanagić I, Malikić S, Ford M, et al. Allelic decomposition and exact genotyping of highly polymorphic and structurally variant genes. Nat Commun 2018; 9(1):828.
[104] Twist GP, Gaedigk A, Miller NA, et al. Erratum: Constellation: a tool for rapid, automated phenotype assignment of a highly polymorphic pharmacogene, CYP2D6, from whole-genome sequences. NPJ Genom Med 2017;2:16039.
[105] Twist GP, Gaedigk A, Miller NA, et al. Constellation: a tool for rapid, automated phenotype assignment of a highly polymorphic pharmacogene, CYP2D6, from whole-genome sequences. NPJ Genom Med 2016;1: 15007 [Erratum in: NPJ Genom Med 2017;2:16039].
[106] GitHub.PharmGKB/PharmCAT. Available at: https://github.com/PharmGKB/PharmCAT.
[107] Hicks JK, Crews KR, Hoffman JM, et al. A clinician-driven automated system for integration of pharmacogenetic interpretations into an electronic medical record. Clin Pharmacol Ther 2012;92(5):563–6.
[108] Goldspiel BR, Flegel WA, DiPatrizio G, et al. Integrating pharmacogenetic information and clinical decision

support into the electronic health record. J Am Med Inform Assoc 2014;21(3):522–8.
[109] Welch BM, Kawamoto K. The need for clinical decision support integrated with the electronic health record for the clinical application of whole genome sequencing information. J Pers Med 2013;3(4):306–25.
[110] Overby CL, Kohane I, Kannry JL, et al. Opportunities for genomic clinical decision support interventions. Genet Med 2013;15(10):817–23.
[111] Nishimura AA, Shirts BH, Dorschner MO, et al. Development of clinical decision support alerts for pharmacogenomic incidental findings from exome sequencing. Genet Med 2015;17(11):939–42.
[112] Blagec K, Koopmann R, Crommentuijn-van Rhenen M, et al. Implementing pharmacogenomics decision support across seven European countries: The Ubiquitous Pharmacogenomics (U-PGx) project. J Am Med Inform Assoc 2018;25(7):893–8.
[113] Cavallari LH, Pratt VM. Building evidence for clinical use of pharmacogenomics and reimbursement for testing. Adv Mol Pathol 2018;1:125–34.
[114] Khoury MJ. Dealing with the evidence dilemma in genomics and personalized medicine. Clin Pharmacol Ther 2010;87(6):635–8.
[115] Altman RB. Pharmacogenomics: "noninferiority" is sufficient for initial implementation. Clin Pharmacol Ther 2011;89(3):348–50.
[116] Pirmohamed M, Hughes DA. Pharmacogenetic tests: the need for a level playing field. Nat Rev Drug Discov 2013;12(1):3–4.
[117] van der Wouden CH, Swen JJ, Samwald M, et al. A brighter future for the implementation of pharmacogenomic testing. Eur J Hum Genet 2016;24(12):1658–60.
[118] Ji Y, Si Y, McMillin GA, et al. Clinical pharmacogenomics testing in the era of next generation sequencing: challenges and opportunities for precision medicine [review]. Expert Rev Mol Diagn 2018;18(5):411–21.
[119] Schwarz UI, Gulilat M, Kim RB. The role of next-generation sequencing in pharmacogenetics and pharmacogenomics [review]. Cold Spring Harb Perspect Med 2019;9(2) [pii:a033027].

Advances in Molecular Pathology 2 (2019) 133–142
ADVANCES IN MOLECULAR PATHOLOGY

Consumer-initiated Genetic Testing and Pharmacogenomics

Ann M. Moyer, MD, PhD*, Linnea M. Baudhuin, PhD
Department of Laboratory Medicine and Pathology, Mayo Clinic, 200 First Street Southwest, Rochester, MN 55905, USA

KEYWORDS

• Genetic testing • Pharmacogenetics • Pharmacogenomics • Consumer-initiated • Direct-to-consumer • Hereditary disorder • Personalized medicine

KEY POINTS

- Consumer-initiated genetic testing, which is advertised and sold directly to the public, has emerged for purposes including disease risk, disease carrier status, pharmacogenomics, ancestry, and entertainment.
- Early studies have not been conclusive as to whether consumer-initiated genetic testing leads to healthy changes in diet and lifestyle.
- Although a medical professional is not required for consumer-initiated testing, results may affect medical care; individuals may encounter barriers when bringing unsolicited results to their regular providers.
- Early studies have shown a low percentage of unsupervised medication changes among consumers undergoing consumer-initiated pharmacogenomic testing, but this may equate to a large number of individuals as testing becomes more widespread.
- Both consumers and health care providers should be aware of the differences between traditional medical and consumer-initiated genetic tests as well as limitations and risks of consumer-initiated genetic testing, which include privacy risks, inaccuracies, and incompleteness of testing.

INTRODUCTION: WHAT IS CONSUMER-INITIATED TESTING?

Consumer-initiated genetic testing for diverse purposes, including medical insights (eg, carrier status, disease risk, pharmacogenomics), general wellness, ancestry, and entertainment (infotainment), is increasing with more than 15 million genetic data records housed by major companies in this space [1]. Much of this testing is driven by the public's growing interest in genetics as well as the hope of personalized health care. Traditional genetic testing is provider initiated and designed to diagnose disease, identify individuals at risk because of a family history of disease, detect individuals who are carriers for recessive disease for family planning purposes, or to predict and avoid adverse medication reactions or lack of efficacy of medications (pharmacogenomics). Therefore, traditional genetic tests are often performed on selected patient populations and not widely available to all individuals who may be interested in genetic testing. In contrast, consumer-initiated testing is advertised and sold directly to the public, providing an opportunity for testing to those who are often generally healthy and may not be eligible for traditional testing. In addition, the cost of consumer-initiated testing is often much lower than traditional provider-initiated diagnostic testing, also contributing

Disclosure: The authors have nothing to disclose.

*Corresponding author, *E-mail address:* Moyer.Ann@Mayo.edu

https://doi.org/10.1016/j.yamp.2019.07.009

to increased accessibility and adoption by the general public.

Consumer-initiated genetic testing was initially offered in the early 2000s. However, after the US Government Accountability Office investigated the practices of those early direct-to-consumer (DTC) testing companies, they thought that the advertising claims exaggerated the benefits of testing and released a report with their findings [2]. This led the US Food and Drug Administration (FDA) to send letters to the DTC testing companies in 2010 informing them that their products represented medical devices, which had not been FDA approved, and later in 2013 to send letters stating that testing must be discontinued until they received FDA approval [3,4]. As of 2019, only 1 company, 23andMe, has obtained marketing authorization from the FDA for DTC testing [5]. At present, 23andMe is authorized to offer carrier screening for Bloom syndrome, a genetic health risk test (hereditary thrombophilia, alpha-1 antitrypsin deficiency, late-onset Alzheimer disease, Parkinson disease, Gaucher disease, factor XI deficiency, celiac disease, glucose-6-phosphate dehydrogenase deficiency, hereditary hemochromatosis, and early-onset primary dystonia), a genetic health risk report for *BRCA1/BRCA2* (selected variants), and pharmacogenetic reports [5–7]. In addition, the FDA indicated that they would exempt additional future genetic health risk tests that 23andMe offers, as well as those of other companies after submission of their first premarket notification; however, they also indicated that diagnostic tests that often lead to major treatment decisions were not part of the scope of the exemption [6]. In order to gain FDA approval for medically related DTC tests, manufacturers must show that the information is understandable by consumers.

In addition to the DTC testing offered by 23andMe, a new model of consumer-initiated testing has emerged (Fig. 1). Unlike the traditional DTC testing, which touts consumer empowerment and proposes that these tests can eliminate the need for physician and/or genetic counselor involvement [3], other consumer-initiated tests are available with which the consumer may request testing via a Web site, but a provider who is affiliated with the testing company reviews the information provided by the consumer and places the order. This type of testing that is ordered by a health care provider, even if not the patient's regular provider, is usually in the category of laboratory-developed tests, which as a matter of policy are typically not reviewed by the FDA [5].

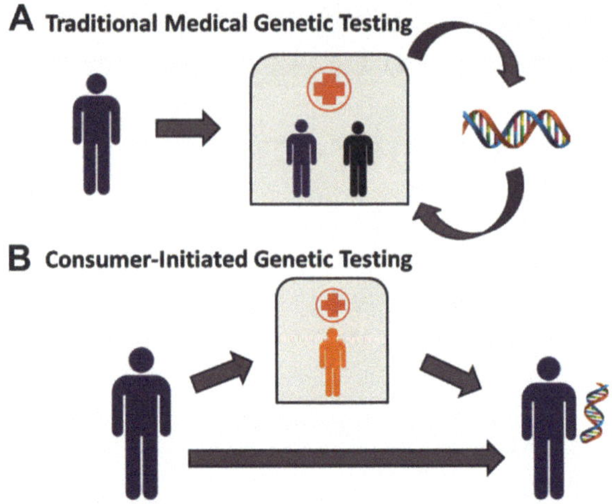

FIG. 1 Types of genetic testing. In traditional medical genetic testing (**A**), the consumer/patient (*blue figure*) presents to a provider (*black figure*) who orders genetic testing when indicated. The results (depicted by the DNA symbol) are returned to the provider who then discusses them with the consumer/patient. Consumer-initiated genetic testing (**B**) has 2 pathways. The consumer may order testing through an intermediary provider (*orange figure*) or directly. The results are returned to the patient, who may take them to the patient's usual provider, and/or may have an option to speak with a genetic counselor through the genetic testing company.

PROS AND CONS OF CONSUMER-INITIATED TESTING

Although there are many purported potential benefits of consumer-initiated testing, from both a personal and societal standpoint, some investigators have argued that the benefits of these tests are limited [8]. Patients having increased access to their own genetic data, whether it is for health or entertainment purposes, has often been cited as a benefit of consumer-initiated testing. It has also been maintained that consumer-initiated genetic testing may lead to healthy changes in diet and/or lifestyle. In a recent study of 1002 participants who had received personal genomic testing, modest and mostly positive changes in diet and exercise were noted, regardless of the genetic test results [9]. Although these results were consistent with 1 prior study that also found positive health behavior changes [10], other studies have found no association with diet or exercise changes [11–15]. In the studies with positive impact, it is possible that the changes observed were caused by selection bias, with participants choosing to obtain genetic testing as part of a larger goal of improving health and diet. For example, most studies have been conducted on early adopters who tend to be white, more highly educated, and of better overall health than the general population. In addition, many studies have had low participation rates, small sample sizes, short follow-up, and self-reported behavioral changes, and included tests with limited or no demonstrated utility, among other limitations [16]. Thus, ascertaining the true health-related impact of these tests on an unbiased population has been challenging.

Whether or not obtaining consumer-initiated genetic test results induces anxiety or regret in consumers is not well characterized. However, in a recent study, only 2% of the respondents who had undergone consumer-initiated genetic testing expressed regret for their decision to pursue testing, with 1% indicating that the decision had harmed them, although the nature of the harm was not reported [17]. In addition, approximately 40% of participants in the same study were disappointed that their results were less informative than they had expected. Concern has also been raised as to whether testing and return of results may increase anxiety of consumers, although limited research suggests that this may primarily be a concern for a small subset of consumers [18–20]. Although experience with genetic testing may help consumers learn more about genetics, consumers reported lower confidence in genetic knowledge after undergoing personal DTC genetic testing [21].

Consumer-initiated genetic testing is often performed by people to learn more about their ancestry. However, each ancestry-related genetic testing company draws on its own proprietary set of genetic variants to determine consumer ethnicity, and vastly different results have been obtained from one company to another [22]. This variation arises because there is no complete database of human DNA samples that is globally representative. Most genetic variant databases comprise white samples, and thus matches produced for nonwhite people are less accurate. Also, because genetic markers are from modern populations, generalizations have to be made with respect to populations from hundreds of years ago. Furthermore, claims by genetic testing companies to determine ancestry may affect the identity of ethnic groups. For example, US tribal communities have raised concerns about DNA testing being used to establish membership or even tribal enrollment without consideration of the nongenetic social, political, and cultural aspects that are also important contributors to their identity [23].

Consumers interested in genealogy may undergo testing to determine how their research aligns with their genetic results, or genetic testing may be a tool when research has hit a dead end, such as with adoptees from agencies with no paper trail. In some cases, family secrets have been uncovered, including infidelity, adoption, and conception with assistance from donor sperm or eggs [24,25]. Such findings can have significant psychological consequences and alter people's sense of identity.

Although a medical professional is not required for consumer-initiated testing, many individuals who undergo such testing receive results that may affect medical care, but they may encounter barriers when bringing results to their regular providers. Primary care providers, who may be the most likely to encounter patients bringing unsolicited genetic testing results to appointments, have expressed concerns about the ethical, legal, and social implications of genetic testing and skepticism about consumer-initiated testing [26,27]. In addition, clinicians may not be confident in their basic genetics knowledge and may be uncomfortable or unprepared for using genetic information in patient care [27–30]. In a 2016 study of 1026 consumers who underwent DTC testing, 63% planned to share their results with a health care provider, but at 6 months after testing only 27% reported having done so; among those individuals, 35% were very satisfied with the discussion, whereas 18% were not at all satisfied [31]. In addition to primary care, some patients schedule an appointment for genetic counseling. In a study of 1026 individuals who received DTC test results, 4% made or planned to make an appointment with a genetic counselor, whereas 38% indicated that they would have met with a genetic counselor had an in-person appointment option been available. In general, those seeking genetic counseling were younger, more frequently had children, and were more likely to have previous experience with genetic testing [32].

Consumer privacy and nondiscrimination have recently emerged as additional concerns related to DTC genetic testing, particularly since the 2018 story of the identification of the so-called Golden State killer broke [1,8]. Police were able to identify the suspect by matching DNA from the crime scene with genetic data in a public genealogy database, GEDmatch, where the relatives of the suspect had deposited data. Although DTC testing companies must follow consumer privacy protection laws and provide disclosures regarding privacy policies, there are privacy concerns among the public. Recent studies have found that 74% of consumers thought that it was very important that law enforcement procurement of genetic testing data be illegal, whereas, in a different study, 80% of respondents supported police searches of genetic data on public Web sites to identify perpetrators of violent crimes and 78% supported searches for crimes against children [1,33,34]. Although the Combined DNA Index System (CODIS) database historically used by law enforcement contains genetic information from convicted and suspected criminals and is enriched in data from racial and ethnic minority populations, public genealogy databases contain data primarily from white populations, so perhaps cross-referencing these public databases may reduce bias in law enforcement arrests [35].

Genomic data that have been deidentified can be reidentified with available genomic software [36]. Thus, consumers who make their deidentified data available to the public may incorrectly assume that their data will always be anonymous. Although consumer reidentification is likely rare, sensitive medical information about consumers and their relatives can be revealed if reidentification occurs. It is unclear whether consumers fully appreciate the extent of the risks to themselves and their families if their genomic data were to become reidentified and whether they factor those risks into their choice to undergo DTC testing [8]. Furthermore, consumers may not fully appreciate that data breaches may occur, such as the cyberattacks that have been attempted on the 100,000 Genomes Project data [37].

KEY DIFFERENCES BETWEEN CONSUMER-INITIATED AND TRADITIONAL MEDICAL GENETIC TESTING

The main difference between consumer-initiated genetic testing and clinical diagnostic genetic testing is that a specific clinical question prompts diagnostic testing, whereas most individuals undergoing consumer-initiated testing are ostensibly healthy and there is no specific clinical indication. As such, diagnostic panel-based testing typically involves a robust set of genes, including the complete coding regions and relevant noncoding regions, known to be important in the disease of interest. The goal of this type of testing is to maximize sensitivity and minimize false-negative results. In some cases, exome or genome sequencing is used in place of a targeted multigene panel, allowing broader coverage, although potentially sacrificing sensitivity of genes that are not as deeply covered. These tests typically report variants classified by the American College of Medical Genetics and Genomics (ACMG) and the Association for Molecular Pathology (AMP) standards and guidelines for the interpretation of sequence variants as pathogenic, likely pathogenic, or variant of uncertain significance (VUS) [38]. In contrast, consumer-initiated testing may be less complete, including only certain relevant genes, regions of genes, or targeted single nucleotide variants [39]. Testing may interpret all variants in the included genes or may only interpret a few well-curated variants; variant assessment is typically automated to reduce the costs of testing. Some laboratories chose to only report variants classified as pathogenic for the highest clinical specificity. Other laboratories also include likely pathogenic variants, which may increase sensitivity but also leads to more false-positive results [39]. In general, consumer-initiated tests do not report VUS [39,40]. It is important for both diagnostic and consumer-initiated tests to clearly indicate the genes/regions included in tests, as well as the reporting strategy. An additional consideration for consumer-initiated testing is that use of the word negative is generally discouraged to describe cases in which no pathogenic or likely pathogenic variants are detected because this may lead to false reassurance of the consumer. Instead, aligning the language with other sections of the report that address posttest residual risk is recommended [39].

DTC and most consumer-initiated genetic tests are not considered diagnostic and only offer information on genetic risks for limited conditions and variants. For some included conditions, the variants tested are enriched in an affected population compared with healthy cohorts but may not be sufficient to cause disease because other factors, such as environment and lifestyle, may influence individual risk. In general, the genes associated with disease are not comprehensively sequenced and not all genes related to disease are included. An example of a DTC genetic test that does not tell the whole story and may lead to false reassurance or false anxiety in the consumer is 23andMe's test for hereditary colon cancer, which received FDA clearance in January 2019 [41]. This test only includes the 2 most common genetic variants influencing *MUTYH*-associated polyposis. However, most colorectal cancers do not have an underlying genetic cause. Thus, testing negative for these variants does not mean an individual will not develop colorectal cancer, nor does it imply that an individual will not develop hereditary colorectal cancer, because Lynch syndrome is the most common type of hereditary colorectal cancer, and 23andMe's test does not include genetic variants for Lynch syndrome. Another example of a limited genetic test is the DTC 23andMe test for Parkinson disease, which includes only 1 variant in *LRRK2* and 1 variant in *GBA* [42]. Although the 23andMe Web site does clearly indicate that other genes are involved and that other variables affect risk, how closely consumers read or understand these types of disclaimers is not known.

Another limitation to DTC testing is that specific tests are often ethnicity specific. For example, in its *BRCA1* and *BRCA2* analyses for hereditary breast and ovarian cancer, the 23andMe test examines only 3 pathogenic variants common in individuals of Ashkenazi Jewish descent (about 11 million people worldwide), but there are more than 2000 reported mutations in these genes. Thus, for the 7.7 billion people who do not have Ashkenazi Jewish heritage, this test is highly unlikely to be relevant [43]. Furthermore, these non-Ashkenazi individuals who do not have one of these 3 variants may incorrectly think that they are free from *BRCA* mutations when, in fact, this test had not begun to address their risk. These largely incomplete genetic tests for inherited disorders are of limited clinical value and may create misperceptions among consumers who are not aware of what was missing from the test [44].

ACCURACY CONCERNS

Concerns about the accuracy of DTC testing have arisen. The disclaimers in DTC testing typically indicate that the information is not to be used for medical decision making; however, consumers still expect and deserve accurate results. A recent study evaluated 49 patient samples that were received by a clinical laboratory for confirmation of genetic variants reported in DTC raw data and found that 40% of the variants reported across multiple genes were false-positives [45]. Among the false-positive findings, 94.1% were in cancer susceptibility genes, including 8 *BRCA1/2* variants, 3 *TP53* variants, 2 *MLH1* variants, a common *CHEK2* pathogenic European founder variant, and 1 variant in *ATM*. As mentioned in a response by the testing company, these variants were not included in the genetic health report produced for the consumer, but were in the raw data, which may be requested by the consumer [46]. The raw data may include variants in genes that would be diagnostic and, in some cases, actionable if reported in a clinical diagnostic setting; however, the raw data often include a disclaimer indicating that the information is neither validated nor intended for medical use. Despite these warnings, third-party services are available with which the consumer can upload the raw data and receive an interpretation [47]. As such, the investigators of the original study suggest that accuracy of the raw data is as important as the data included in the DTC report and that this is an important issue that providers and consumers should recognize [48].

In addition to concerns regarding false-positive results, there may be discrepancies in how the third-party services interpret some variants compared with how the variants would be classified by a clinical laboratory using the ACMG/AMP guidelines for variant interpretation [38]. The same clinical laboratory performing confirmatory studies noted that 8 variants in 5 genes (*ATM*, *BRCA1*, *BRCA2*, *COL3A1*, and *COL5A1*) had been classified as increased risk by a third-party interpretation service, whereas these variants are found at high frequencies in the general population and would be classified as benign by most clinical laboratories [45]. Many variant interpretation services do not provide clinical-grade variant interpretations. Often, these services query public databases, such as dbSNP (Single Nucleotide Polymorphism Database), and then report the classification provided in the database rather than using the systematic approach outlined in the ACMG/AMP guidelines to assess the probability that the variant causes disease. As such, discrepancies are expected but can be misleading to the patient and/or provider [47,49]. Before a medical provider acts on a result from DTC testing, a confirmatory test should be ordered from a reputable clinical diagnostic laboratory [45].

CONSUMER-INITIATED PHARMACOGENOMICS

Although many DTC and consumer-initiated genetic tests involve traits, ancestry, and disease risk prediction, some tests are either exclusively for pharmacogenomics or include pharmacogenomic information. Pharmacogenomic testing provides information to predict likelihood of medication response and/or risk for adverse medication reaction to aid in medication selection or dosing. Most of the genes tested encode enzymes that metabolize medications; however, genes encoding drug targets, transporters, and human leukocyte antigen molecules may also be tested.

Pharmacogenomic testing has the potential to significantly affect patients, given that most individuals take 1 or more medications over a lifetime and that several recent studies have shown that greater than 90% of individuals have at least 1 variant that would be actionable if a relevant medication were to be prescribed [50–53]. In late 2018, the FDA authorized marketing of a DTC pharmacogenetic report by 23andMe [54]. In the announcement, the FDA indicated that medical decisions should be made after discussing the results with a health care provider rather than by a consumer independently and that the test results should be confirmed using clinical pharmacogenetics testing. Shortly after granting 23andMe marketing approval for their pharmacogenetic report, the FDA issued a safety communication warning both patients and providers that many genetic tests claiming to predict medication response have not been reviewed by the FDA and that recommendations for some medications may not be supported by sufficient evidence [55].

CHALLENGES OF CONSUMER-INITIATED PHARMACOGENOMIC TESTING

DTC pharmacogenomic testing presents a few unique challenges. First, as stated by the FDA, consumers should not alter medication therapy independently from a health care provider. Many tests feature colorful reports that appear easy to interpret on first glance. As such, it has been suggested that, if consumers were to receive information that a medication may be harmful to them, they may decide to discontinue the medication until they can make an appointment to discuss the result. A study of 961 patients who underwent DTC pharmacogenomic testing found that, among the 875 participants with at least 1 result suggesting an increased risk of adverse medication reaction or decreased likelihood of response, less than 1% of consumers (9 out of 875) reported an unsupervised medication change within the first 6 months after receiving results [56]. Although this is reassuring in some respects, scaling up the testing to hundreds of thousands or millions of individuals and applying a 0.9% rate of unsupervised medication changes could have a significant impact. In addition, some participants may have been unwilling to admit unsupervised changes, so this may represent an underestimate. Overall, less than 6% of participants changed a prescription (unsupervised or in consultation with a health care provider) in response to testing, indicating that many individuals within this population may not have been taking relevant medications for which testing revealed an actionable result.

Consumer-initiated testing sometimes does involve a provider as an intermediary (see Fig. 1); however, this individual is most often not the patient's typical prescriber and may not be involved beyond placing the test order. As such, it is unclear whether these models of consumer-initiated testing have similar rates of unsupervised medication changes. Similar to other genetic testing, many providers are not comfortable with pharmacogenomic results, potentially presenting a barrier to clinical use of the information. A study of 481 DTC pharmacogenomic test recipients and 844 participants awaiting results found that the result recipients used more physician visits and their providers were more likely to order additional tests, whereas there were no differences in anxiety or distress related to follow-up tests [57].

A second challenge facing consumer-initiated pharmacogenomic testing is that results are typically returned as a pdf file and not integrated into discrete results in the electronic health record (EHR). For optimal effectiveness of preemptive pharmacogenomic testing, which is performed before the point in time when results are needed, the results need to be readily available at the time a medication is prescribed for which results are actionable. This requirement is typically accomplished by use of clinical decision support alerts, which require structured data [58,59]. In some EHRs, providers are able to manually enter information from tests that do not automatically populate discrete fields via an interface; however, manual entry is subject to data entry error and is generally not recommended for laboratory results without careful quality control measures. Even with mechanisms in place for easy deposit of data from DTC pharmacogenomic tests, there may be drawbacks. Test results must be clinically confirmed before use, so entry of these data may lead to confusion as to whether the information is from the initial test or the confirmatory test. In addition, testing is not currently standardized and DTC/consumer-initiated tests may not include the same genes or alleles as clinical testing, which may lead to discrepancies in results [59–61].

Similar to other consumer-initiated genetic tests, pharmacogenomic tests may also be limited in the variants or alleles detected. Although this may lead to false-negative results for hereditary conditions, it may also lead to inappropriate medication recommendations in pharmacogenomics. Recently, an AMP working group published guidelines establishing a minimum set of alleles that should be included in testing for *CYP2C19* and *CYP2C9* [62,63]. Alleles were recommended in tier 1 if they were well-characterized variants that were known to have an impact on drug response, an appreciable minor allele frequency in a population, and publicly available reference materials; tier 2 alleles met at least 1 but not all criteria required for inclusion in tier 1. A comparison of the alleles included in the only currently approved DTC pharmacogenomic test against the recommendations for these two genes is included in Fig. 2.

<table>
<tr><th></th><th colspan="2">CYP2C19</th><th colspan="2">CYP2C9</th></tr>
<tr><th></th><th>AMP Recommendation</th><th>DTC (23andMe)</th><th>AMP Recommendation</th><th>DTC (23andMe)</th></tr>
<tr><td rowspan="6">Tier 1</td><td rowspan="2">*2</td><td rowspan="2">✓</td><td>*2</td><td>✓</td></tr>
<tr><td>*3</td><td>✓</td></tr>
<tr><td rowspan="2">*3</td><td rowspan="2">✓</td><td>*5</td><td>✓</td></tr>
<tr><td>*6</td><td>✓</td></tr>
<tr><td rowspan="2">*17</td><td rowspan="2">✓</td><td>*8</td><td>x</td></tr>
<tr><td>*11</td><td>x</td></tr>
<tr><td rowspan="9">Tier 2</td><td>*4A</td><td>x</td><td rowspan="3">*12</td><td rowspan="3">x</td></tr>
<tr><td>*4B</td><td>x</td></tr>
<tr><td>*5</td><td>x</td></tr>
<tr><td>*6</td><td>x</td><td rowspan="3">*13</td><td rowspan="3">x</td></tr>
<tr><td>*7</td><td>x</td></tr>
<tr><td>*8</td><td>x</td></tr>
<tr><td>*9</td><td>x</td><td rowspan="3">*15</td><td rowspan="3">x</td></tr>
<tr><td>*10</td><td>x</td></tr>
<tr><td>*35</td><td>x</td></tr>
</table>

FIG. 2 Comparison between minimum set of *CYP2C19* and *CYP2C9* alleles recommended by AMP for inclusion in clinical testing and the alleles included in the 23andMe DTC test for these genes. Recommended alleles are listed by tier, with tier 1 indicating the allele results in altered function, is present at an appreciable minor allele frequency in a population, and reference materials are available. Tier 2 alleles met at least 1, but not all 3, criteria required for tier 1. A tick (✓) and green shading indicates the allele is included in the DTC test, whereas an x and red shading indicates that it is not included. (*AMP recommendation data from* Pratt VM, Del Tredici AL, Hachad H, et al. Recommendations for clinical CYP2C19 genotyping allele selection: a report of the Association for Molecular Pathology. J Mol Diagn. 2018;20(3):269-76; and Pratt VM, Cavallari LH, Del Tredici AL, et al. Recommendations for clinical CYP2C9 genotyping allele selection: a joint recommendation of the Association for Molecular Pathology and College of American Pathologists. J Mol Diagn. 2019 [published online ahead of print]; https://doi.org/10.1016/j.jmoldx.2019.04.003.)

SUMMARY

Rapid advances in genetic knowledge, decreasing costs of testing, and growing public interest in personalized medicine have led to the emergence of DTC and consumer-initiated genetic testing. Although this represents an exciting time for consumers to have easier access to their personal genetic information, it also signals a major change for the medical community in terms of the knowledge and types of questions with which a patient may now present. It is essential for providers to be knowledgeable about the types of testing available, including which results may and may not be used for medical decisions, and to be prepared to answer questions or have resources available when patients bring test results along to appointments. Furthermore, both consumers and health care providers should be aware of the limitations and risks of consumer-initiated genetic testing.

REFERENCES

[1] Hendricks-Sturrup RM, Prince AER, Lu CY. Direct-to-consumer genetic testing and potential loopholes in protecting consumer privacy and nondiscrimination. JAMA 2019. https://doi.org/10.1001/jama.2019.3384.

[2] U.S. Government Accountability Office. Direct-to-consumer genetic tests: misleading test results are further complicated by deceptive marketing and other questionable practices: congretional testimony. Available at: http://www.gao.gov/assets/130/125079.pdf. Accessed May 27, 2019.

[3] Annas GJ, Elias S. 23andMe and the FDA. N Engl J Med 2014;370(11):985–8.

[4] Green RC, Farahany NA. Regulation: the FDA is overcautious on consumer genomics. Nature 2014;505(7483): 286–7.

[5] U.S. Food and Drug Administration. Direct-to-consumer tests. Available at: https://www.fda.gov/medical-devices/vitro-diagnostics/direct-consumer-tests. Accessed May 27, 2019.

[6] U.S. Food and Drug Administration. FDA allows marketing of first direct-to-consumer tests that provide genetic risk information for certain conditions. Available at: https://www.fda.gov/newsevents/newsroom/pressannouncements/ucm551185.htm. Accessed May 25, 2019.

[7] Wynn J, Chung WK. 23andMe paves the way for direct-to-consumer genetic health risk tests of limited clinical utility. Ann Intern Med 2017;167(2):125–6.

[8] Park JY, Risher MT, Caulfield T, et al. Privacy in direct-to-consumer genetic testing. Clin Chem 2019;65(5):612–7.

[9] Nielsen DE, Carere DA, Wang C, et al. Diet and exercise changes following direct-to-consumer personal genomic testing. BMC Med Genomics 2017;10(1):24.

[10] Kaufman DJ, Bollinger JM, Dvoskin RL, et al. Risky business: risk perception and the use of medical services among customers of DTC personal genetic testing. J Genet Couns 2012;21(3):413–22.

[11] Bloss CS, Schork NJ, Topol EJ. Effect of direct-to-consumer genomewide profiling to assess disease risk. N Engl J Med 2011;364(6):524–34.

[12] Bloss CS, Wineinger NE, Darst BF, et al. Impact of direct-to-consumer genomic testing at long term follow-up. J Med Genet 2013;50(6):393–400.

[13] Gray SW, Gollust SE, Carere DA, et al. Personal genomic testing for cancer risk: results from the impact of personal genomics study. J Clin Oncol 2017;35(6):636–44.

[14] Li SX, Ye Z, Whelan K, et al. The effect of communicating the genetic risk of cardiometabolic disorders on motivation and actual engagement in preventative lifestyle modification and clinical outcome: a systematic review and meta-analysis of randomised controlled trials. Br J Nutr 2016;116(5):924–34.

[15] Hollands GJ, French DP, Griffin SJ, et al. The impact of communicating genetic risks of disease on risk-reducing health behaviour: systematic review with meta-analysis. BMJ 2016;352:i1102.

[16] Janssens AC. The hidden harm behind the return of results from personal genome services: a need for rigorous and responsible evaluation. Genet Med 2015;17(8):621–2.

[17] Roberts JS, Gornick MC, Carere DA, et al. Direct-to-consumer genetic testing: user motivations, decision making, and perceived utility of results. Public Health Genomics 2017;20(1):36–45.

[18] Broady KM, Ormond KE, Topol EJ, et al. Predictors of adverse psychological experiences surrounding genome-wide profiling for disease risk. J Community Genet 2018;9(3):217–25.

[19] Egglestone C, Morris A, O'Brien A. Effect of direct-to-consumer genetic tests on health behaviour and anxiety: a survey of consumers and potential consumers. J Genet Couns 2013;22(5):565–75.

[20] Francke U, Dijamco C, Kiefer AK, et al. Dealing with the unexpected: consumer responses to direct-access BRCA mutation testing. PeerJ 2013;1:e8.

[21] Carere DA, Kraft P, Kaphingst KA, et al. Consumers report lower confidence in their genetics knowledge following direct-to-consumer personal genomic testing. Genet Med 2016;18(1):65–72.

[22] Agro C, Denne L. Twins get some 'mystifying' results when they put 5 DNA ancestry kits to the test. Available at: https://www.cbc.ca/news/technology/dna-ancestry-kits-twins-marketplace-1.4980976. Accessed June 11, 2019.

[23] Walajahi H, Wilson DR, Hull SC. Constructing identities: the implications of DTC ancestry testing for tribal communities. Genet Med 2019. https://doi.org/10.1038/s41436-018-0429-2.

[24] Crawshaw M. Direct-to-consumer DNA testing: the fallout for individuals and their families unexpectedly learning of their donor conception origins. Hum Fertil (Camb) 2018;21(4):225–8. Available at: https://www.apa.org/monitor/2018/06/cover-genetic-testing. Accessed May 29, 2019.

[25] Pappas S. Genetic testing and family secrets. Monitor on Psychology 2018;49(6):44.

[26] Hamilton JG, Abdiwahab E, Edwards HM, et al. Primary care providers' cancer genetic testing-related knowledge, attitudes, and communication behaviors: a systematic review and research agenda. J Gen Intern Med 2017;32(3):315–24.

[27] Powell KP, Cogswell WA, Christianson CA, et al. Primary care physicians' awareness, experience and opinions of direct-to-consumer genetic testing. J Genet Couns 2012; 21(1):113–26.

[28] Mikat-Stevens NA, Larson IA, Tarini BA. Primary-care providers' perceived barriers to integration of genetics services: a systematic review of the literature. Genet Med 2015;17(3):169–76.

[29] Pet DB, Holm IA, Williams JL, et al. Physicians' perspectives on receiving unsolicited genomic results. Genet Med 2019;21(2):311–8.

[30] Powell KP, Christianson CA, Cogswell WA, et al. Educational needs of primary care physicians regarding direct-to-consumer genetic testing. J Genet Couns 2012;21(3):469–78.
[31] van der Wouden CH, Carere DA, Maitland-van der Zee AH, et al. Consumer perceptions of interactions with primary care providers after direct-to-consumer personal genomic testing. Ann Intern Med 2016;164(8):513–22.
[32] Koeller DR, Uhlmann WR, Carere DA, et al, PGen Study Group. Utilization of genetic counseling after direct-to-consumer genetic testing: findings from the impact of Personal Genomics (PGen) Study. J Genet Couns 2017;26(6):1270–9.
[33] Bollinger JM, Green RC, Kaufman D. Attitudes about regulation among direct-to-consumer genetic testing customers. Genet Test Mol Biomarkers 2013;17(5):424–8.
[34] Guerrini CJ, Robinson JO, Petersen D, et al. Should police have access to genetic genealogy databases? Capturing the Golden State Killer and other criminals using a controversial new forensic technique. PLoS Biol 2018;16(10):e2006906.
[35] Kim J, Edge MD, Algee-Hewitt BFB, et al. Statistical detection of relatives typed with disjoint forensic and biomedical loci. Cell 2018;175(3):848–58.e6.
[36] Schwab AP, Luu HS, Wang J, et al. Genomic privacy. Clin Chem 2018;64(12):1696–703.
[37] Jay J. Hackers mounting cyber-attacks to access DNA data of thousands of Brits. Available at: https://www.teiss.co.uk/threats/hackers-dna-data-brits/. Accessed June 11, 2019.
[38] Richards S, Aziz N, Bale S, et al. Standards and guidelines for the interpretation of sequence variants: a joint consensus recommendation of the American College of Medical Genetics and Genomics and the Association for Molecular Pathology. Genet Med 2015;17(5):405–24.
[39] Lu JT, Ferber M, Hagenkord J, et al. Evaluation for genetic disorders in the absence of a clinical indication for testing: elective genomic testing. J Mol Diagn 2019;21(1):3–12.
[40] Adams MC, Evans JP, Henderson GE, et al. The promise and peril of genomic screening in the general population. Genet Med 2016;18(6):593–9.
[41] Ducharme J. 23andMe has a new genetic cancer test. But the results don't tell you the whole story. Available at: https://time.com/5510557/23andme-colorectal-cancer-test/. Accessed June 11, 2019.
[42] 23andMe. Available at: https://www.23andme.com/topics/health-predispositions/parkinsons-disease/. Accessed: May 28, 2019.
[43] Why you should be careful about 23andMe's health test. Available at: https://www.nytimes.com/interactive/2019/02/01/opinion/23andme-cancer-dna-test-brca.html. Accessed June 11, 2019.
[44] Baudhuin LM. The FDA and 23andMe: violating the first amendment or protecting the rights of consumers? Clin Chem 2014;60(6):835–7.
[45] Tandy-Connor S, Guiltinan J, Krempely K, et al. False-positive results released by direct-to-consumer genetic tests highlight the importance of clinical confirmation testing for appropriate patient care. Genet Med 2018;20(12):1515–21.
[46] Wu S, Pollard J, Chowdry A, et al. Addressing the accuracy of direct-to-consumer genetic testing. Genet Med 2019;21(3):758–9.
[47] Badalato L, Kalokairinou L, Borry P. Third party interpretation of raw genetic data: an ethical exploration. Eur J Hum Genet 2017;25(11):1189–94.
[48] Tandy-Connor S, Krempely K, Pesaran T, et al. Advocating for the consumer: clinical confirmation of all direct-to-consumer raw data alterations remains critical. Genet Med 2019;21(3):760–1.
[49] Dorschner MO, Amendola LM, Turner EH, et al. Actionable, pathogenic incidental findings in 1,000 participants' exomes. Am J Hum Genet 2013;93(4):631–40.
[50] Van Driest SL, Shi Y, Bowton EA, et al. Clinically actionable genotypes among 10,000 patients with preemptive pharmacogenomic testing. Clin Pharmacol Ther 2014;95(4):423–31.
[51] Ji Y, Skierka JM, Blommel JH, et al. Preemptive pharmacogenomic testing for precision medicine: a comprehensive analysis of five actionable pharmacogenomic genes using next-generation DNA sequencing and a customized CYP2D6 genotyping cascade. J Mol Diagn 2016;18(3):438–45.
[52] Mostafa S, Kirkpatrick CMJ, Byron K, et al. An analysis of allele, genotype and phenotype frequencies, actionable pharmacogenomic (PGx) variants and phenoconversion in 5408 Australian patients genotyped for CYP2D6, CYP2C19, CYP2C9 and VKORC1 genes. J Neural Transm (Vienna) 2019;126(1):5–18.
[53] Bush WS, Crosslin DR, Owusu-Obeng A, et al. Genetic variation among 82 pharmacogenes: The PGRNseq data from the eMERGE network. Clin Pharmacol Ther 2016;100(2):160–9.
[54] U.S. Food and Drug Administration. FDA authorizes first direct-to-consumer test for detecting genetic variants that may be associated with medication metabolism. Available at: https://www.fda.gov/news-events/press-announcements/fda-authorizes-first-direct-consumer-test-detecting-genetic-variants-may-be-associated-medication. Accessed May 29, 2019.
[55] U.S. Food and Drug Administration. The FDA warns against the use of many genetic tests with unapproved claims to predict patient response to specific medications: FDA safety communication. Available at: https://www.fda.gov/medical-devices/safety-communications/fda-warns-against-use-many-genetic-tests-unapproved-claims-predict-patient-response-specific#actions. Accessed May 29, 2019.

[56] Carere DA, VanderWeele TJ, Vassy JL, et al. Prescription medication changes following direct-to-consumer personal genomic testing: findings from the Impact of Personal Genomics (PGen) Study. Genet Med 2017; 19(5):537–45.

[57] Bloss CS, Schork NJ, Topol EJ. Direct-to-consumer pharmacogenomic testing is associated with increased physician utilisation. J Med Genet 2014;51(2):83–9.

[58] Caraballo PJ, Sutton JA, Moyer AM, et al. Technical challenges and opportunities when implementing pharmacogenomics decision support integrated in the electronic health record. Stud Health Technol Inform 2017;245: 1255.

[59] Moyer AM, Caraballo PJ. The challenges of implementing pharmacogenomic testing in the clinic. Expert Rev Pharmacoecon Outcomes Res 2017;17(6): 567–77.

[60] Moyer AM, Rohrer Vitek CR, Giri J, et al. Challenges in ordering and interpreting pharmacogenomic tests in clinical practice. Am J Med 2017;130(12):1342–4.

[61] Bousman CA, Jaksa P, Pantelis C. Systematic evaluation of commercial pharmacogenetic testing in psychiatry: a focus on CYP2D6 and CYP2C19 allele coverage and results reporting. Pharmacogenet Genomics 2017;27(11): 387–93.

[62] Pratt VM, Del Tredici AL, Hachad H, et al. Recommendations for clinical CYP2C19 genotyping allele selection: a report of the Association for Molecular Pathology. J Mol Diagn 2018;20(3):269–76.

[63] Pratt VM, Cavallari LH, Del Tredici AL, et al. Recommendations for clinical CYP2C9 genotyping allele selection: a joint recommendation of the Association for Molecular Pathology and College of American Pathologists. J Mol Diagn 2019. https://doi.org/10.1016/j.jmoldx.2019.04.003.

Informatics

Advances in Molecular Pathology 2 (2019) 143–152

ADVANCES IN MOLECULAR PATHOLOGY

Machine Learning in Biology and Medicine

Javad Noorbakhsh, PhD[a,1], Harshpreet Chandok, MS[b,1], R. Krishna Murthy Karuturi, PhD[b,*], Joshy George, PhD[b,*]

[a]The Jackson Laboratory for Genomic Medicine, 10 Discovery Drive, Farmington, CT 06032, USA; [b]Computational Sciences, The Jackson Laboratory for Genomic Medicine, 10 Discovery Drive, Farmington, CT 06032, USA

KEYWORDS

• Computational biology • Medicine • Machine learning • Supervised learning • Unsupervised learning • Reinforcement learning • Lifelong learning

KEY POINTS

- Understanding complex biological processes in a cell is critical to improve the understanding of the biology of most diseases and will help to optimally intervene to mitigate the disease.
- The state of the cells involved in the disease can be characterized using multimodal imaging and next-generation sequencing technologies.
- Commonly, the phenotype information of the disease is in clinical records as unstructured text.
- Machine learning is a technology that enables us to understand the relationship between the state of the cells and the phenotype of the disease.
- In this review, the authors introduce common machine learning paradigms and illustrate how they can be used for the progress in biology and medicine.

INTRODUCTION

Humans, like other multicellular organisms, are made up of many cells, the fundamental units of life. The cells in a complex multicellular organism are organized into tissues, which are groups of similar cells that work together on a specific task. Organs are structures made up of 2 or more tissues organized to carry out a particular function. The cells in a tissue have specific functions, and the molecular processes in the cells are regulated to achieve this functionality. A disease condition happens when the regulatory process breaks down [1–6]. The breakdown in the regulatory mechanisms can happen in several ways, including single nucleotide mutations, insertions and deletions, copy number changes, epigenetic modifications, and changes in the chromatin conformations [7]. It is important to identify the alterations responsible for the disruption of these biochemical processes before an optimal intervention can be made.

Recent advances in the next-generation sequencing (NGS) technologies and multimodal imaging enable us to comprehensively profile the genomic, epigenetic, and protein profiles of the normal and diseased tissues

Disclosure Statement: The work was partially supported by the National Cancer Institute of the National Institutes of Health under Award Number P30CA034196.

[1] Equal contribution.

*Corresponding authors. *E-mail addresses:* krishna.karuturi@jax.org; joshy.george@jax.org
twitter: @JavadNoorbakhsh (J.N.); @harshpreet_22 (H.C.); @karuturi_murthy (K.K.); @gjoshy (J.G.)

https://doi.org/10.1016/j.yamp.2019.07.010 www.advancesinmolecularpathology.com
2589-4080/19/

[8–10]. Together these molecular profiles comprise the genotype of the disease. Clinical practices and research leveraging electronic health records (EHRs) are widely implemented [11,12] and therefore provide a comprehensive characterization of the phenotype of the disease [13].

Using machine learning (ML) algorithms, we can integrate large scale heterogeneous data (e.g. clinical, imaging, and genomic data), and allow researchers to better understand the genetic basis of disease and identify the optimal therapeutic approach. Several research programs have been designed to take advantage of this approach, as exemplified by the *All of Us* research program, which aims to collect genome sequence data from 1 million participants to become a critical component of the precision medicine research platform [9,14].

Given such massive datasets, one could in principle integrate molecular markers and other clinical correlates of disease to devise rules to identify appropriate clinical decision. However, as the number of scenarios increases, defining rules to accurately address all scenarios becomes very demanding, ineffiecient, and innaccurate. ML approaches, on the other hand, do not depend on rules defined by human experts. Instead, they process data in raw form and are programmed to learn to perform the task of identifying these rules. Usually, the tasks are not well-defined and a concise relationship between input and output may not be known. Instead several examples of input/output pairs are presented to the algorithm. The computational method then adjusts its parameters in order to provide the best approximation of the relationship implicit in the input/output examples. This approach has been successfully applied in solving important clinical challenges, such as detection of retinopathy [15], melanoma [16], and Parkinson disease [17], and in predicting readmission risk [18].

In this review, we initially introduce the major categories of ML with their application in biology and medicine. We, then discuss deep learning and text mining as separate topics, and discuss the significant impact that these methods have made in the medical research recently. We, then review some of the successful applications of ML to complex problems in biology and medicine.

MACHINE LEARNING PARADIGM

There are 3 basic types of learning paradigms in ML: supervised learning, unsupervised learning, and reinforcement learning (RL).

Supervised Learning

The supervised learning method can be used to design a predictor using samples with known class labels (training data) to predict the class of a new sample. For example, the gene expression profile of a tumor sample can be used to predict the prognosis of the patient using a predictor built from gene expression profiles of tumor samples with known patient prognosis [19]. The supervised learning process is called a classification when the output labels are categorical (eg, good vs poor prognosis), and called regression when the output is continuous (eg, number of months survived). Linear and logistic regressions are examples of supervised learning algorithms. The predictor (to be precise, function to predict) learned could be a straight line or a very complex curve in a very high dimensional space depending on the nature of the data provided. There are several hundred different classification algorithms have been developed [20], as the No Free Lunch theorem guarantees that there is no such thing as an optimal classification algorithm that works for all datasets and clinical decisions to be modeled [21].

One important question that arises in supervised learning is the performance of the classification model in classifying a new sample. Empirical learning of classifiers attempts to infer a prediction model from only a finite set of samples. Therefore, a complicated model can learn not only the real patterns but also the noise in the training data to the extent that it negatively impacts the performance of the model on new data, a phenomenon called overfitting. When this happens, the average prediction error estimated during training could be much lower than the error on unknown samples. Regularization is a way to balance the classification error and the complexity of the model, to favor simpler over unnecessarily complicated models, thus imposing Occam's razor on the solution.

Cross-validation is a strategy to test the model's ability to predict new data that was not used in estimating it, in order to flag problems like overfitting or selection bias and to give an insight on how the model will generalize to an independent dataset. Typically, this involves partitioning the data into mutually exclusive subsets, developing the classifier model on one subset and validating the analysis on the remaining subset. To reduce variability, multiple rounds of cross-validation are performed using different partitions, and the validation results are combined over the rounds to give an estimate of the model's predictive performance [22,23].

Often, the cross-validation procedure is also used to tune the hyperparameters (parameters that govern learning of the predictor) of the classification model. If this is indeed the case, then one risks the possibility of optimistically biasing the error estimation. One way to overcome this problem is to use a nested cross-validation methodology whereby inner cross-validation is used to tune the parameters and select the best model. Second, outer cross-validation is used to evaluate the model selected by the inner cross-validation and select hyperparameters for best prediction performance [24].

Supervised learning methods have been successfully used in the design of prognostic and predictive biomarkers. A variety of factors influence a patient's clinical outcome, including intrinsic characteristics of the patient, the disease, and the effects of any treatments that the patient receives. The treatment-independent characteristics are called prognostic factors, whereas the biomarkers that can identify the response to a therapeutic regimen are called predictive biomarkers. Prognostic biomarkers identify the patients who are to be treated aggressively, and predictive biomarkers help to identify the optimal therapy for the patient. In addition, prognostic markers can also reveal the biology of the disease process. In cancer, these outcomes are usually death, recurrence of disease, or both. For such studies, distinct study phases have been proposed and usually begin with exploratory studies to identify promising prognostic markers and move toward larger, preferably prospective, confirmatory studies [25]. Phase 1 studies are early exploratory analyses to generate hypotheses and to identify potential markers for further investigation. Phase 2 studies continue the exploratory investigation and assess the relationship between marker and prognosis. Phase 3 studies are large, confirmatory studies that state prior hypotheses and should certainly be protocol driven to ensure the highest level of evidence [26].

The method used to derive the prognostic markers can have a strong influence on the results and on the interpretation of the study. Successful ML methods used in the design of prognostic markers include regression models and classification and regression trees [27]. Other approaches, for example, artificial neural networks (ANN), are sometimes used for the analysis of marker studies [28,29]. An exemplary application of supervised learning method is the 70-gene-panel–based predictor to identify low-risk patients accurately in early-stage breast cancer, thereby relieving them from the side effects of unnecessary chemotherapy [30].

Unsupervised Learning

Unsupervised learning is a class of algorithms used to draw inferences on underlying organization and associations among the samples without relevant labels. Cluster analysis, association rule mining, and dimensionality reduction methods are all part of the unsupervised analysis.

Cluster analysis is a method that groups the samples into distinct groups such that the samples in the same group are more similar to each other than samples in other groups. There are several clustering algorithms available with different pros and cons. The most commonly used clustering algorithms in biomedical research are the K-means, hierarchical clustering, and self-organizing maps [31].

It is often assumed that the clusters identified are truly meaningful in the sense that they correspond to a real underlying grouping. However, in reality, there is no agreed definition of what a true cluster is, and the interpretation strongly depends on the context and aim of the research [32].

Association rule learning is an unsupervised analysis method for discovering interesting relations among features characterizing samples based on a chosen measure of interestingness [33]. The final goal is to help machine mimic the human brain's feature extraction and association capabilities from uncategorized data. Association rule learning algorithms have been successfully used to detect multimorbidity and comorbidity in old age [34].

Unsupervised learning has been most used in identifying homogeneous subgroups of biological samples. In most diseases, the clinical outcome and therapeutic effectiveness are heterogeneous, and therefore, it is important to identify homogeneous subgroups of patients to identify the biological determinants of the disease and effectiveness of therapy. This approach has been very successful in the treatment of patients with breast cancer [35–37], but there is a growing realization that such an approach would be beneficial for all cancer types [38–41].

Another application of unsupervised learning algorithms is in the analysis of single-cell RNA-seq data to identify novel cell types in a tissue [42–44].

Reinforcement Learning

RL is an approach that is categorized between supervised and unsupervised learning. It does not rely on a set of labeled training data and so is not a supervised learning algorithm, but it is also not unsupervised learning because it relies on the reward that the learning algorithm needs to maximize. The learning approach is to find the right actions to take in different situations to maximize the reward.

RL method has been successfully applied to optimizing antiretroviral therapy in human immunodeficiency virus [45] and in determining the best approach to managing sepsis [46]. Unlike the supervised learning method that produces one-time predictions, the decision made by the RL algorithm affects both the patient's future health and the patient's future treatment option.

In recent times, it is fortunate to have many available treatment options for any given disease condition, and figuring out the best treatment policy to use for a particular patient is challenging for clinicians. In theory, this is a problem that can be addressed using RL algorithm. In a normal RL context to evaluate a policy, one would simply have the agent make decisions and then compute the average reward based on the outcome. Such an approach would not be ethical because of using human subjects in training RL algorithm. Therefore, it is necessary to learn from observational historical data. In RL literature, this is referred to as "Off-Policy Evaluation," and there are many RL algorithms that can learn the optimal policy effectively in this context [47]. Despite this challenge, RL algorithms are being used to solve major challenges in health care [48].

TEXT MINING FOR INFERENCE FROM LITERATURE

The ever-increasing number of scientific publications in the MEDLINE database, which holds millions of references of life sciences-related articles, is a wealth for scientists to garner relevant information. However, getting access to the most relevant information can be tedious because of the lack of intelligent search tools. For example, we have the ability to identify the genomic alterations associated with cancer using sequencing technology at reasonable costs. However, identifying the clinically relevant mutations from the list can be challenging. There are databases for manually curated lists of disease-related and therapeutically targetable genomic alterations, but these are time consuming to construct and often incomplete [49].

ML-based natural language processing (NLP) techniques can be used to extract structured information from unstructured text [50] and then can be curated and categorized based on related terms or keywords [51]. These structured data can then be used as features for ML algorithms to predict disease progression and drug-drug interactions [52].

There are several applications that use NLP technique in health care. For example, DeepPhe is an open source implementation of an NLP method for obtaining phenotype-related information of patients with cancer from EHRs [53]. Another NLP-based approach demonstrated superior performance in the identification of a contralateral breast cancer event from clinical reports [52]. An NLP-based approach is also used to organize and classify cancer-related literature into biologically meaningful categories that can help scientists retrieve the desired information efficiently [54].

However, as the ML or Artificial Intelligence (AI) system gets deployed using the initial dataset for training, the datasets also get updated frequently because of the advances in technology. Efforts are being applied to produce datasets (eg, Dream Challenge [55]) to establish standards for benchmarking, testing, and evaluating the performances of various cancer-related algorithms by overcoming the issues of data sharing, security, and standardization.

DEEP LEARNING

Deep learning or deep neural networks (DNN) is another ML technique, which has gained significant momentum in recent years. DNNs are a class of artificial neural networks (ANN) with a large number of hidden layers and specific activation functions.

The basic building block of an ANN is a neuron, which receives a set of values as input, and produces a single output based on them. The most common form of such a function is achieved by summing the linear combination of all the inputs, each scaled by a corresponding weight, and passing the output through a nonlinear function. A set of such neurons forms a layer, and several such layers are interposed between the input layer and the output layer. The layers between the input and output layers are called hidden layers, and when the number of the hidden layer is many more than one, it is technically referred to as a DNN.

DNNs have become one of the most used ML methods owing to improvements in computing speed combined with their data-driven approach, and a lack of the need for feature engineering. They have in particular been very successful at image classification, speech recognition, and NLP [56–58].

Convolutional neural networks (CNN), a type of DNN, have gained popularity in computer vision because of their ability to summarize local image features in each layer and feed it to the next layer for further abstraction. The basic idea of a CNN is that features in certain data types (such as images) are hierarchical on different length scales. For example, on a small scale, an image is constituted of lines and edges with different contrast. On an intermediate scale, it contains texture structure (eg, furry vs smooth). A higher length scale may correspond to an eye or an ear, and at the larger scales, objects such as faces could be recognized. CNN is structured such that each neuron is specialized in some specific feature depending on its depth in the network. To achieve this, neurons within layers are assumed to have a spatial organization in relation to each other (eg, 2-dimensional or 3-dimensional). The weights of each neuron are set locally by connecting it to the corresponding neuron in the previous layer and its neighboring neurons. By using similar local weights for all neurons within each layer, this approach dramatically reduces the number of model parameters and overcomes overfitting.

CNNs are suitable for processing visual and other 2-dimensional data and have demonstrated superior results in both image and speech applications [59–61]. They can be trained with standard backpropagation and are easier to train than other regular, deep, feed-forward neural networks. In addition to imaging applications in health care, CNNs are also used to call mutation detections by converting sequencing data to images [62,63].

DNNs tend to have many layers with a large number of parameters. In general, there should be 10 times more training cases than the Vapnik-Chervonenkis (VC) dimension of the hypothesis set. In the case of a DNN, the VC dimension is equal to the number of weights. Therefore, one should have 10 times the number of training cases than the weights [64]. A sample size smaller than this can result in overfitting and therefore will not generalize well. Given the cost of labeling data, several procedures have been developed to mitigate this issue. The most common approach is to use a regularization approach that forces some parameters of the model to zero. A dropout is an approach to regularization in neural networks that helps to reduce interdependent learning among the neurons. Using network architectures that are aware of the features in the data also can reduce the number of parameters. For example, in CNNs, parameter space is significantly reduced by using the same parameters for all the neurons within the same layer. Other approaches to compensate for the dearth of data are to use data augmentation (eg, image rotation, normalization, reflection, and distortion), use of attention-based classification, multi-instance learning, and weakly supervised learning.

One major drawback of using DNNs is the "black-box" feature or a lack of clarity on why the network has made the decision. That is, even when a network learns some task very well, it is not very easy to understand how the network has reached its conclusions. In recent years, many efforts have been put into exploring the procedure through which the network learns. One approach is to convert the weights of the neural network into an image format for visualization that may yield insights into the logic of the decision. Another approach is to find a set of inputs that maximize the output of specific neurons. By repeating such an approach, it has been shown that certain neurons in the network become specialized to respond to specific inputs [65].

There have been significant advances in use of DNN for clinical applications. For example, deep learning was used to predict anticancer drug combination outcome directly from gene expression data in cell line experiments [66]. CNNs have also been extensively used for image analysis in clinical settings. For example, they have been used for classification of skin lesions into malignant and benign and have achieved dermatologist-level accuracies [67]. In another work, Khosravi and colleagues [68] applied a CNN framework to blastocyst images from in vitro fertilization cases and outperformed individual embryologists in predicting embryo quality for successful pregnancy.

LIFELONG LEARNING

The classic ML paradigm starts with a labeled dataset to which a learning algorithm is applied to produce a model without considering any previously learned knowledge. This approach may need a large number of training examples depending on the complexity of the learning algorithm, and can be quite limited; especially in the clinical setting, where data points are continuously being acquired. Therefore, it is necessary to do lifelong ML or continuous learning, which tries to mimic "human learning" to build a lifelong learning machine. Ideally, this approach should also be able to discover new tasks and learn on the job in open environments in a self-supervised manner. One could argue that without the lifelong learning capability, ML systems will probably never be truly intelligent [69].

CAVEATS IN THE APPLICATION OF MACHINE LEARNING

ML depends on the quality, objectivity, and size of the data sets used to generate the model, and a lack of truly random or comprehensive data can result in bias.

TABLE 1
Machine Learning Paradigms, Algorithms, and Their Applications

Learning Category	ML Method	Characteristics	Scope of Applications	References
Supervised learning	K-Nearest Neighbor	Does not involve training (lazy learning)	Image classification, predicting the molecular subtype of cancers	Li et al [74], 2012
	Naïve Bayes	Assumes features are independent (conditioned on class membership)	Cancer type predictions	Banu & Thirumalai-kolunduoubramanian [75], 2018
	Decision Trees	Provides interpretable rules of classification	Prognostic markers, predictive markers	Geurts et al [76], 2009
	Support Vector Machines	Linear and nonlinear classification. Maximum-margin criteria provide robust generalization ability	Prognostic markers, predictive markers	Wu et al [77], 2017
	Neural Networks	Capable of learning complex problems with little fine-tuning, computationally intensive; tends to be difficult to interpret	Cancer risk prediction, identifying new chemotypes	Mueller et al [78], 2012
	Deep Learning	Essentially, neural networks with many hidden layers	Ideal for computer vision applications (pathology images) and text mining (EHR)	Angermueller et al [55], 2016; Tang et al [79], 2019; Webb [80], 2018
Unsupervised learning	K-means clustering	Partitions the observations in predefined k clusters in which each observation belongs to the cluster with the nearest mean	RNA-seq analysis, sequence clustering, image cytometry	Nugent & Meila [81], 2010
	Hierarchical clustering	Provides hierarchical organization of samples and clusters enable better visualization of the structure in the data	Very popular in biological domain because of the excellent visualization capabilities	Ronan et al [82], 2016
	Spectral clustering	Global and local structure of the similarities among samples determines the clustering	Single-cell RNA-sequencing data analysis	Zheng et al [14], 2019; Kiselev et al [42], 2017
RL	Q-learning	Finds a policy that maximizes the expected value of the total reward over all successive steps starting from the current state	Behavioral ecology	Frankenhuis et al [83], 2019
	Temporal difference	Learn by bootstrapping from the current estimate of the value function	Models for learning in biological systems	Neftci & Averbeck [84], 2019

(continued on next page)

TABLE 1
(*continued*)

Learning Category	ML Method	Characteristics	Scope of Applications	References
Others	Generative Adversarial Networks	Two neural networks contest with each other to generate new data with the same statistics as the training set	Understanding the organization of biological systems. generating realistic datasets	Wang et al [85], 2018
	Text mining	A set of techniques that models and structures the information content of textual sources for obtaining information	Extracting information for EHR	Ohno-Machado et al [86], 2013

Eliminating harmful biases is essential because ML is often applied to decisions with serious implications, such as diagnostics and therapeutic interventions in medical environments. The data should be representative of different races, genders, backgrounds, and cultures that could be adversely affected. Scientists developing the algorithms should shape data samples in a way that minimizes bias. Left unchecked, feeding biased data to self-learning systems can lead to unintended and sometimes dangerous outcomes. An example of bias introduced in an ML application is the Correctional Offender Management Profiling for Alternative Sanctions, a machine-learning system that makes recommendations for criminal sentencing, by predicting which people are likely to reoffend. Its training model includes race as an input parameter, but not more extensive data points like past arrests. As a result, it has an inherent racial bias that made it unjust and unethical [70]. Such biases can be an issue even without the involvement of ML algorithms as exemplified by the gender bias in the diagnosis and treatment of coronary heart disease [71], but ML approaches designed with the help of such datasets may exacerbate the problem as policymaking always lags behind innovation.

Modern ML algorithms require far more data for learning because of the large number of parameters in their models. As algorithms make inferences based on these big datasets, there is a higher likelihood of sensitive information being unintentionally included. In addition, sensitive information can be predicted about individuals based on the shared information, thereby threatening individual privacy. The current solution to this problem is to limit access to data which inevitably thwarts innovations in the field. A better solution to this problem needs to be found. A variety of approaches can be used to detect and mitigate the problem of bias in ML systems by designing algorithms that can detect [72] and mitigate biases [73].

SUMMARY

The impact of ML in biology and medicine is accelerating at an increasing pace and is already generating actionable insights (Table 1). Personalized predictive health care is the future of medicine, and ML will play an integral part of this goal. The increased use of such systems will generate more data that can be used to generate better models, and continuous learning algorithms will improve at a much faster pace. The future of biology and medicine looks very promising with deep profiling of patients and advances in machine learning.

REFERENCES

[1] Davies KE, Nowak KJ. Molecular mechanisms of muscular dystrophies: old and new players. Nat Rev Mol Cell Biol 2006;7(10):762–73.

[2] Heineke J, Molkentin JD. Regulation of cardiac hypertrophy by intracellular signalling pathways. Nat Rev Mol Cell Biol 2006;7(8):589–600.

[3] Guggino WB, Stanton BA. New insights into cystic fibrosis: molecular switches that regulate CFTR. Nat Rev Mol Cell Biol 2006;7(6):426–36.

[4] Kudlow BA, Kennedy BK, Monnat RJ Jr. Werner and Hutchinson Gilford progeria syndromes: mechanistic basis of human progeroid diseases. Nat Rev Mol Cell Biol 2007;8(5):394–404.

[5] Muoio DM, Newgard CB. Molecular and metabolic mechanisms of insulin resistance and β-cell failure in type 2 diabetes. Nat Rev Mol Cell Biol 2008;9(3):193–205.

[6] Golemis EA, Scheet P, Beck TN, et al. Molecular mechanisms of the preventable causes of cancer in the United States. Genes Dev 2018;32(13–14):868–902.

[7] Byun JA, Melacini G. NMR methods to dissect the molecular mechanisms of disease-related mutations (DRMs): understanding how DRMs remodel functional free energy landscapes. Methods 2018;148:19–27.
[8] Carter TC, He MM. Challenges of identifying clinically actionable genetic variants for precision medicine. J Healthc Eng 2016;2016.
[9] Collins FS, Varmus H. A new initiative on precision medicine. N Engl J Med 2015;372(9):793–5.
[10] Kitchen RR, Rozowsky JS, Gerstein MB, et al. Decoding neuroproteomics: integrating the genome, translatome and functional anatomy. Nat Neurosci 2014;17(11):1491–9.
[11] Overby CL, Pathak J, Gottesman O, et al. A collaborative approach to developing an electronic health record phenotyping algorithm for drug-induced liver injury. J Am Med Inform Assoc 2013;20(e2):e243–52.
[12] Gottesman O, Kuivaniemi H, Tromp G, et al. The Steele R, Nigam N, Electronic Medical Records and Genomics (eMERGE) Network: past, present, and future. Genet Med 2013;15(10):761–71.
[13] Rasmussen-Torvik LJ, Stallings SC, Gordon AS, et al. Design and anticipated outcomes of the eMERGE-PGx project: a multicenter pilot for preemptive pharmacogenomics in electronic health record systems. Clin Pharmacol Ther 2014;96(4):482–9.
[14] Zheng R, Li M, Liang Z, et al. SinNLRR: a robust subspace clustering method for cell type detection by nonnegative and low rank representation. Bioinformatics 2019 [pii:btz139].
[15] Brown JM, Campbell JP, Beers A, et al. Automated diagnosis of plus disease in retinopathy of prematurity using deep convolutional neural networks. JAMA Ophthalmol 2018;136(7):803–10.
[16] Haenssle HA, Fink C, Schneiderbauer R, et al. Man against machine: diagnostic performance of a deep learning convolutional neural network for dermoscopic melanoma recognition in comparison to 58 dermatologists. Ann Oncol 2018;29(8):1836–42.
[17] Zhan A, Mohan S, Tarolli C, et al. Using smartphones and machine learning to quantify Parkinson disease severity: the mobile Parkinson disease score. JAMA Neurol 2018;75(7):876–80.
[18] Benuzillo J, Caine W, Evans RS, et al. Predicting readmission risk shortly after admission for CABG surgery. J Card Surg 2018;33(4):163–70.
[19] Cuzick J, Swanson GP, Fisher G, et al. Prognostic value of an RNA expression signature derived from cell cycle proliferation genes in patients with prostate cancer: a retrospective study. Lancet Oncol 2011;12(3):245–55.
[20] Ferńandez-Delgado M, Cernadas E, Barro SE. Do we need hundreds of classifiers to solve real world classification problems? J Mach Learn Res 2014;15:3133–81.
[21] Wolpert DH, Macready WG. No free lunch theorems for optimization. IEEE Trans Evol Comput 1997;1:67–82.
[22] Molinaro AM, Simon R, Pfeiffer RM. Prediction error estimation: a comparison of resampling methods. Bioinformatics 2005;21(15):3301–7.
[23] Varma S, Simon R. Bias in error estimation when using cross-validation for model selection. BMC Bioinformatics 2006;7:91.
[24] Cawley GC, Talbot NLC. On over-fitting in model selection and subsequent selection bias in performance evaluation. J Mach Learn Res 2010;11:2079–107.
[25] Ransohoff DF. How to improve reliability and efficiency of research about molecular markers: roles of phases, guidelines, and study design. J Clin Epidemiol 2007; 60(12):1205–19.
[26] Kattan MW. Judging new markers by their ability to improve predictive accuracy. J Natl Cancer Inst 2003; 95(9):634–5.
[27] Zlobec I, Steele R, Nigam N, et al. A predictive model of rectal tumor response to preoperative radiotherapy using classification and regression tree methods. Clin Cancer Res 2005;11(15):5440–3.
[28] Zafeiris D, Rutella S, Ball GR. An artificial neural network integrated pipeline for biomarker discovery using Alzheimer's disease as a case study. Comput Struct Biotechnol J 2018;16:77–87.
[29] Bertolaccini L, Solli P, Pardolesi A, et al. An overview of the use of artificial neural networks in lung cancer research. J Thorac Dis 2017;9(4):924–31.
[30] Cardoso F, van't Veer LJ, Bogaerts J, et al. 70-gene signature as an aid to treatment decisions in early-stage breast cancer. N Engl J Med 2016;375(8):717–29.
[31] D'Haeseleer P. How does gene expression clustering work? Nat Biotechnol 2005;23(12):1499–501.
[32] Hennig C. What are the true clusters? Pattern Recognit Lett 2015;64(15):53–62.
[33] Hipp J, Güntzer U, Nakhaeizadeh G. Algorithms for association rule mining—a general survey and comparison. SIGKDD Explor 2000;2(2):58–64.
[34] Held FP, Blyth F, Gnjidic D, et al. Association rules analysis of comorbidity and multimorbidity: the :concord health and aging in men project. J Gerontol A Biol Sci Med Sci 2016;71(5):625–31.
[35] Perou CM, Sørlie T, Eisen MB, et al. Molecular portraits of human breast tumours. Nature 2000;406(6797):747–52.
[36] Sorlie T, Perou CM, Tibshirani R, et al. Gene expression patterns of breast carcinomas distinguish tumor subclasses with clinical implications. Proc Natl Acad Sci U S A 2001;98(19):10869–74.
[37] Dai X, Li T, Bai Z, et al. Breast cancer intrinsic subtype classification, clinical use and future trends. Am J Cancer Res 2015;5(10):2929–43.
[38] Cancer Genome Atlas Research Network. Comprehensive genomic characterization defines human glioblastoma genes and core pathways. Nature 2008;455(7216):1061–8.
[39] Tothill RW, Tinker AV, George J, et al. Novel molecular subtypes of serous and endometrioid ovarian cancer linked to clinical outcome. Clin Cancer Res 2008; 14(16):5198–208.
[40] Cancer Genome Atlas Network. Comprehensive molecular characterization of human colon and rectal cancer. Nature 2012;487(7407):330–7.

[41] Cancer Genome Atlas Research Network. Comprehensive genomic characterization of squamous cell lung cancers. Nature 2012;489(7417):519–25.
[42] Kiselev VY, Kirschner K, Schaub MT, et al. SC3: consensus clustering of single-cell RNA-seq data. Nat Methods 2017;14(5):483–6.
[43] Xu C, Su Z. Identification of cell types from single-cell transcriptomes using a novel clustering method. Bioinformatics 2015;31(12):1974–80.
[44] Butler A, Hoffman P, Smibert P, et al. Integrating single-cell transcriptomic data across different conditions, technologies, and species. Nat Biotechnol 2018;36(5): 411–20.
[45] Parbhoo S, Bogojeska J, Zazzi M, et al. Combining kernel and model based learning for HIV therapy selection. AMIA Jt Summits Transl Sci Proc 2017;2017:239–48.
[46] Komorowski M, Celi LA, Badawi O, et al. The artificial intelligence clinician learns optimal treatment strategies for sepsis in intensive care. Nat Med 2018;24(11):1716–20.
[47] Gottesman O, Johansson F, Meier J, et al. Evaluating reinforcement learning algorithms in observational health settings. arxiv 2018.
[48] Liu Y, Logan B, Liu N, et al. Deep reinforcement learning for dynamic treatment regimes on medical registry data. Healthc Inform 2017;2017:380–5.
[49] Patterson SE, Statz CM, Yin T, et al. Utility of the JAX Clinical Knowledgebase in capture and assessment of complex genomic cancer data. NPJ Precis Oncol 2019;3:2.
[50] Roden DM, Denny JC. Integrating electronic health record genotype and phenotype datasets to transform patient care. Clin Pharmacol Ther 2016;99(3):298–305.
[51] Sebastiani F. Machine learning in automated text categorization. ACM Comput Surv 2002;34(1):1–47.
[52] Zeng Z, Li X, Espino S, et al. Contralateral breast cancer event detection using nature language processing. AMIA Annu Symp Proc 2018;2017:1885–92.
[53] Savova GK, Tseytlin E, Finan S, et al. DeepPhe: a natural language processing system for extracting cancer phenotypes from clinical records. Cancer Res 2017; 77(21):e115–8.
[54] Baker S, Ali I, Silins I, et al. Cancer Hallmarks Analytics Tool (CHAT): a text mining approach to organize and evaluate scientific literature on cancer. Bioinformatics 2017;33(24):3973–81.
[55] Angermueller C, Pärnamaa T, Parts L, et al. Deep learning for computational biology. Mol Syst Biol 2016;12(7):878.
[56] LeCun Y, Bengio Y, Hinton G. Deep learning. Nature 2015;521(7553):436–44.
[57] Goodfellow IJ, Erhan D, Carrier PL, et al. Challenges in representation learning: a report on three machine learning contests. Neural Netw 2015;64:59–63.
[58] Bengio Y, Lee H. Editorial introduction to the neural networks special issue on deep learning of representations. Neural Netw 2015;64:1–3.
[59] LeCun Y, Boser B, Denker JS, et al. Backpropagation applied to handwritten zip code recognition. Neural Comput 1989;1(4):541–51.
[60] He K, Zhang X, Ren S, et al. Deep Residual Learning for Image Recognition. IEEE Conference on Computer Vision and Pattern Recognition (CVPR), 2016.
[61] Tizhoosh HR, Pantanowitz L. Artificial intelligence and digital pathology: challenges and opportunities. J Pathol Inform 2018;9:38.
[62] Sahraeian SME, Liu R, Lau B, et al. Deep convolutional neural networks for accurate somatic mutation detection. Nat Commun 2019;10(1):1041.
[63] Poplin R, Chang PC, Alexander D, et al. A universal SNP and small-indel variant caller using deep neural networks. Nat Biotechnol 2018;36(10):983–7.
[64] Abu-Mostafa YS, Magdon-Ismail M, Lin H-T. Learning from data 2012.
[65] Yosinski J, Clune J, Nguyen A, et al. Understanding neural networks through deep visualization. arxiv.org; 2015.
[66] Preuer K, Lewis RP, Hochreiter S, et al. DeepSynergy: predicting anti-cancer drug synergy with deep learning. Bioinformatics 2018;34(9):1538–46.
[67] Esteva A, Kuprel B, Novoa RA, et al. Dermatologist-level classification of skin cancer with deep neural networks. Nature 2017;542(7639):115–8.
[68] Khosravi P, Kazemi E, Zhan Q, et al. Deep learning enables robust assessment and selection of human blastocysts after in vitro fertilization. NPJ Digit Med 2019;2(1).
[69] Parisi GI, Kemker R, Part JL, et al. Continual lifelong learning with neural networks: a review. Arxiv 2019.
[70] Larson J, Surya M, Lauren K, et al. How we analyzed the COMPAS recidivism algorithm 2016. Available at: https://www.propublica.org/article/how-we-analyzed-the-compas-recidivism-algorithm.
[71] Beery TA. Gender bias in the diagnosis and treatment of coronary artery disease. Heart Lung 1995;24(6): 427–35.
[72] Chen I, Johansson FD, Sontag D. Why is my classifier discriminatory? Arxiv 2018, Advances in Neural Information Processing Systems 31; 2018. p. 3543–54.
[73] Amini A, Soleimany A, Schwarting W, et al. Uncovering and mitigating algorithmic bias through learned latent structure. In AAAI/ACM Conference on Artificial Intelligence, Ethics and Society. 2019. Honolulu, Hawaii.
[74] Li C, Zhang S, Zhang H, et al. Using the K-nearest neighbor algorithm for the classification of lymph node metastasis in gastric cancer. Comput Math Methods Med 2012;2012:876545.
[75] Banu AB, Thirumalaikolundusubramanian P. Comparison of Bayes classifiers for breast cancer classification. Asian Pac J Cancer Prev 2018;19(10):2917–20.
[76] Geurts P, Irrthum A, Wehenkel L. Supervised learning with decision tree-based methods in computational and systems biology. Mol Biosyst 2009;5(12):1593–605.
[77] Wu T, Wang Y, Jiang R, et al. A pathways-based prediction model for classifying breast cancer subtypes. Oncotarget 2017;8(35):58809–22.
[78] Mueller R, Dawson ES, Meiler J, et al. Discovery of 2-(2-benzoxazoyl amino)-4-aryl-5-cyanopyrimidine as negative allosteric modulators (NAMs) of metabotropic

glutamate receptor 5 (mGlu(5)): from an artificial neural network virtual screen to an in vivo tool compound. ChemMedChem 2012;7(3):406–14.
[79] Tang B, Pan Z, Yin K, et al. Recent advances of deep learning in bioinformatics and computational biology. Front Genet 2019;10:214.
[80] Webb S. Deep learning for biology. Nature 2018; 554(7693):555–7.
[81] Nugent R, Meila M. An overview of clustering applied to molecular biology. Methods Mol Biol 2010;620: 369–404.
[82] Ronan T, Qi Z, Naegle KM. Avoiding common pitfalls when clustering biological data. Sci Signal 2016; 9(432):re6.
[83] Frankenhuis WE, Panchanathan K, Barto AG. Enriching behavioral ecology with reinforcement learning methods. Behav Processes 2019;161:94–100.
[84] Neftci EO, Averbeck BB. Reinforcement learning in artificial and biological systems. Nat Mach Intell 2019;1(3): 133–43.
[85] Wang X, Dizaji KG, Huang H. Conditional generative adversarial network for gene expression inference. Bioinformatics 2018;34(17):1603–11.
[86] Ohno-Machado L, Nadkarni P, Johnson K. Natural language processing: algorithms and tools to extract computable information from EHRs and from the biomedical literature. J Am Med Inform Assoc 2013; 20(5):805.

Solid Tumors

Advances in Molecular Pathology 2 (2019) 153–162
ADVANCES IN MOLECULAR PATHOLOGY

Clinical Use of Cell-Free DNA in Tumor Diagnostics

Tejus A. Bale, MD, PhD, Maria E. Arcila, MD*
Diagnostic Molecular Pathology Laboratory, Department of Pathology, Memorial Sloan Kettering Cancer Center, 1275 York Avenue, New York, NY 10065, USA

KEYWORDS
• Cell-free DNA • cfDNA • Circulating tumor DNA • ctDNA • Liquid biopsy

KEY POINTS

- Molecular testing of tumor derived cell-free DNA offers many advantages over tissue-based analysis.
- Several clinical applications for cell-free DNA testing have been identified and are entering into clinical use.
- The diversity of cell-free DNA specimen types and clinical scenarios results in a high degree of complexity.
- Careful consideration of cost, sensitivity, and specificity, as well as technologic limitations and preanalytic factors must be used in test selection and development.

INTRODUCTION

The detection of DNA fragments shed by cells into body fluids, commonly referred to as cell-free DNA (cfDNA), has led to the rapid adoption of cfDNA based testing platforms. Originally centering on cfDNA of fetal origin detected in maternal plasma samples, the discovery of freely circulating DNA molecules that could be analyzed for gender and chromosomal abnormalities transformed the arena of prenatal screening [1–3]. Not long after unforeseen maternal cancer diagnoses were revealed among rare patients undergoing DNA-based prenatal testing, opportunities afforded by tumor-derived cfDNA, bearing the mutational signature of its cancer of origin, were recognized [4–7].

Molecular testing has taken on an essential role in cancer management as tumor-specific mutations continue to guide therapy and predict outcome. However, major limitations are posed by the reliance of this testing on tumor tissue. As clinicians and pathologists are keenly aware, tumor tissue may be of limited quantity or purity. Surgery, and its associated risks, may not be feasible or indicated, and rarely, if ever attempted at multiple timepoints to keep pace with tumor evolution and the development of treatment resistance. The promise of liquid biopsies opens new avenues for cancer diagnostics and tumor monitoring that may dramatically improve the usefulness of molecular testing [8–10].

SIGNIFICANCE

As cells die, DNA fragments are shed into the extracellular space where, under normal homeostatic conditions in healthy individuals, they are thought to be cleared rapidly. In the context of cancer, however, the balance shifts; higher cell turnover and necrosis of malignant cells leads to increased release of nucleic acids mediated by phagocytes [11]. Evidence also exists to

Disclosure Statement: The authors have nothing to disclose.

*Corresponding author, *E-mail address:* arcilam@mskcc.org

https://doi.org/10.1016/j.yamp.2019.07.011

suggest tumor cells actively release nucleic acids, potentially as a means of influencing distant cellular niches [12–14]. These 2 mechanisms are referred to as passive and active, respectively. Although concentrations vary among patients and stage/type of cancer, a comparison of circulating plasma DNA found means approximately 14 times greater among patients with solid tumors as compared with controls, with significantly higher levels among patients with metastatic disease [7]. However, analysis of cfDNA is not limited to that shed into the bloodstream, also known as circulating tumor DNA (ctDNA). Indeed, the list of body fluid specimen types from which cfDNA can be readily detected with clinical usefulness continues to expand, including cerebrospinal fluid (CSF) [15–17], vitreous fluid [18,19], saliva [20–22], sputum [22,23], stool [24–26], urine [27–30], effusions [31,32], cyst fluids [33,34], breast discharge [35,36], and many others (Figs. 1 and 2).

Advantages of Cell-Free DNA Testing

The allure of liquid biopsy grows increasingly apparent as molecular pathology becomes essential for the accurate diagnosis of cancer and necessary for optimal treatment selection. Many applications of cfDNA testing offer advantages not afforded by traditional tissue biopsy:

- Sampling of surgically inaccessible sites [37].
- Serial sampling [38–40].

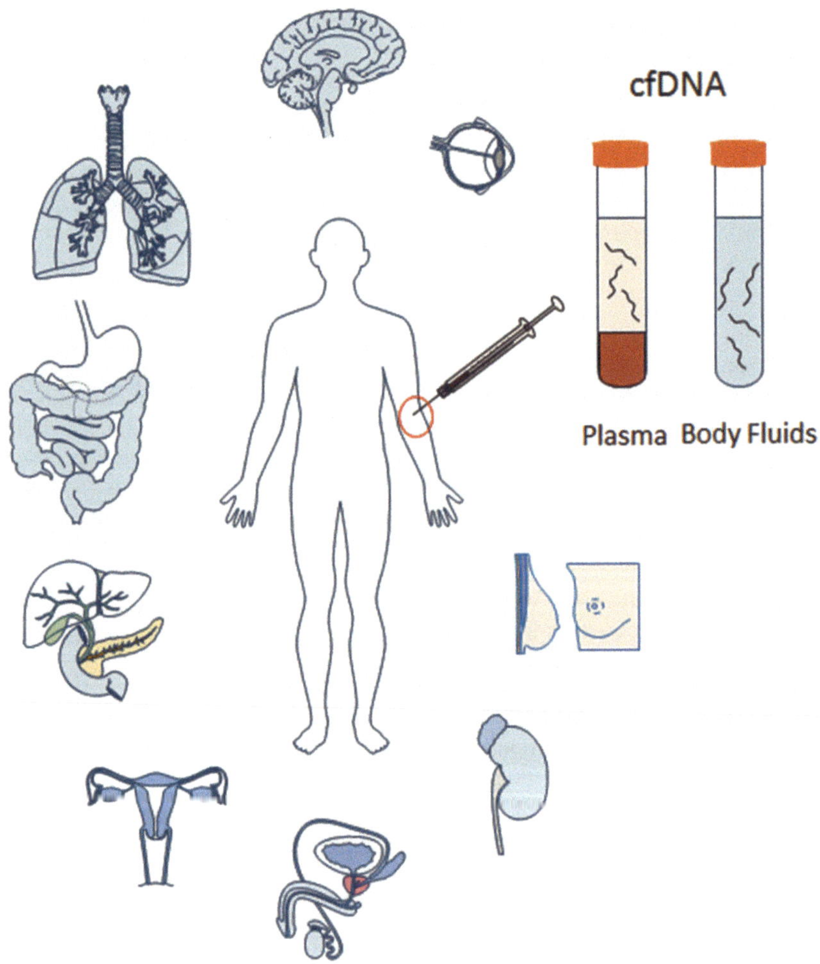

FIG. 1 cfDNA is released from both normal and tumor cells from all organs in the body. These small cfDNA fragments are released into circulation as well as into other body fluids, including the CSF, vitreous fluid, saliva, sputum, stool, urine, effusions, cyst fluids, breast discharge and many others. cfDNA may be isolated from all body fluids for subsequent testing.

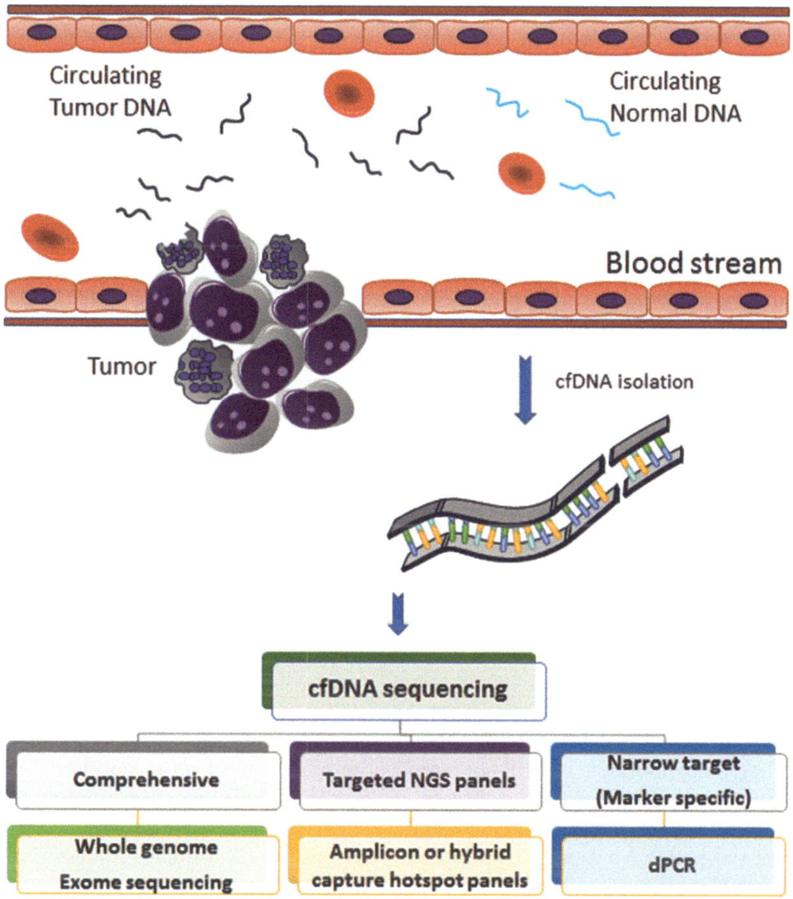

FIG. 2 Origin of circulating cfDNA and methods of testing. Circulating cfDNA may be released by apoptotic and necrotic cells, as well as through the secretion of living cells both normal and tumor derived. In patients with cancer, the fraction of tumor-derived cfDNA comprises ctDNA and may represent a very small proportion. After isolation, cfDNA may be sequenced using a broad range of methods, ranging from highly comprehensive (whole genome, whole exome) to intermediate target next-generation sequencing panels (eg, amplicon and hybrid capture based) and narrow single gene testing (eg, digital polymerase chain reaction [dPCR]). NGS, next-generation sequencing.

- More accurate representation of tumor heterogeneity and evolution [15,41].
- Reduced artifact from chemical processing [42,43].
- Early screening for cancer [44,45].

Clinical Applications in Cancer Molecular Diagnostics

- Diagnosis: Although many previous studies have established the ability to detect known mutations from previously characterized tissue biopsies in cfDNA [46–48], recent studies have established that the sensitivity of cfDNA assays is sufficient for the de novo calling of mutations [15,16,47,49], this being a necessary attribute ahead of clinical validation. Although many tumor types can share common mutation signatures, and tumor type prediction based on mutations remains a largely subjective clinical endeavor, recent studies clearly indicate that cfDNA analysis, at least in some clinical scenarios, can and will supplant tissue biopsy for tumor diagnosis [37,50].
- Molecular stratification: Critical to cancer management is the ability to detect clinically actionable mutations and biomarkers. Notably, the success of molecular pathology in the arena of non-small cell lung cancer has extended to liquid biopsy. Tumor

genotyping is high priority and standard of care to guide therapy in patients with non-small cell lung cancer; specific mutations in epidermal growth factor receptor (EGFR) being well-known to confer sensitivity to certain EGFR inhibitors. The technical difficulty of tissue sampling, coupled with established high correlation of tumor mutations with those detected in ctDNA from plasma, has resulted in quick clinical translation of EGFR hotspot testing from cfDNA [51–53]. Similarly, more comprehensive next-generation sequencing (NGS) applications have been readily used in cfDNA from CSF and lung fine needle aspiration [16,54]. Applications of ctDNA testing for risk stratification in hematologic malignancies are also under investigation [55,56].

- Resistance mechanism detection: The relatively noninvasive nature of liquid biopsies allows for serial sampling, and multiple testing opportunities throughout the course of disease. Several studies have established that cfDNA can facilitate rapid cancer genotyping at diagnosis and after drug resistance. cfDNA efficiently detects the EGFR T790M resistance mutation among patients with lung cancer, which would result in a change in treatment [37,54,57–59]. Although molecular diagnostics performed on traditional biopsy specimens is limited by tissue sampling, contributions to cfDNA are made from multiple tumor sites, including disease sites not at the level of radiographic detection. These factors combine to make cfDNA a superior means to screen for known and novel resistance mechanisms [32,43,60–62]. Studies have also established that ctDNA is more reflective of disease across tissue compartments, including lymph nodes and bone marrow, as well as more indicative of clonal dynamics throughout course of disease in the context of chronic lymphocytic leukemia and myeloid malignancies [63–67].
- Minimal residual disease: The challenge of minimal residual disease tumor monitoring has been the need for highly sensitive, patient- and mutation-specific assays. Recent advances in cfDNA technologies are beginning to demonstrate that this may be clinically feasible in the near future for both solid tumors and hematologic malignancies [68–72].
- Prognostic value of cfDNA: Beyond tumor-specific mutations, the potential for cfDNA to predict treatment response and prognosis is emerging. Although not ready for clinical use, several studies have linked the higher percentages of ctDNA to increased tumor stage, size, metastatic burden, and decreased survival [50,73–77]. The presence of tumor-derived cfDNA in CSF was associated with higher disease burden and adverse outcome among patients with glioma [77]. Pretreatment cfDNA and ctDNA have been associated with decreased recurrence-free survival and treatment resistance in numerous cancer types [50,77–80], whereas low pretreatment values generally correlate with better outcomes [78,81–85]. These collective findings imply that, with rigorous validation and control of preanalytical factors, cfDNA may serve as an easily detectable prognostic clinical biomarker.

Technical Considerations

Several technical considerations must be considered with regards to specimen type, disease, clinical application, and testing platform. For example, despite the mechanisms discussed elsewhere in this article, typically only a small fraction of the ctDNA in plasma originates from tumor, whereas the vast majority is derived from leukocytes. Although polymerase chain reaction (PCR)-based applications can readily overcome this challenge, the ability to call mutations with high confidence when present at less than 1% of reads has been a long-standing impediment to the clinical deployment of NGS assays for ctDNA, because this approximates the error rate of most standard NGS platforms. However, in recent years developments in techniques and methodologies have greatly improved sensitivity and specificity of mutation detection. Some of these advancements are reviewed here.

- Size selection: cfDNA molecules show a size distribution with a dominant peak at 166 bp with an approximately 10-bp periodicity, consistent with nucleosomal structure [77]. It is well-established that cfDNA originating from tumor cells are shorter in fragment length (usually <167 bp) as compared with background cfDNA from nonmalignant cells [86–90]. Sensitivity for ctDNA has been achieved by several methodologies that apply size selection for these short cfDNA fragments: these include physical sorting, that is, electrophoresis [91–94] and/or in silico methodologies, which use filtering algorithms to enrich for the appropriate fragment size [94–97].
- Molecular barcoding: Despite the comprehensiveness of NGS assays, the false positive rate owing to errors introduced during PCR amplification steps of library preparation compiled with that of sequencing prohibits calling variants present at a frequency of less than 1%. One strategy to overcome

this limitation involves the use of unique molecular identifiers to tag individual template molecules, also known as a molecular barcode [98–100]. These identifiers allow PCR duplicates originating from the same template DNA molecule to be grouped together. Each group of duplicates is collapsed into a single consensus sequence. This process in turn allows for a bioinformatic approach to correct errors of PCR and sequencing. This development alone, or in combination with, ultra-deep sequencing or other techniques, has greatly improved detection of low frequency variants in cfDNA, including de novo mutation calling at mean allele fractions of 0.1% [100–102].

- Emerging technologies: Recent advances in single-molecule level sequencing (ie, nanopore, third-generation NGS), have shown that technology originally developed for long-read sequencing may be adaptable and applicable to ultra-short DNA reads including cfDNA [103–106]. Although significant limitations remain (namely a required minimum mutant allele fraction of 10%), this technology could expand cfDNA testing for a number of applications, particularly in resource-limited settings. Other emerging techniques to surmount the issue of low signal-to-noise ratio include the use of CRISPR-associated proteins (Cas 9, Cas13a), the high specificity of which can be leveraged for targeted capture of mutant cfDNA at low abundance [107,108].

It is noteworthy that the challenges of detection of ctDNA in plasma do not necessarily plague detection of ctDNA from other specimen types. The relatively acellular nature of other body fluids, including CSF, results in a low background level of normal cfDNA. For example, somatic alterations in tumor-derived cfDNA have been detected in CSF in the majority of patients with primary and metastatic brain tumors [15,16,109,110]. Despite low cfDNA yields after extraction from CSF, the relative fraction of tumor-derived cfDNA is generally high, enabling mutation detection even at relatively low sequence coverage (<100×) [16]. Moreover, patients with a brain tumor are among those with a high risk for surgical biopsy, often with disease that is genomically highly heterogeneous and multifocal [15,62]. This notion, coupled with typically undetectable tumor ctDNA from central nervous system tumors in plasma, has catapulted CSF cfDNA testing into the clinical arena [15,37,111].

A note on test selection: Approaches to cfDNA testing can vary depending on the application and specific clinical scenario (see Fig. 2). Although the technological advances described herein have extended cfDNA testing to highly comprehensive approaches including whole-exome sequencing [112,113], the relative advantages of a blanket approach over more targeted testing should be carefully considered. For example, highly targeted assays based on digital PCR offer the advantage of allowing absolute quantitation and accurate determination of sensitivity reached at each patient-specific sample based on the number of molecules captured [114–116]. Although lacking in the ability of large NGS-based testing for detection of known and novel markers, using a targeted approach for known markers can generate testing with high clinical impact and a reliable and rapid turnaround time. In general, the more comprehensive the assay, the more technical and bioinformatics support will be required. Based on the capabilities of an individual laboratory and testing volumes, extensive batching of samples may be required, and components of the testing may need to be centralized. These factors ultimately could impact the time to test result.

FUTURE CONSIDERATIONS AND AVENUES TO INVESTIGATE

Many of the inherent biologic factors affecting cfDNA remain to be fully understood. For example, although fetal cfDNA half-life is thought to be relatively short (minutes to hours), that of cancer-derived cfDNA is unclear, particularly in the context of disease type, location, and treatment status among other factors [81,117–119]. Notably, the sensitivity of CSF for the detection of mutations in primary brain tumors is lower among low grade tumors and those without extension into the CSF space [17]. Biologic factors affecting the individual patient have been shown to alter cfDNA levels. For example, the role of kidney function, hydration status, and tumor type is likely to affect any ctDNA that is passed on to the urine, altering the performance of cfDNA tests. Further adding to the complexity surrounding cfDNA testing are the host of preanalytical factors that can alter a sample's yield, quality, and overall usefulness [120–122]. Optimal specimen processing time, preservative selection, and centrifugation protocols are required to generate reliably consistent and reproducible results ahead of clinical testing [123–125]. While expert guidelines for clinical use of cfDNA are awaited, just as in other areas of molecular diagnostics, all aspects of assay performance will be subject to regulatory requirements for clinical validation under the Clinical Laboratory Improvement Amendments (CLIA). Given the range of cfDNA specimen types and applications, a one-size-fits-all approach is not feasible. A balance between cost, sensitivity, and specificity requires strong consideration when designing and implementing cfDNA testing.

Another major consideration is the clinical interpretation of data and the incorporation of cfDNA analysis results into clinical practice. Although tumor-derived cfDNA has been well-established to be highly concordant with tissue-based diagnostics, broad clinical implementation has yet to be fully realized. Increased incorporation of cfDNA technologies into clinical trials will likely not only increase the quantity and quality of data generated from these trials, but will also establish the real-world clinical feasibility and usefulness of this type of testing and increase their adoption into the standard of care [126,127].

Meanwhile, there is continued expansion of cell-free analytes and testing paradigms. The use of cell-free RNA may offer the capacity to detect diagnostic, prognostic, and even targetable gene fusions; this is a point of weakness in most cfDNA sequencing methods [123,128–130]. There is also growing interest in querying the methylation status of cfDNA. This process applies to specific genes [131,132], as well as harnessing this information to identify the source tissue of cfDNA fragments. This latter application has great potential for determining tissue of origins in tumors of unknown primary as well as for detection of early-stage cancers, the low mutational load of which may confound the sensitivity of other means of detection [45].

SUMMARY

Testing of cfDNA in cancer affords new opportunities for minimally invasive tumor diagnosis and prognostication. These data can possibly result at an earlier timepoint in the course of disease, with fewer risks to the patient and with a more comprehensive sampling of alterations across tumor sites. Throughout the duration of treatment, these techniques can be used for repeat sampling, opening up new possibilities for the monitoring of response to therapy, resistance detection, and early detection of tumor recurrence. Because headway is still being made in terms of optimal techniques, expert guidelines, and widespread clinical adoption, the importance of a gold standard tissue biopsy has not been immediately diminished. Nonetheless, the advantages of cfDNA testing are becoming widely recognized, and will increasingly exist side by side as complementary and in some cases alternative techniques to traditional diagnostics, as they already do in many laboratory settings.

REFERENCES

[1] Lo YM, Corbetta N, Chamberlain PF, et al. Presence of fetal DNA in maternal plasma and serum. Lancet 1997; 350(9076):485–7.

[2] Liao GJ, Chan KC, Jiang P, et al. Noninvasive prenatal diagnosis of fetal trisomy 21 by allelic ratio analysis using targeted massively parallel sequencing of maternal plasma DNA. PLoS One 2012;7(5):e38154.

[3] Dello Russo C, Cesta A, Longo S, et al. Validation of extensive next-generation sequencing method for monogenic disorder analysis on cell free fetal DNA: noninvasive prenatal diagnosis. J Mol Diagn 2019;21(4):572–9.

[4] Tada M, Omata M, Kawai S, et al. Detection of ras gene mutations in pancreatic juice and peripheral blood of patients with pancreatic adenocarcinoma. Cancer Res 1993;53(11):2472–4.

[5] Bianchi DW, Chudova D, Sehnert AJ, et al. Noninvasive prenatal testing and incidental detection of occult maternal malignancies. JAMA 2015;314(2):162–9.

[6] Ji X, Li J, Huang Y, et al. Identifying occult maternal malignancies from 1.93 million pregnant women undergoing noninvasive prenatal screening tests. Genet Med 2019. [Epub ahead of print].

[7] Leon SA, Shapiro B, Sklaroff DM, et al. Free DNA in the serum of cancer patients and the effect of therapy. Cancer Res 1977;37(3):646–50.

[8] Siravegna G, Marsoni S, Siena S, et al. Integrating liquid biopsies into the management of cancer. Nat Rev Clin Oncol 2017;14(9):531–48.

[9] Stewart CM, Kothari PD, Mouliere F, et al. The value of cell-free DNA for molecular pathology. J Pathol 2018; 244(5):616–27.

[10] Krishnamurthy N, Spencer E, Torkamani A, et al. Liquid biopsies for cancer: coming to a patient near you. J Clin Med 2017;6(1) [pii:E3].

[11] Jahr S, Hentze H, Englisch S, et al. DNA fragments in the blood plasma of cancer patients: quantitations and evidence for their origin from apoptotic and necrotic cells. Cancer Res 2001;61(4):1659–65.

[12] Stroun M, Lyautey J, Lederrey C, et al. About the possible origin and mechanism of circulating DNA apoptosis and active DNA release. Clin Chim Acta 2001;313(1–2):139–42.

[13] Stroun M, Maurice P, Vasioukhin V, et al. The origin and mechanism of circulating DNA. Ann N Y Acad Sci 2000;906:161–8.

[14] D'Asti E, Chennakrishnaiah S, Lee TH, et al. Extracellular vesicles in brain tumor progression. Cell Mol Neurobiol 2016;36(3):383–407.

[15] Miller AM, Shah RH, Pentsova EI, et al. Tracking tumour evolution in glioma through liquid biopsies of cerebrospinal fluid. Nature 2019;565(7741):654–8.

[16] Pentsova EI, Shah RH, Tang J, et al. Evaluating cancer of the central nervous system through next-generation sequencing of cerebrospinal fluid. J Clin Oncol 2016; 34(20):2404–15.

[17] Wang Y, Springer S, Zhang M, et al. Detection of tumor-derived DNA in cerebrospinal fluid of patients with primary tumors of the brain and spinal cord. Proc Natl Acad Sci U S A 2015;112(31):9704–9.
[18] Berry JL, Xu L, Murphree AL, et al. Potential of aqueous humor as a surrogate tumor biopsy for retinoblastoma. JAMA Ophthalmol 2017;135(11):1221–30.
[19] Hiemcke-Jiwa LS, Ten Dam-van Loon NH, Leguit RJ, et al. Potential diagnosis of vitreoretinal lymphoma by detection of MYD88 mutation in aqueous humor with ultrasensitive droplet digital polymerase chain reaction. JAMA Ophthalmol 2018;136(10):1098–104.
[20] Wang Y, Springer S, Mulvey CL, et al. Detection of somatic mutations and HPV in the saliva and plasma of patients with head and neck squamous cell carcinomas. Sci Transl Med 2015;7(293):293ra104.
[21] Perdomo S, Avogbe PH, Foll M, et al. Circulating tumor DNA detection in head and neck cancer: evaluation of two different detection approaches. Oncotarget 2017; 8(42):72621–32.
[22] Hyun KA, Gwak H, Lee J, et al. Salivary exosome and cell-free DNA for cancer detection. Micromachines (Basel) 2018;9(7) [pii:E340].
[23] Wu Z, Yang Z, Li CS, et al. Differences in the genomic profiles of cell-free DNA between plasma, sputum, urine, and tumor tissue in advanced NSCLC. Cancer Med 2019;8(3):910–9.
[24] Caldas C, Hahn SA, Hruban RH, et al. Detection of K-ras mutations in the stool of patients with pancreatic adenocarcinoma and pancreatic ductal hyperplasia. Cancer Res 1994;54(13):3568–73.
[25] Kisiel JB, Yab TC, Taylor WR, et al. Stool DNA testing for the detection of pancreatic cancer: assessment of methylation marker candidates. Cancer 2012;118(10): 2623–31.
[26] van Lanschot MC, Carvalho B, Coupe VM, et al. Molecular stool testing as an alternative for surveillance colonoscopy: a cross-sectional cohort study. BMC Cancer 2017;17(1):116.
[27] Stasik S, Salomo K, Heberling U, et al. Evaluation of TERT promoter mutations in urinary cell-free DNA and sediment DNA for detection of bladder cancer. Clin Biochem 2019;64:60–3.
[28] Hayashi Y, Fujita K, Matsuzaki K, et al. Diagnostic potential of TERT promoter and FGFR3 mutations in urinary cell-free DNA in upper tract urothelial carcinoma. Cancer Sci 2019;110(5):1771–9.
[29] Togneri FS, Ward DG, Foster JM, et al. Genomic complexity of urothelial bladder cancer revealed in urinary cfDNA. Eur J Hum Genet 2016;24(8):1167–74.
[30] Birkenkamp-Demtroder K, Nordentoft I, Christensen E, et al. Genomic alterations in liquid biopsies from patients with bladder cancer. Eur Urol 2016;70(1):75–82.
[31] Husain H, Nykin D, Bui N, et al. Cell-Free DNA from ascites and pleural effusions: molecular insights into genomic aberrations and disease biology. Mol Cancer Ther 2017;16(5):948–55.
[32] Hummelink K, Muller M, Linders TC, et al. Cell-free DNA in the supernatant of pleural effusion can be used to detect driver and resistance mutations, and can guide tyrosine kinase inhibitor treatment decisions. ERJ Open Res 2019;5(1) [pii:00016-2019].
[33] Singhi AD, McGrath K, Brand RE, et al. Preoperative next-generation sequencing of pancreatic cyst fluid is highly accurate in cyst classification and detection of advanced neoplasia. Gut 2018;67(12):2131–41.
[34] Volckmar AL, Endris V, Gaida MM, et al. Next generation sequencing of the cellular and liquid fraction of pancreatic cyst fluid supports discrimination of IPMN from pseudocysts and reveals cases with multiple mutated driver clones: first findings from the prospective ZYSTEUS biomarker study. Genes Chromosomes Cancer 2019;58(1):3–11.
[35] Carolis S, Pellegrini A, Santini D, et al. Liquid biopsy in the diagnosis of HPV DNA in breast lesions. Future Microbiol 2018;13:187–94.
[36] de Groot JS, Moelans CB, Elias SG, et al. DNA promoter hypermethylation in nipple fluid: a potential tool for early breast cancer detection. Oncotarget 2016;7(17): 24778–91.
[37] Huang TY, Piunti A, Lulla RR, et al. Detection of Histone H3 mutations in cerebrospinal fluid-derived tumor DNA from children with diffuse midline glioma. Acta Neuropathol Commun 2017;5(1):28.
[38] Khan KH, Cunningham D, Werner B, et al. Longitudinal liquid biopsy and mathematical modeling of clonal evolution forecast time to treatment failure in the PROSPECT-C phase II colorectal cancer clinical trial. Cancer Discov 2018;8(10):1270–85.
[39] Krebs MG, Metcalf RL, Carter L, et al. Molecular analysis of circulating tumour cells-biology and biomarkers. Nat Rev Clin Oncol 2014;11(3):129–44.
[40] Coombes RC, Page K, Salari R, et al. Personalized detection of circulating tumor DNA antedates breast cancer metastatic recurrence. Clin Cancer Res 2019;25(14): 4255–63.
[41] Thierry AR, Pastor B, Jiang ZQ, et al. Circulating DNA demonstrates convergent evolution and common resistance mechanisms during treatment of colorectal cancer. Clin Cancer Res 2017;23(16): 4578–91.
[42] Damodaran S, Berger MF, Roychowdhury S. Clinical tumor sequencing: opportunities and challenges for precision cancer medicine. Am Soc Clin Oncol Educ Book 2015;e175–82.
[43] Wong SQ, Li J, Tan AY, et al. Sequence artefacts in a prospective series of formalin-fixed tumours tested for mutations in hotspot regions by massively parallel sequencing. BMC Med Genomics 2014;7:23.
[44] Molparia B, Nichani E, Torkamani A. Assessment of circulating copy number variant detection for cancer screening. PLoS One 2017;12(7):e0180647.
[45] Shen SY, Singhania R, Fehringer G, et al. Sensitive tumour detection and classification using plasma

cell-free DNA methylomes. Nature 2018;563(7732):579–83.

[46] Cohen PA, Flowers N, Tong S, et al. Abnormal plasma DNA profiles in early ovarian cancer using a non-invasive prenatal testing platform: implications for cancer screening. BMC Med 2016;14(1):126.

[47] Cohen JD, Li L, Wang Y, et al. Detection and localization of surgically resectable cancers with a multi-analyte blood test. Science 2018;359(6378):926–30.

[48] Berchtold D, Akovbiantz A. The nonresectable pancreatic tumor, an interdisciplinary problem. The surgeon's viewpoint. Schweiz Med Wochenschr 1988;118(20):773–4 [in German].

[49] Martinez-Ricarte F, Mayor R, Martinez-Saez E, et al. Molecular diagnosis of diffuse gliomas through sequencing of cell-free circulating tumor DNA from cerebrospinal fluid. Clin Cancer Res 2018;24(12):2812–9.

[50] Bettegowda C, Sausen M, Leary RJ, et al. Detection of circulating tumor DNA in early- and late-stage human malignancies. Sci Transl Med 2014;6(224):224ra224.

[51] Qian X, Liu J, Sun Y, et al. Circulating cell-free DNA has a high degree of specificity to detect exon 19 deletions and the single-point substitution mutation L858R in non-small cell lung cancer. Oncotarget 2016;7(20):29154–65.

[52] Leighl NB, Page RD, Raymond VM, et al. Clinical utility of comprehensive cell-free DNA analysis to identify genomic biomarkers in patients with newly diagnosed metastatic non-small cell lung cancer. Clin Cancer Res 2019. [Epub ahead of print].

[53] Li BT, Janku F, Jung B, et al. Ultra-deep next-generation sequencing of plasma cell-free DNA in patients with advanced lung cancers: results from the Actionable Genome Consortium. Ann Oncol 2019;30(4):597–603.

[54] Guibert N, Tsukada H, Hwang DH, et al. Liquid biopsy of fine-needle aspiration supernatant for lung cancer genotyping. Lung Cancer 2018;122:72–5.

[55] Roschewski M, Dunleavy K, Pittaluga S, et al. Circulating tumour DNA and CT monitoring in patients with untreated diffuse large B-cell lymphoma: a correlative biomarker study. Lancet Oncol 2015;16(5):541–9.

[56] Roschewski M, Staudt LM, Wilson WH. Dynamic monitoring of circulating tumor DNA in non-Hodgkin lymphoma. Blood 2016;127(25):3127–32.

[57] Ho HL, Huang CC, Ku WH, et al. Liquid biopsy for detection of EGFR T790M mutation in non-small cell lung cancer: an experience of proficiency testing in Taiwan. J Chin Med Assoc 2019;82(6):473–6.

[58] Su KY, Tseng JS, Liao KM, et al. Mutational monitoring of EGFR T790M in cfDNA for clinical outcome prediction in EGFR-mutant lung adenocarcinoma. PLoS One 2018;13(11):e0207001.

[59] Yang K, Li J, Zhao J, et al. Developing ultrasensitive library-aliquot-based droplet digital PCR for detecting T790M in plasma-circulating tumor DNA of non-small-cell-lung-cancer patients. Anal Chem 2018;90(19):11203–9.

[60] Otsubo K, Sakai K, Takeshita M, et al. Genetic profiling of non-small cell lung cancer at development of resistance to first- or second-generation EGFR-TKIs by CAPP-Seq analysis of circulating tumor DNA. Oncologist 2019 [pii:theoncologist.2019-0101].

[61] Macias M, Alegre E, Alkorta-Aranburu G, et al. The dynamic use of EGFR mutation analysis in cell-free DNA as a follow-up biomarker during different treatment lines in non-small-cell lung cancer patients. Dis Markers 2019;2019:7954921.

[62] Brastianos PK, Carter SL, Santagata S, et al. Genomic characterization of brain metastases reveals branched evolution and potential therapeutic targets. Cancer Discov 2015;5(11):1164–77.

[63] Yeh P, Hunter T, Sinha D, et al. Circulating tumour DNA reflects treatment response and clonal evolution in chronic lymphocytic leukaemia. Nat Commun 2017;8:14756.

[64] Yeh P, Dickinson M, Ftouni S, et al. Molecular disease monitoring using circulating tumor DNA in myelodysplastic syndromes. Blood 2017;129(12):1685–90.

[65] Kis O, Kaedbey R, Chow S, et al. Circulating tumour DNA sequence analysis as an alternative to multiple myeloma bone marrow aspirates. Nat Commun 2017;8:15086.

[66] Oberle A, Brandt A, Voigtlaender M, et al. Monitoring multiple myeloma by next-generation sequencing of V(D)J rearrangements from circulating myeloma cells and cell-free myeloma DNA. Haematologica 2017;102(6):1105–11.

[67] Rustad EH, Coward E, Skytoen ER, et al. Monitoring multiple myeloma by quantification of recurrent mutations in serum. Haematologica 2017;102(7):1266–72.

[68] Chin RI, Chen K, Usmani A, et al. Detection of solid tumor molecular residual disease (MRD) using circulating tumor DNA (ctDNA). Mol Diagn Ther 2019;23(3):311–31.

[69] Zhong L, Chen J, Huang X, et al. Monitoring immunoglobulin heavy chain and T-cell receptor gene rearrangement in cfDNA as minimal residual disease detection for patients with acute myeloid leukemia. Oncol Lett 2018;16(2):2279–88.

[70] Nakamura S, Yokoyama K, Yusa N, et al. Circulating tumor DNA dynamically predicts response and/or relapse in patients with hematological malignancies. Int J Hematol 2018;108(4):402–10.

[71] Lin SY, Orozco JIJ, Hoon DSB. Detection of minimal residual disease and its clinical applications in melanoma and breast cancer patients. Adv Exp Med Biol 2018;1100:83–95.

[72] Chaudhuri AA, Chabon JJ, Lovejoy AF, et al. Early detection of molecular residual disease in localized lung cancer by circulating tumor DNA profiling. Cancer Discov 2017;7(12):1394–403.

[73] Thierry AR, Mouliere F, Gongora C, et al. Origin and quantification of circulating DNA in mice with human

colorectal cancer xenografts. Nucleic Acids Res 2010; 38(18):6159–75.
[74] Lochowska BA, Nowak D, Bialasiewicz P. Cell-free tumour DNA as a diagnostic and prognostic biomarker in non-small cell lung carcinoma. Adv Respir Med 2019;87(2):118–22.
[75] Kamat AA, Bischoff FZ, Dang D, et al. Circulating cell-free DNA: a novel biomarker for response to therapy in ovarian carcinoma. Cancer Biol Ther 2006;5(10): 1369–74.
[76] Mirtavoos-Mahyari H, Ghafouri-Fard S, Khosravi A, et al. Circulating free DNA concentration as a marker of disease recurrence and metastatic potential in lung cancer. Clin Transl Med 2019;8(1):14.
[77] Parkinson CA, Gale D, Piskorz AM, et al. Exploratory analysis of TP53 mutations in circulating tumour DNA as biomarkers of treatment response for patients with relapsed high-grade serous ovarian carcinoma: a retrospective study. PLoS Med 2016; 13(12):e1002198.
[78] Dawson SJ, Tsui DW, Murtaza M, et al. Analysis of circulating tumor DNA to monitor metastatic breast cancer. N Engl J Med 2013;368(13):1199–209.
[79] Spindler KL, Pallisgaard N, Vogelius I, et al. Quantitative cell-free DNA, KRAS, and BRAF mutations in plasma from patients with metastatic colorectal cancer during treatment with cetuximab and irinotecan. Clin Cancer Res 2012;18(4):1177–85.
[80] Romanel A, Gasi Tandefelt D, Conteduca V, et al. Plasma AR and abiraterone-resistant prostate cancer. Sci Transl Med 2015;7(312):312re310.
[81] Diehl F, Schmidt K, Choti MA, et al. Circulating mutant DNA to assess tumor dynamics. Nat Med 2008;14(9): 985–90.
[82] Riediger AL, Dietz S, Schirmer U, et al. Mutation analysis of circulating plasma DNA to determine response to EGFR tyrosine kinase inhibitor therapy of lung adenocarcinoma patients. Sci Rep 2016;6:33505.
[83] Gray ES, Rizos H, Reid AL, et al. Circulating tumor DNA to monitor treatment response and detect acquired resistance in patients with metastatic melanoma. Oncotarget 2015;6(39):42008–18.
[84] Newman AM, Bratman SV, To J, et al. An ultrasensitive method for quantitating circulating tumor DNA with broad patient coverage. Nat Med 2014;20(5): 548–54.
[85] Forshew T, Murtaza M, Parkinson C, et al. Noninvasive identification and monitoring of cancer mutations by targeted deep sequencing of plasma DNA. Sci Transl Med 2012;4(136):136ra168.
[86] Diehl F, Li M, Dressman D, et al. Detection and quantification of mutations in the plasma of patients with colorectal tumors. Proc Natl Acad Sci U S A 2005; 102(45):16368–73.
[87] Mouliere F, Robert B, Arnau Peyrotte E, et al. High fragmentation characterizes tumour-derived circulating DNA. PLoS One 2011;6(9):e23418.
[88] Underhill HR, Kitzman JO, Hellwig S, et al. Fragment length of circulating tumor DNA. PLoS Genet 2016; 12(7):e1006162.
[89] Tsui NB, Jiang P, Chow KC, et al. High resolution size analysis of fetal DNA in the urine of pregnant women by paired-end massively parallel sequencing. PLoS One 2012;7(10):e48319.
[90] Cheng THT, Jiang P, Tam JCW, et al. Genomewide bisulfite sequencing reveals the origin and time-dependent fragmentation of urinary cfDNA. Clin Biochem 2017;50(9):496–501.
[91] Li Y, Zimmermann B, Rusterholz C, et al. Size separation of circulatory DNA in maternal plasma permits ready detection of fetal DNA polymorphisms. Clin Chem 2004;50(6):1002–11.
[92] Jorgez CJ, Bischoff FZ. Improving enrichment of circulating fetal DNA for genetic testing: size fractionation followed by whole gene amplification. Fetal Diagn Ther 2009;25(3):314–9.
[93] Hahn T, Drese KS, O'Sullivan CK. Microsystem for isolation of fetal DNA from maternal plasma by preparative size separation. Clin Chem 2009;55(12): 2144–52.
[94] Hellwig S, Nix DA, Gligorich KM, et al. Automated size selection for short cell-free DNA fragments enriches for circulating tumor DNA and improves error correction during next generation sequencing. PLoS One 2018; 13(7):e0197333.
[95] Yu SC, Chan KC, Zheng YW, et al. Size-based molecular diagnostics using plasma DNA for noninvasive prenatal testing. Proc Natl Acad Sci U S A 2014;111(23): 8583–8.
[96] Garrigou S, Perkins G, Garlan F, et al. A study of hypermethylated circulating tumor DNA as a universal colorectal cancer biomarker. Clin Chem 2016;62(8): 1129–39.
[97] Mouliere F, Chandrananda D, Piskorz AM, et al. Enhanced detection of circulating tumor DNA by fragment size analysis. Sci Transl Med 2018;10(466) [pii: eaat4921].
[98] Schmitt MW, Kennedy SR, Salk JJ, et al. Detection of ultra-rare mutations by next-generation sequencing. Proc Natl Acad Sci U S A 2012;109(36):14508–13.
[99] Kou R, Lam H, Duan H, et al. Benefits and challenges with applying unique molecular identifiers in next generation sequencing to detect low frequency mutations. PLoS One 2016;11(1):e0146638.
[100] Kinde I, Wu J, Papadopoulos N, et al. Detection and quantification of rare mutations with massively parallel sequencing. Proc Natl Acad Sci U S A 2011;108(23): 9530–5.
[101] Phallen J, Sausen M, Adleff V, et al. Direct detection of early-stage cancers using circulating tumor DNA. Sci Transl Med 2017;9(403) [pii:eaan2415].
[102] Newman AM, Lovejoy AF, Klass DM, et al. Integrated digital error suppression for improved detection of circulating tumor DNA. Nat Biotechnol 2016;34(5):547–55.

[103] Wilson BD, Eisenstein M, Soh HT. High-fidelity nanopore sequencing of ultra-short DNA targets. Anal Chem 2019;91(10):6783–9.
[104] Wei S, Weiss ZR, Williams Z. Rapid multiplex small DNA sequencing on the MinION nanopore sequencing platform. G3 (Bethesda) 2018;8(5):1649–57.
[105] Norris AL, Workman RE, Fan Y, et al. Nanopore sequencing detects structural variants in cancer. Cancer Biol Ther 2016;17(3):246–53.
[106] Cheng SH, Jiang P, Sun K, et al. Noninvasive prenatal testing by nanopore sequencing of maternal plasma DNA: feasibility assessment. Clin Chem 2015;61(10): 1305–6.
[107] Aalipour A, Dudley JC, Park SM, et al. Deactivated CRISPR Associated Protein 9 for Minor-Allele Enrichment in Cell-Free DNA. Clin Chem 2018;64(2):307–16.
[108] Gootenberg JS, Abudayyeh OO, Lee JW, et al. Nucleic acid detection with CRISPR-Cas13a/C2c2. Science 2017;356(6336):438–42.
[109] Pan W, Gu W, Nagpal S, et al. Brain tumor mutations detected in cerebral spinal fluid. Clin Chem 2015; 61(3):514–22.
[110] Swinkels DW, de Kok JB, Hanselaar A, et al. Early detection of leptomeningeal metastasis by PCR examination of tumor-derived K-ras DNA in cerebrospinal fluid. Clin Chem 2000;46(1):132–3.
[111] De Mattos-Arruda L, Mayor R, Ng CKY, et al. Cerebrospinal fluid-derived circulating tumour DNA better represents the genomic alterations of brain tumours than plasma. Nat Commun 2015;6:8839.
[112] Manier S, Park J, Capelletti M, et al. Whole-exome sequencing of cell-free DNA and circulating tumor cells in multiple myeloma. Nat Commun 2018;9(1):1691.
[113] Toledo RA, Garralda E, Mitsi M, et al. Exome sequencing of plasma DNA portrays the mutation landscape of colorectal cancer and discovers mutated VEGFR2 receptors as modulators of antiangiogenic therapies. Clin Cancer Res 2018;24(15):3550–9.
[114] Demaree B, Weisgerber D, Dolatmoradi A, et al. Direct quantification of EGFR variant allele frequency in cell-free DNA using a microfluidic-free digital droplet PCR assay. Methods Cell Biol 2018;148:119–31.
[115] Russo IJ, Ju Y, Gordon NS, et al. Toward personalised liquid biopsies for urothelial carcinoma: characterisation of ddPCR and urinary cfDNA for the detection of the TERT 228 G>A/T mutation. Bladder Cancer 2018; 4(1):41–8.
[116] Stallard S, Savelieff MG, Wierzbicki K, et al. CSF H3F3A K27M circulating tumor DNA copy number quantifies tumor growth and in vitro treatment response. Acta Neuropathol Commun 2018;6(1):80.
[117] Lo YM, Zhang J, Leung TN, et al. Rapid clearance of fetal DNA from maternal plasma. Am J Hum Genet 1999; 64(1):218–24.
[118] Yu SC, Lee SW, Jiang P, et al. High-resolution profiling of fetal DNA clearance from maternal plasma by massively parallel sequencing. Clin Chem 2013;59(8): 1228–37.
[119] Kustanovich A, Schwartz R, Peretz T, et al. Life and death of circulating cell-free DNA. Cancer Biol Ther 2019;20(8):1057–67.
[120] Barra GB, Santa Rita TH, de Almeida Vasques J, et al. EDTA-mediated inhibition of DNases protects circulating cell-free DNA from ex vivo degradation in blood samples. Clin Biochem 2015;48(15):976–81.
[121] Sherwood JL, Corcoran C, Brown H, et al. Optimised pre-analytical methods improve KRAS mutation detection in circulating tumour DNA (ctDNA) from patients with non-small cell lung cancer (NSCLC). PLoS One 2016;11(2):e0150197.
[122] Barrett AN, Zimmermann BG, Wang D, et al. Implementing prenatal diagnosis based on cell-free fetal DNA: accurate identification of factors affecting fetal DNA yield. PLoS One 2011;6(10):e25202.
[123] Sorber L, Zwaenepoel K, Jacobs J, et al. Circulating cell-free DNA and RNA analysis as liquid biopsy: optimal centrifugation protocol. Cancers (Basel) 2019;11(4) [pii:E458].
[124] Ward Gahlawat A, Lenhardt J, Witte T, et al. Evaluation of storage tubes for combined analysis of circulating nucleic acids in liquid biopsies. Int J Mol Sci 2019; 20(3) [pii:E704].
[125] Zhao Y, Li Y, Chen P, et al. Performance comparison of blood collection tubes as liquid biopsy storage system for minimizing cfDNA contamination from genomic DNA. J Clin Lab Anal 2019;33(2):e22670.
[126] Buono G, Gerratana L, Bulfoni M, et al. Circulating tumor DNA analysis in breast cancer: is it ready for prime-time? Cancer Treat Rev 2019;73:73–83.
[127] Ulrich BC, Paweletz CP. Cell-free DNA in oncology: gearing up for clinic. Ann Lab Med 2018;38(1):1–8.
[128] Mellert HS, Alexander KE, Jackson LP, et al. A blood-based test for the detection of ROS1 and RET fusion transcripts from circulating ribonucleic acid using digital polymerase chain reaction. J Vis Exp 2018;(134):e57079.
[129] Asano N, Matsuzaki J, Ichikawa M, et al. A serum microRNA classifier for the diagnosis of sarcomas of various histological subtypes. Nat Commun 2019;10(1):1299.
[130] Gawronski AR, Lin YY, McConeghy B, et al. Structural variation and fusion detection using targeted sequencing data from circulating cell free DNA. Nucleic Acids Res 2019;47(7):e38.
[131] Henriksen SD, Madsen PH, Larsen AC, et al. Cell-free DNA promoter hypermethylation in plasma as a predictive marker for survival of patients with pancreatic adenocarcinoma. Oncotarget 2017;8(55):93942–56.
[132] Sturgeon SR, Balasubramanian R, Schairer C, et al. Detection of promoter methylation of tumor suppressor genes in serum DNA of breast cancer cases and benign breast disease controls. Epigenetics 2012; 7(11):1258–67.

Advances in Molecular Pathology 2 (2019) 163–175
ADVANCES IN MOLECULAR PATHOLOGY

Practical Concepts, Current Challenges, and Technological Advances in Clinical Next-Generation Sequencing Assays for Solid Tumors

Mir B. Alikhan, MD*, Mustafa Al-Kawaaz, MD, Karen Kaul, MD, PhD, Linda Sabatini, PhD
NorthShore University HealthSystem, Department of Pathology, 2650 Ridge Avenue, Evanston, IL 60201, USA

KEYWORDS
• Next-generation sequencing • Solid tumors • Gene testing panels • Tumor mutation burden • Liquid biopsy
• Microsatellite instability

KEY POINTS

- Next-generation sequencing (NGS) has revolutionized the detection of multiple types of genetic alterations to aid in the diagnosis, prognosis, and therapy options for cancer.
- Complexity of NGS testing requires careful gene panel selection, extensive validation, sophisticated bioinformatics processes, and scrupulous variant interpretation.
- Despite the success of NGS, much work is required to widely adopt new biomarkers such as tumor mutation burden and liquid biopsies.
- As NGS testing enters the mainstream, issues of reimbursement and Food and Drug Administration approval are still outstanding and need to be resolved to minimize patient stress and harm.

INTRODUCTION

The genetics of cancer is complex. The hope that cancer develops from a single key driver alteration, such as the translocation between chromosomes 9 and 22 in chronic myeloid leukemia [1], was found not to be the case. Rather, tumorigenesis is often a stepwise process [2] with acquisition of mutations in key genes. These are broadly classified into 2 groups: activating mutations in oncogenes that promote the growth and survival of tumor cells as well as inactivating mutations in tumor suppressor genes that would remove the inhibition of cell proliferation. Although the cause of many of these mutations is not always clear, certain risk factors have been identified, including inherited/germline mutations, environmental factors (smoking, alcohol use), and infections (such as human papillomavirus) [3].

The "holy grail" of molecular oncology involves the identification of an alteration in the genome of tumor cells that distinguishes it from normal cells. Ideally, this specific change would allow targeted therapy, such as trastuzumab (Herceptin) in ERBB2 (human epidermal growth factor receptor 2 [HER2])-amplified breast cancer [4], to effectively eliminate tumor cells while sparing host tissue, leading to decreased toxicity. For many reasons, this has been elusive, partly due to

Disclosures: The authors have nothing to disclose.

*Corresponding author, *E-mail address:* malikhan2@northshore.org

https://doi.org/10.1016/j.yamp.2019.07.012
2589-4080/19/

the complexity of the mutational landscape seen in cancer. Understanding this genomic complexity first required the sequencing of the normal human genome. Its characterization was painstakingly accomplished in 2003 after nearly 15 years of work as part of the Human Genome Project [5,6]. This, the largest international scientific collaboration to date, used Sanger sequencing to determine the sequence of the nearly 3-billion base pairs in the human genome at a cost of about $3 billion. Soon after the completion of this project, there was rapid development in sequencing technologies and computational algorithms, starting with pyrosequencing methods and later massive parallel sequencing (or next-generation sequencing [NGS]) that dramatically reduced the cost and time of sequencing. With the data from the Human Genome Project publicly available, discovery and identification of causative mutations in tumors accelerated.

In 2005, The Cancer Genome Atlas was initiated as a large-scale project to catalog the genetic alterations in neoplasia [7]. Through this and other publicly available databases, researchers, clinicians, and pathologists can identify, record, retrieve, and reference a trove of molecular data critical for clinical decision-making. This necessity was made evermore apparent when, in 2015, US President Barack Obama launched the Precision Medicine Initiative [8], a comprehensive set of policy goals directed toward the identification of genetic changes in cancer and the tools needed to target those changes. With the understanding of the complexity of tumor genetics and the fact that tumors, even those with similar morphology, can be significantly different genetically, a specific mutational profile can be constructed for each tumor. This allows identification of potentially druggable mutations and those with diagnostic and/or prognostic significance.

With new and emerging technologies in sequencing, individualized tumor profiling has become technically simpler, faster, and cheaper than ever before. Rather than interrogating multiple genes on separate assays, a single run can encompass the sequencing of dozens of genes for multiple patients. As detection methods become more sensitive, further headway is being made toward screening for genetic alterations in small biopsies and even in peripheral blood (in the form of circulating cell-free tumor DNA and circulating tumor cells), making the entire process of genetic testing and disease monitoring easier for patients.

Despite these substantial advancements, much work is still needed to attain the "holy grail" in cancer. The sheer volume of data generated even by profiling a single tumor requires standardization in terms of which variants are significant, particularly in targeted therapies and clinical trials that may positively alter a patient's disease outcome. Newer biomarkers, such as tumor mutational burden, also need standardization and criteria from the community regarding the significance of such alterations, both on a biological level as well as for therapeutic purposes. Finally, the cost of these technologies is not insignificant, and reimbursement remains insufficient for NGS testing; there is legitimate concern over the patient's out-of-pocket expense and whether this testing is cost effective overall. As new therapies emerge and informative genetic alterations increasingly become standardized, the drive for payers to cover testing and therapeutics will hopefully accelerate, alleviating at least some of the concerns borne by patients after the stressful diagnosis of cancer.

TECHNICAL CONSIDERATIONS

History of Sequencing

Nucleic acid sequencing has come a long way since the advent of the chain termination method developed by Sanger and colleagues [9] in 1977. Although this method is quite accurate and is able to sequence long fragments of DNA, it is very time consuming and expensive. The initial steps toward more efficient sequencing came in the form of pyrosequencing. This was marketed in 2005 by 454 Life Sciences and subsequently acquired by Roche. The technique developed by Rothberg, Margulies and colleagues [10] involved DNA fragmentation followed by emulsion polymerase chain reaction (ePCR), loading onto a flow cell, and subsequent sequencing based on luminescence signal generation. This was followed by the development of a solid-phase isothermal bridge amplification and sequencing by fluorescent reversible chain termination by Solexa in 2006. This technology was acquired by Illumina and now dominates the commercial NGS market. Another significant technology is sequencing by hydrogen ion sensing, also developed by Rothberg and colleagues [11] for Ion Torrent Systems, later acquired by ThermoFisher Scientific. This was marketed in 2010 and also uses emulsion PCR as the amplification step. Further details on the chemistries and methodologies of these platforms are discussed shortly.

Next-Generation Sequencing Sample Preparation

Regardless of the method used, the general process of NGS is similar (Fig. 1). Following DNA extraction, random fragmentation of the template can occur,

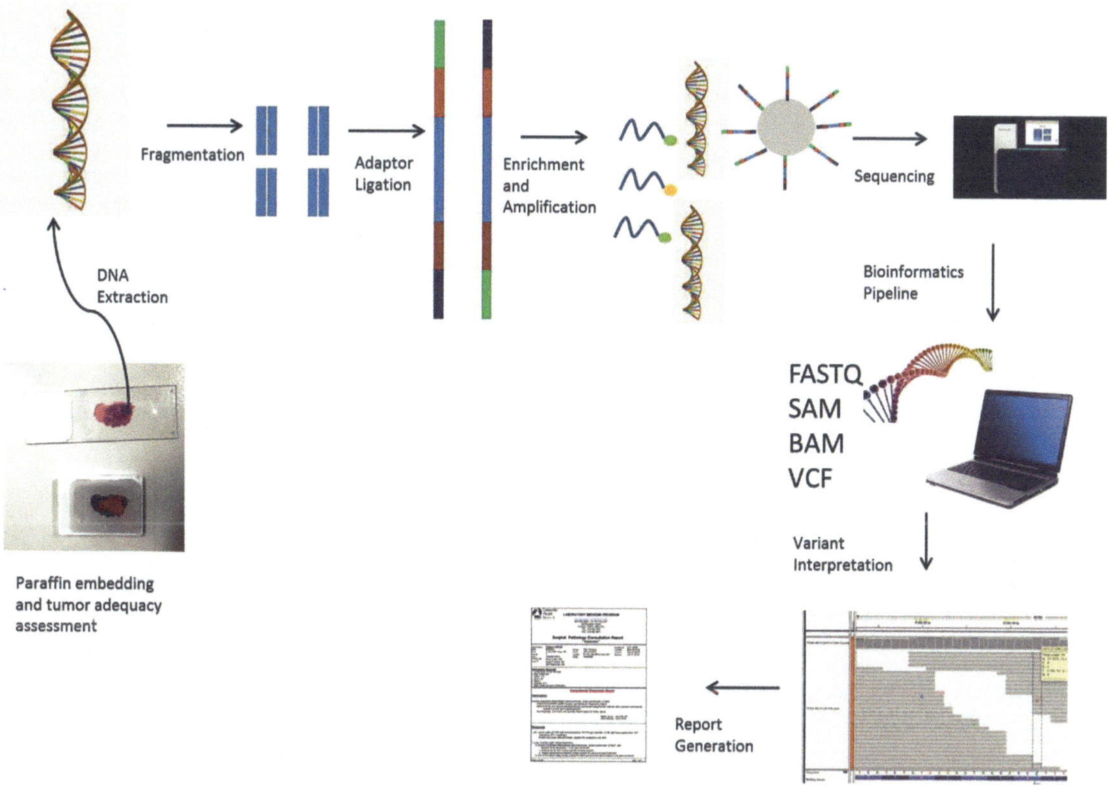

FIG. 1 General workflow for NGS testing from assessment of tumor adequacy (*left*) to report generation (*bottom right*).

particularly for hybrid-capture–based sequencing. This can be achieved inherently in formalin fixed tissues, given the propensity for the chemical to cross-link and fragment DNA [12]. Another method involves fragmentation by acoustic waves, marketed most popularly by Covaris. This yields overlapping DNA fragments, which are then ligated to platform-specific adapters that allow their identification while subjected to multiplex testing. This library of DNA fragments is then amplified, either by ePCR or by isothermal bridge amplification.

Sequencing on most platforms available today is in the form of short-read outputs, usually with read lengths of 100 to 600 base-pairs. This allows for greater accuracy and is cheaper than the alternative of long-read sequencing. The latter has the advantage of detecting long repetitive sequences in the DNA but is more expensive and not as accurate [13]. Platforms that use the long-read technology include systems by Oxford Nanopore Technologies and Pacific BioSciences (now part of Illumina).

Bioinformatics

Sequencing nucleic acids generates a voluminous amount of data, composed of not only the nucleotide present at a particular genomic coordinate (a "call") but also the many parameters associated with that call. This complexity requires a bioinformatics pipeline (Fig. 2). Each platform has specific algorithms that calculate the probability of a true call based on signal-to-noise ratio [14]. This can be computed by a quality metric termed the Phred score. The sequence reads for each fragment along with the quality score for each call are compiled in a text-based file format termed an FASTQ file. The sequence reads are then aligned to the reference genome. Many software tools are available to aid in alignment, such as Novoalign. Following alignment, an SAM (sequence alignment map) or BAM (the binary version of SAM) file is generated that is used for subsequent steps. Further processing and variant calling is accomplished by other open-source software tools such as Genome Analysis Toolkit or

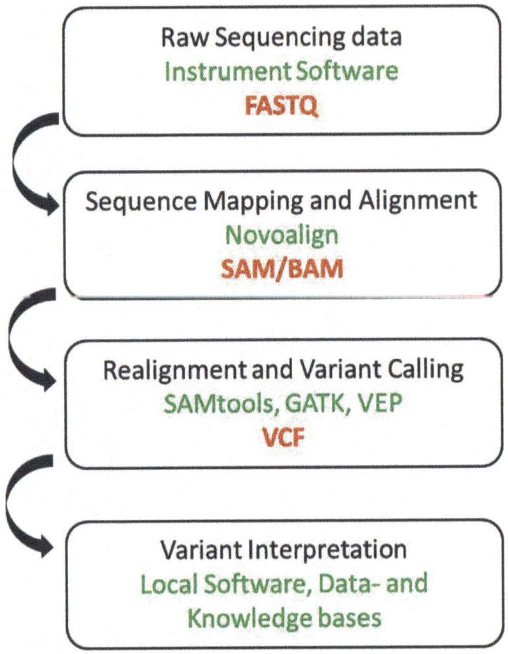

FIG. 2 Bioinformatics processing steps. The process (*black text*) requires specialized software (examples in *green*) to generate a specific file type for the next step in analysis (*red*).

SAMtools. These generate a variant call format file that contains information regarding the chromosome position, reference base, and alternate call. The final process is annotation of the variant. Software with annotation function, such as ANNOVAR or VEP, can give information regarding the location of the variant (intron vs exon) and the consequence of the change (eg, synonymous vs nonsynonymous). Algorithms that predict the biological function of the variant are also available, such as Sorting Intolerant from Tolerant (SIFT).

Variant Calling

Despite all the tools available in the form of databases, knowledge bases, algorithms, and bioinformatics tools, the clinical interpretation of each variant in the context of the patient's individual tumor is still an arduous process. Synthesizing these data and organizing it in a form that is useful for clinicians is a difficult task. A multitude of databases, such as cBioPortal, OncoKB, and COSMIC (Catalogue Of Somatic Mutations In Cancer) and online tools such as the IARC p53 database (http://p53.iarc.fr/) and MyCancerGenome aid in interpretation. Differentiating between germline mutation, variants of unknown significance, and clinically significant mutations can be difficult. Prediction algorithms such as SIFT and PolyPhen rely on evolutionary conservation of the locus or on pathway associations. These can be incorporated into local bioinformatics algorithms for ease of use. Despite these tools, interpretation can still be challenging and time consuming. To aid in interpretation, the Association for Molecular Pathology, in conjunction with the College of American Pathologists and the American Society of Clinical Oncology have issued guidelines and tiers for variant interpretation in cancer [15]. These should be incorporated in every report.

Commercially Available Next-Generation Sequencing Panels

Currently, several NGS panels are available. ThermoFisher offers a 52-gene Oncomine Focus assay as well as a larger 161-gene panel. Illumina offers a variety of panels targeting from 15 (TruSight Tumor 15) to 1385 (TruSight RNA Pan-Cancer) cancer-associated genes. Some institutions have developed their own custom panels such as FoundationOne CDx and MSK-IMPACT (by Memorial Sloan Kettering Cancer Center), which are also available and are approved by Food and Drug Administration (FDA), as are the Oncomine Dx Target Test (comprising of 23 genes specific for non–small cell lung cancer) and the Praxis Extended RAS Panel. Although many cancer driver genes are included in these panels, there is still considerable debate as to the utility of sequencing dozens of genes for which there is no current therapeutic benefit nor is the prognostic prediction clear. One major study to document the efficacy of such panels is the IMPACT trial (Initiative for Molecular Profiling and Advanced Cancer Therapy). About 35% of patients queried over the 10-year course of the study had a targetable genetic alteration for which directed therapy was given. The median overall survival was slightly longer in the matched-therapy group versus the nonmatched (9.3 vs 7.3 months). Progression-free survival was also slightly better [16]. Another recent study of 640 patients came to similar conclusions [17]. It is controversial whether such benefits significantly outweigh the costs of larger panels. However, as our knowledge of the significance of cancer mutations grows exponentially, it will certainly be helpful to have the data on hand to help design and study further therapeutic targets.

QUALITY CONSIDERATIONS

Guidelines for Next-Generation Sequencing Validation

As with any assay in clinical pathology, NGS testing should be thoroughly validated and continuously monitored for optimal performance. The complexity of NGS can be realized when considering that within a single NGS run, thousands of reactions are taking place for multiple patients simultaneously. In addition, the bioinformatics pipeline associated with the run must also be robust and thoroughly validated. With this in mind, guidelines have been published, most notably a joint consensus recommendation by both the Association for Molecular Pathology and the College of American Pathologists [18].

Selection of Gene Panel and Enrichment Method

Although conceptually, the entire genome of a tumor can be sequenced (whole genome sequencing [WGS]), this is impractical due to expense, low overall sequence coverage (about 30X), and low clinical utility. Whole exome sequencing, which entails interrogation of just 2% of the entire genome, is mostly used in cancer research studies, such as determination of tumor mutational burden. Although much less expensive than WGS and providing more coverage, it is still beyond the reach of most clinical laboratories.

Targeted gene panels are the most widely used application of NGS today. The validation process of such a panel begins with selection of a gene panel. For many laboratories, this has become easier due to commercially available gene panels as discussed previously. However, such panels need to be constantly updated, as the rapid development of disease-gene association discoveries and new therapies often require additions to existing panels.

Once the targets for the NGS panel are chosen, the laboratory must choose the enrichment method, which is often either amplicon-based or hybridization-capture–based (Fig. 3) [19]. Both have their advantages and disadvantages, and the laboratory should assess each method to determine which is best for their needs. Amplification-based methods often require less DNA input and have a simplified, quicker workflow but suffer from higher rates of false variant calls. These, however, can be adjusted for using bioinformatic parameters. Hybridization-capture–based methods allow for better uniformity in sequencing but require more DNA input and longer processing times [20]. Once selected, the capture method should be evaluated with pilot studies to ensure proper performance. False calls, such as co-amplification or co-capture of pseudogenes, should be evaluated. Analytics such as coverage, quality of reads, and allelic read percentages should be assessed. Bioinformatic parameters should be optimized to exclude, for example, false-positive calls from homologous regions.

Initial Validation

Following optimization of wet-bench processes and bioinformatic algorithms, validation with multiple samples should be carried out. Although it may be difficult to validate the presence of rare variants, it should be noted that NGS validation is a methods-based validation. Thus, specific variants, particularly rare ones, need not be validated individually. Rather, the types of variants should be validated (single nucleotide variants, indels, etc.). In terms of sample size for validation, the recommendations suggest at least 59 samples for adequate statistical confidence for quality metrics and assay performance.

Assay Monitoring

Continuous monitoring should be carried out at regular intervals. Control samples should be tested with every run to ensure proper assay performance from run to run and for the early detection of any false negatives

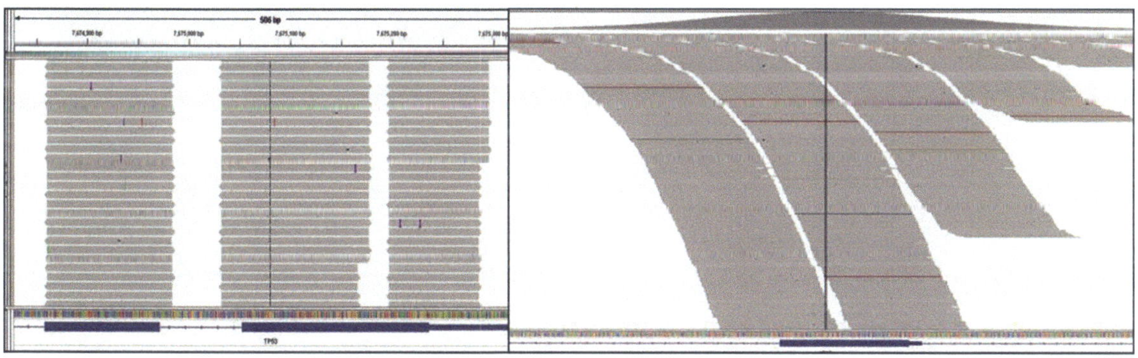

FIG. 3 Comparison of output between amplicon-based sequencing (*left*) versus hybrid-capture–based (*right*) as shown in Integrated Genomics Viewer.

or false positives that may appear. Quality metrics such as coverage, uniformity, quality scores, read length, etc. should be evaluated for each run (Fig. 4). Proficiency testing is another method of continuous validation. Because of regular updates of bioinformatics software and hardware, significant updates to the bioinformatics pipeline also require at least an abbreviated revalidation. This is also the case whenever NGS reagents are updated. The cost of such validation and revalidation is not insignificant and must be budgeted accordingly before bringing NGS testing in-house.

PLATFORMS

Multiple platforms are currently available for clinical NGS (Table 1). These platforms differ in their sequencing chemistry, and these differences result in particular strengths and weaknesses inherent to each. When making a choice as to which platform to bring in-house, the laboratory should keep the following considerations in mind: sample size, types of samples (small biopsies vs resection specimens only), types of genetic changes desired to be detected, DNA versus RNA sequencing, required read length and fidelity, and overall coverage.

Illumina

Illumina currently offers the most used platform in clinical genomics. It uses sequencing by synthesis (SBS) technology using reversible termination detected by fluorescent dyes.

Chemistry

The chemistry involves DNA polymerase incorporating dNTPs with a fluorescent label to a DNA template through sequential cycles of synthesis. Errors resulting from sequencing for homopolymer regions are

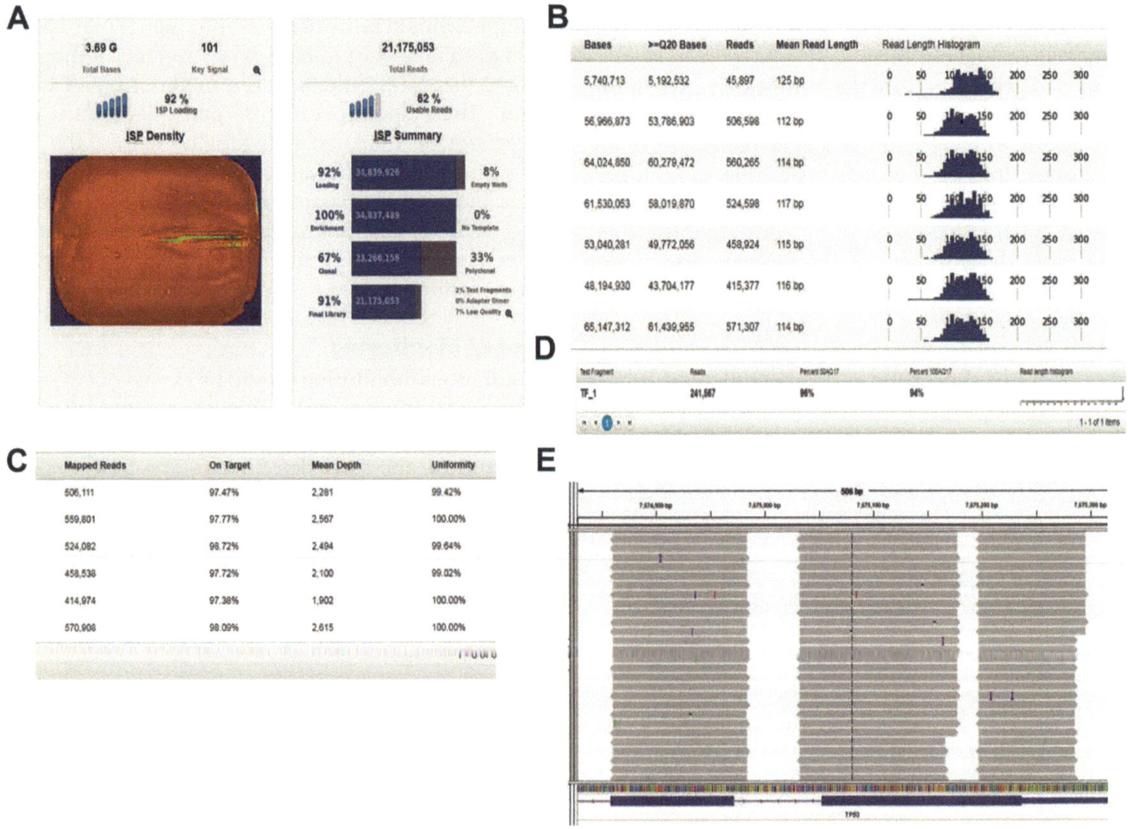

FIG. 4 Quality metrics, sequencing run—Ion S5. (**A**) Chip loading with % templated beads, % clonal versus polyclonal templates, % low-quality reads. (**B**) Read length histograms with percentage greater than or equal to Q20 bases. (**C**) Depth of coverage with % on-target reads and % uniformity. (**D**) Quality metrics for spiked test fragments. (**E**) Aligned reads visualized in Integrative Genomics Viewer.

TABLE 1
Next-Generation Sequencing Platforms and Characteristics

Platform	Read Length	Run Time	Maximum Output	Reads per Run
Illumina				
iSeq	2 × 150	9–17 h	1.2 Gb	4 million
MiniSeq	2 × 150	4–24 h	7.5 Gb	25 million
MiSeq	2 × 300	4–55 h	15 Gb	25 million
NextSeq	2 × 150	12–30 h	120 Gb	400 million
HiSeq	2 × 150	1–3.5 d	1800 Gb	6 billion
NovaSeq	2 × 250	13–44 h	6000 Gb	20 billion
Ion/ThermoFisher				
PGM	200–400	2–7 h	30 Mb–2 Gb	400,000–5 million
S5	200–600	3–21 h	300 Mb–50 Gb	2–130 million
Proton	200	2.5 h	15 Gb	80 million
Pacific Biosciences				
RS II	15,000	4 h	1 Gb	55,000
Sequel II	50,000	1–3 h	5–10 Gb	2 million
Oxford Nanopore				
MinION	Up to 2 Mb	Up to 48 h	50 Gb	1 million
PromethION	Up to 2 Mb	Up to 72 h	Up to 12 Tb	~20 million

Data based on reports by vendor.
Abbreviations: Gb, gigabases; Mb, megabases; Tb, terabases.

extensively reduced by this technology due to the addition of one base at a time and because the addition of the subsequent base does not take place without the removal of the terminator group [21]

Strengths and weaknesses

This technology is superior in sequencing of challenging areas such as GC-rich strands and repetitive areas such as homopolymers. The major weakness in comparison to other platforms is the requirement of relatively larger amounts of input DNA, making it difficult to use the Illumina platform for many small biopsies and cytology preparations.

Ion Torrent

Ion Torrent sequencing is also sequencing by synthesis. However, it uses changes in pH generated by DNA polymerization to detect the addition of bases rather than fluorescent dyes.

Chemistry

In this platform, the formation of the covenant bond by the addition of dNTP results in the release of a hydrogen ion and a pyrophosphate group. dNTPs are added when they match the leading strand. The technology provides information regarding the sequence by monitoring hydrogen ion release every time a unique dNTP is added to the reaction, leading to change in pH. The method is susceptible to errors in homopolymer regions due to the addition of multiple bases in one cycle, resulting in the release of more hydrogen ions.

Strengths and weaknesses

The main weakness is the lower accuracy in homopolymer areas. Ion torrent sequencers can successfully sequence with lower DNA content giving it an edge in cases where tumor cells are relatively scant. This is particularly important when analyzing cell-free DNA or circulating tumor DNA.

Other Technologies

Pacific biosciences

This platform uses a single-stranded circular DNA formed by ligation of hairpin ends to a targeted double stranded DNA of interest. A polymerase interacts with the circular DNA fragment and starts the replication process. The nucleotides are labeled with a fluorescent tag.

The PacBio technology is more often used in the research areas such as human medical research, ecology, and infectious disease. With the long-read sequencing, PacBio can be used in whole genome, targeted, complex populations; RNA sequencing; and epigenetics [22]. However, they suffer from high error rates of greater than 10%.

Oxford nanopore

Nanopore sequencing technology takes advantage of the unique changes in voltage for each nucleotide because DNA is threaded through ion channels (often protein nanopores) embedded in an electrically resistant layer, such as a lipid bilayer. The currently available sequencers have the ability to generate large numbers of very long reads at low cost and in real time, albeit with a relatively high error rate. The long reads make them a good fit for applications such as de novo assembly, sequencing through repetitive regions of a genome, establishing haplotype blocks, among others, although their portability has made them a practical choice for sequencing directly in the field [23].

CLINICAL APPLICATIONS OF NEXT-GENERATION SEQUENCING

Driver Mutations

The primary clinical utility in the genetic testing of tumor samples is the detection of driver mutations that affect tumor initiation, growth, and progression. However, most of the genetic alterations acquired by tumors are passenger mutations that do not significantly contribute to a growth advantage for the neoplasm [24]. The identification of driver mutations is a significant area of ongoing research [25–27]. Ideally, targeting the driver mutation would most potently eliminate the tumor. This is the premise behind such intense study to identify and target the drivers. The fruits of this collective labor can be summarized by their inclusion in the National Comprehensive Cancer Network guidelines for the treatment of various tumors, completing the pathway from the laboratory bench to the patient bedside [28].

Genetic Alterations and Targeted Therapies

Historically, simple mutations (single nucleotide variants [SNVs] and small insertions and deletions) were detected using PCR or Sanger sequencing. Larger alterations, such as translocations and copy number alterations, required the use of FISH, comparative genomics (such as array comparative genomic hybridization), or immunohistochemistry. Now, with the ability of NGS to use RNA sequencing protocols, all 4 types of alterations can potentially be detected. One of the more developed areas in the detection of therapeutically significant alterations is lung adenocarcinoma. Significant genes include EGFR, ALK, ROS1, and BRAF. Patients with EGFR mutations, most commonly exon 19 deletions and a missense mutation in exon 21 (L858R), are eligible to receive EGFR-tyrosine kinase inhibitors such as gefitinib, erlotinib, and others. Targeted therapy is also available for patients with tumors harboring BRAF V600E mutations, such as dabrafenib, in combination with trametinib. Those with anaplastic lymphoma kinase (ALK) rearrangements are candidates for initial therapy with ALK inhibitors such as alectinib and crizotinib. Crizotinib is also approved for use with ROS1-rearranged tumors and patients with tumors showing amplification or exon 14 skipping of the MET gene. Recently, the FDA has approved larotrectinib for use in cancers harboring fusions involving NTRK genes. This approval was tumor agnostic, signaling one of the first therapies to be used across tumor types.

In addition to these important targets, other predictive markers are also worth testing: the presence of KRAS mutations such as those involving codon G12 can predict reduced response to anti-EGFR therapies. Thus, their presence would make EGFR-TKIs and EGFR monoclonal antibodies contraindicated for patients with lung cancer and colon cancer, respectively. Importantly, clinical studies are ongoing with promising results for direct inhibition of KRAS [29,30]. Many other genes help predict the aggressiveness of the tumor, such as TP53 mutations. In addition, in patients with prior treatment with EGFR TKIs, NGS analysis may be performed to detect the presence of one of various resistance mutations in the gene (Fig. 5), most commonly T790M, although other mutations are increasingly being identified [31]. Identification of such mutations early in the course of therapy can allow oncologists to switch to third-generation TKIs such as osimertinib [32].

Much progress has also been made in the use of NGS to study cases of breast carcinoma. Trastuzumab (Herceptin), a drug targeting alterations in the driver gene ERBB2 (HER2), was one of the earliest targeted therapies developed, being approved in 1998 [33]. Cases with overexpression of estrogen receptor (ER) often receive endocrine therapy. However, not all patients with ER- or HER2-positive cancers benefit from targeted therapy. A subset of these cases may be due to estrogen receptor 1 (ESR1) mutations, observed in more than

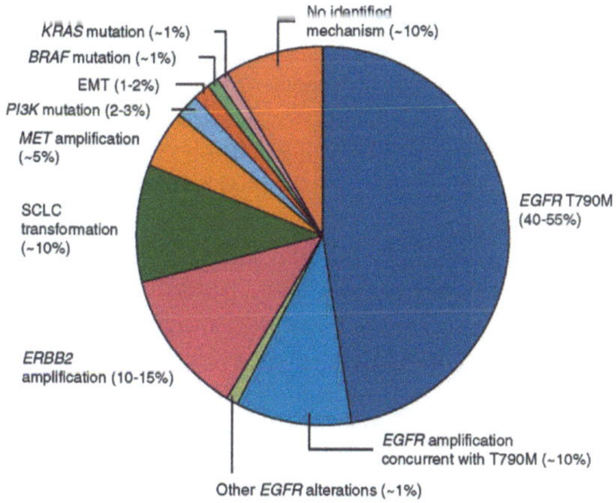

FIG. 5 Mechanisms of acquired resistance to first- and second-generation EGFR TKIs. Frequencies (given in parentheses) are approximations. Only mechanisms that have been detected in patients and reported in at least 2 independent data series are included. (*From* Westover D, Zugazagoitia J, Cho BC, Lovly CM, Paz-Ares L. Mechanisms of acquired resistance to first- and second-generation EGFR tyrosine kinase inhibitors. Ann Oncol. 2018;29(suppl_1):i13; with permission.)

25% of breast carcinomas, which render the ER constitutively active and resistant to endocrine therapy [34]. NGS-based sequencing of ESR1 can now be performed with liquid biopsies using plasma circulating tumor DNA [35]. Clinical trials are ongoing to study drugs targeting tumor with ESR1 mutations, which would allow patients to forgo conventional hormone therapy that may not be beneficial and rather initiate specific treatment of the ESR1 mutation [36].

Another important consideration is mutation in the PIK3CA gene, seen in about 30% to 40% of breast carcinomas. Hotspot mutations in the E542 and E545 codons often have a positive prognostic impact on disease-free survival [37]. Importantly, the FDA has recently approved a targeted therapy, alpelisib, for hormone-receptor positive, HER2-negative breast cancers [38]. Studies showed a promising impact with this targeted therapy, with significantly longer progression-free survival compared with placebo. Although approved for a specific subset of breast carcinoma, one may consider its use in a tumor-agnostic setting, such as in colorectal carcinomas.

Tumor Mutation Burden

Yet another use of NGS that may be tumor agnostic is the calculation of tumor mutational burden (TMB) or tumor mutational load. This is often calculated as the number of somatic, nonsynonymous mutations in the coding regions of the tumor genome. TMB was first explored through whole exome sequencing and found to be particularly high in tumors associated with DNA damage, such as tobacco smoking in lung cancers and ultraviolet radiation in melanomas. The consequence of high TMB would be the production of new proteins (neoantigens) within the tumor cells, which would then be available for presentation to cytotoxic effector cells in the immune system, leading to subsequent activation and tumor cell death. However, cancer cells often develop methods to block immune-mediated apoptosis. For example, overexpression of PD-L1 by the tumor cells serves as a negative regulator of effector T cells, maintaining them in an inactive state and averting apoptosis. Inhibitors of PD-L1 and other targets, also termed immune checkpoint inhibitors, such as pembrolizumab, block PD-L1 and allow activation of immune cells.

It was subsequently discovered that although certain tumors may overexpress PD-L1, as determined by immunohistochemical studies, many of these patients did not benefit from PD-L1 blockade or from drugs that block the CTLA-4 pathway (such as ipilimumab) [39]. In addition, patients without overexpression of PD-L1 had beneficial responses to such therapies. Although the mechanisms of resistance in the former cases are not entirely clear, some investigators began exploring TMB as an alternative or additional biomarker to help predict response to such drugs. Many of these studies focused on lung non–small cell carcinomas and found that high TMB did predict better response to immune checkpoint inhibitors [40].

Calculation of TMB has proved to be problematic. Although the most accurate results would be determined by whole exome sequencing, this is cost-prohibitive, would require high DNA input, and would reduce the overall coverage of the NGS analysis. Many groups have independently determined their own calculations for TMB, the most notable of them being FoundationOne [41]. Investigators from Memorial-Sloan-Kettering have developed a slightly different method of calculating TMB [42]. Both groups found that higher TMB was associated with better survival. However, the challenges in this area include devising the best analytical approach in the calculation of TMB and standardization in the field. As such, investigators are advocating for working groups that would ensure harmonization of best practices and standard criteria for the calculation, validation, and reporting of TMB, including what types of targeted NGS panels to use and what criteria constitutes TMB-high versus indeterminate versus low [43].

In this regard, a consortium has been created with this goal in mind, sponsored by the Friends of Cancer Research. Through their work in the next few years, laboratories around the world performing NGS will hopefully be able to confidently calculate TMB for their patients.

Microsatellite Instability

A related biomarker is microsatellite instability (MSI). Microsatellites are short nucleotide sequences found in tandem repeats throughout the DNA. These are particularly sensitive to mismatch during DNA replication, but these mismatches are corrected through the mismatch repair (MMR) pathway. The pathway involves several proteins encoded by several genes: MLH1, MSH2, MSH6, PMS2, and others. Mutations in these genes render the pathway defective, leading to hypermutability within the genome and possible tumorigenesis. Inherited mutation in these genes is termed Lynch syndrome, or hereditary nonpolyposis colorectal cancer. Sporadic colorectal carcinomas involve the MMR pathway account for about 15% of cases [44], often due to epigenetic silencing by hypermethylation of MLH1.

The clinical significance of MSI is its use as a predictive biomarker, where tumors with high MSI seem to benefit from immune checkpoint inhibitors such as pembrolizumab [45]. This benefit was seen across tumor types and led to FDA approval of the drug for MSI-high tumors in May 2017. Although MSI testing can be performed by immunohistochemistry and PCR, NGS panels that include the relevant regions are often more robust and do not require normal tissue pairs (as is necessary in PCR). As an example, using a 592-gene panel, one group was able to interrogate more than 7000 microsatellite regions, compared with 5 regions in most PCR-based assays [46].

Liquid Biopsy

As a way to reduce patient medical cost, length of stay, and recovery, there is a drive to reduce or eliminate invasive procedures. With this in mind, the concept of circulating tumor cells (CTCs) and cell-free/circulating tumor DNA (ctDNA) is emerging as the next technological feat in molecular diagnostics. With a simple blood draw, tumor cells or their DNA can potentially be detected by sensitive means, most often by testing patient plasma [47]. Its use for the primary diagnosis of new tumors has not been well established. Rather, the clinical utility is best suited for early and rapid detection of recurrences, including those with resistance mutations, without the need for even minimally invasive biopsies. Most studies thus far have focused on breast, lung, prostate, and gastrointestinal tumors.

CellSearch is an FDA-approved antibody-based assay available for clinical use that identifies CTCs by positivity for epithelial markers (epithelial cell adhesion molecule and cytokeratins) and negativity for leukocytes (CD45). CTC count has shown to be prognostically significant in treated tumors [48]. Beyond just the CTC count, studies are ongoing to detect specific genetic alterations in CTCs [49,50]. However, enrichment and detection methods are quite expensive, limiting its widespread use clinically at this time.

Guardant 360 and Guardant Omni are 2 clinically available liquid biopsy assays for ctDNA [51]. The former is a 73-gene panel launched in 2014, whereas the Omni contains 500 genes as well as TMB and was available in 2017. FoundationLiquid also sequences ctDNA. It is a 70-gene panel offered by Foundation Medicine and launched in 2018 that detects SNVs, indels, certain rearrangements, copy-number variations, and MSI from patient plasma [52]. The clinical utility of all 3 are quite similar to that of CTCs: detection of the presence of tumor, particularly from recurrent cancers, as well as mutations that can affect therapy and prognosis, such as resistance mutations. Although these assays claim good sensitivity, further analytical studies and demonstration of clinical effectiveness are needed before their mainstream adoption.

EMERGING TECHNOLOGIES

The impact of NGS technologies is indisputable. However, there is a need and excitement in ongoing development to address significant limitations of current technologies and platforms. In vitro SBS occurs without the benefit of cellular MMR strategies used during normal in vivo DNA replication and hence can be error prone. Direct reads of the DNA base order has been envisioned since the 1960s [53].

After perhaps an early publication from an academic institute reporting on the development of a novel technology, most of the subsequent research and development occurs "under the radar." Hence, this section is likely not comprehensive or entirely accurate (perhaps tomorrow, a truly revolutionary breakthrough will be unveiled with grand fanfare!). Nonetheless, much effort is being applied to the continuous improvement over current sequencing technologies, which is publicly available (Table 2). Hopefully, what is presented here will at least convey the excitement and dramatic advances currently underway.

TABLE 2
Emerging Technologies

Strategy	Company	Website	Emerging Technology
Direct/Nanopore Sequencing	Oxford Nanopore	https://nanoporetech.com/	Protein nanopores embedded in an electrically resistant layer
	Two Pore Guys	https://www.ontera.bio/	DNA sensing using a 2-pore device
	Electronic BioSciences	http://www.electronicbio.com/	Ion current measurements via a mechanically applied pressure differential
Sequencing by Synthesis	Illumina	https://www.illumina.com/	DNA sequencing via fluorescence detection of single-base incorporations
	Ion Torrent	https://www.thermofisher.com/	DNA sequencing via hydrogen ion release during DNA polymerization
	Stratos Genomics	https://www.stratosgenomics.com/	Sequencing by expansion
	GenapSys	http://www.genapsys.com	DNA sequencing via electrical detection of single-base incorporations
	LaserGen	http://www.agilenttechnologies.com/	Reversible terminator chemistry using photocleavable dyes

Nanopore Sequencing

Oxford Nanopore Technologies was the first company to commercially launch a nanopore-based sequencer, as previously discussed. Many innovators, including Oxford Nanopore, are making rapid strides in controlling the rate of DNA moving through the pore (eg, Two Pore Guys) [54], increasing the resolution between bases (eg, Stratos Genomics) [55] and reducing inherent noise (eg, Electronic BioSciences) [56]. When these issues are resolved, nanopore sequencing will be well positioned to revolutionize genomics!

Sequencing by Synthesis

Much effort is underway to continuously improve and expand the current SBS strategies in terms of accuracy, throughput, cost, and read length. Both Illumina and Ion Torrent continue to release new versions of their chemistries and analytical tools. This includes the acquisition of Pacific Biosciences by Illumina in 2018.

Stratos Genomics is developing a hybrid strategy, called sequencing by expansion, in which modified (X-NTP) bases are incorporated during PCR amplification followed by nanopore-based sequencing of the modified/extended strands of DNA for accurate base resolution [55].

GenapSys is developing an SBS strategy, which uses a complementary metal-oxide semiconductor sequencing chip to measure impedance as single nucleotides are incorporated [57]. Sequencing is carried out on microfluidic chips that have a scalable number of detectors, supporting applications ranging from targeted sequencing of specific amplicons to genome-scale data collection. Their goal is a sequencing instrument that is compact, scalable, easy to use, and affordable to purchase and run, enabling a more distributed model for genomics applications.

LaserGen, which was developing a reversible terminator chemistry using photocleavable dyes and terminating groups with the goal of bringing a low cost and accurate SBS platform to the market, was purchased by Agilent in 2018. No information was available with regard to further developments to bring the platform to market.

SUMMARY

NGS is a transformative technology that has radically changed the authors' perspective in regard to the biology of cancer, its diagnosis, and treatment. The fight against cancer is now squarely in the molecular realm, and NGS provides the most potent weapon in discovering the genetic alterations in each tumor that can potentially be targeted. With all the promise that NGS provides, it comes with many challenges. The cost of NGS, although substantially reduced from many years ago, is still considerable, particularly for patients who must also deal with soaring costs associated with the diagnosis and treatment of cancer. In terms of regulations, the speed at which the technology is developing has presented a challenge to government agencies such as the FDA in approving such assays. With newer NGS-based assays such as TMB, MSI testing, and others, specific guidelines need to be drafted to guide the hundreds of laboratories and clinicians who are demanding the regular use of such tests on all their patients. As NGS enters the mainstream, we become closer to offering that "holy grail" for our patients, to effectively and efficiently detect and cure their disease, reduce their suffering, and improve their lives.

REFERENCES

[1] Rowley JD. A new consistent chromosomal abnormality in chronic myelogenous leukaemia identified by quinacrine fluorescence and giemsa staining. Nature 1973; 243(5405):290.

[2] Vogelstein B, Papadopoulos N, Velculescu VE, et al. Cancer genome landscapes. Science 2013;339(6127):1546–58.

[3] Kinzler KW, Vogelstein B. Lessons from hereditary colorectal cancer. Cell 1996;87(2):159–70.

[4] Baselga J, Norton L, Albanell J, et al. Recombinant humanized anti-HER2 antibody (Herceptin) enhances the antitumor activity of paclitaxel and doxorubicin against HER2/neu overexpressing human breast cancer xenografts. Cancer Res 1998;58(13):2825–31.

[5] International Human Genome Sequencing Consortium. Finishing the euchromatic sequence of the human genome. Nature 2004;431(7011):931–45.

[6] Venter JC, Adams MD, Myers EW, et al. The sequence of the human genome. Science 2001;291(5507):1304–51.

[7] Weiss R. NIH Launches cancer genome project. 2005. Available at: http://www.washingtonpost.com/wp-dyn/content/article/2005/12/13/AR2005121301667.html. Accessed May 1, 2019.

[8] FACT SHEET: President Obama's precision medicine initiative. 2015. Available at: whitehouse.gov; https://obamawhitehouse.archives.gov/the-press-office/2015/01/30/fact-sheet-president-obama-s-precision-medicine-initiative. Accessed May 1, 2019.

[9] Sanger F, Nicklen S, Coulson AR. DNA sequencing with chain-terminating inhibitors. Proc Natl Acad Sci U S A 1977;74(12):5463–7.

[10] Margulies M, Egholm M, Altman WE, et al. Genome sequencing in microfabricated high-density picolitre reactors. Nature 2005;437(7057):376–80.

[11] Rothberg JM, Hinz W, Rearick TM, et al. An integrated semiconductor device enabling non-optical genome sequencing. Nature 2011;475(7356):348–52.

[12] Do H, Dobrovic A. Sequence artifacts in DNA from formalin-fixed tissues: causes and strategies for minimization. Clin Chem 2015;61(1):64–71.

[13] Morganti S, Tarantino P, Ferraro E, et al. Complexity of genome sequencing and reporting: Next generation sequencing (NGS) technologies and implementation of precision medicine in real life. Crit Rev Oncol Hematol 2019;133:171–82.

[14] Ledergerber C, Dessimoz C. Base-calling for next-generation sequencing platforms. Brief Bioinform 2011; 12(5):489–97.

[15] Li MM, Datto M, Duncavage EJ, et al. Standards and Guidelines for the Interpretation and Reporting of Sequence Variants in Cancer: A Joint Consensus Recommendation of the Association for Molecular Pathology, American Society of Clinical Oncology, and College of American Pathologists. J Mol Diagn 2017;19(1):4–23.

[16] 2018 ASCO: IMPACT Trial Matches Treatment to Genetic Changes in the Tumor to Improve Survival Across Multiple Cancer Types - The ASCO Post. Available at: https://www.ascopost.com/News/58897. Accessed May 16, 2019.

[17] Dy GK, Nesline MK, Papanicolau-Sengos A, et al. Treatment recommendations to cancer patients in the context of FDA guidance for next generation sequencing. BMC Med Inform Decis Mak 2019;19(1):14.

[18] Jennings LJ, Arcila ME, Corless C, et al. Guidelines for validation of next-generation sequencing-based oncology panels: a joint consensus recommendation of the association for molecular pathology and college of American pathologists. J Mol Diagn 2017;19(3):341–65.

[19] Mamanova L, Coffey AJ, Scott CE, et al. Target-enrichment strategies for next-generation sequencing. Nat Methods 2010;7(2):111–8.

[20] Samorodnitsky E, Jewell BM, Hagopian R, et al. Evaluation of hybridization capture versus amplicon-based methods for whole-exome sequencing. Hum Mutat 2015;36(9):903–14.

[21] Ambardar S, Gupta R, Trakroo D, et al. High throughput sequencing: an overview of sequencing chemistry. Indian J Microbiol 2016;56(4):394–404.

[22] Rhoads A, Au KF. PacBio sequencing and its applications. Genomics Proteomics Bioinformatics 2015;13(5):278–89.

[23] Lu H, Giordano F, Ning Z. Oxford nanopore MinION sequencing and genome assembly. Genomics Proteomics Bioinformatics 2016;14(5):265–79.

[24] Greenman C, Stephens P, Smith R, et al. Patterns of somatic mutation in human cancer genomes. Nature 2007;446(7132):153–8.

[25] Temko D, Tomlinson IPM, Severini S, et al. The effects of mutational processes and selection on driver mutations across cancer types. Nat Commun 2018;9(1):1857.

[26] Poulos RC, Wong YT, Ryan R, et al. Analysis of 7,815 cancer exomes reveals associations between mutational processes and somatic driver mutations. PLoS Genet 2018;14(11):e1007779.

[27] Brown A-L, Li M, Goncearenco A, et al. Finding driver mutations in cancer: Elucidating the role of background mutational processes. PLoS Comput Biol 2019;15(4): e1006981.

[28] Ettinger DS, Aisner DL, Wood DE, et al. NCCN guidelines insights: non-small cell lung cancer, version 5.2018. J Natl Compr Cancer Netw 2018;16(7):807–21.

[29] Christensen J, Fell J, Marx M. Insight towards therapeutic susceptibility of KRAS mutant cancers from MRTX1257, a novel KRAS G12C mutant selective small molecule inhibitor. Presented at the: American Association for Cancer Research. Atlanta, GA, April 3, 2019.

[30] Saiki A, Gaida K, Rex K. Discovery and in vitro characterization of AMG 510–a potent and selective covalent small-molecule inhibitor of KRAS G12C. Presented at the: American Association for Cancer Research. Atlanta, GA, April 2, 2019.

[31] Westover D, Zugazagoitia J, Cho BC, et al. Mechanisms of acquired resistance to first- and second-generation EGFR tyrosine kinase inhibitors. Ann Oncol 2018; 29(suppl_1):i10–9.

[32] Mok TS, Wu Y-L, Papadimitrakopoulou VA. Osimertinib in EGFR T790M-positive lung cancer. N Engl J Med 2017; 376(20):1993–4.

[33] Fischer OM, Streit S, Hart S, et al. Beyond herceptin and gleevec. Curr Opin Chem Biol 2003;7(4):490–5.

[34] Reinert T, Saad ED, Barrios CH, et al. Clinical implications of ESR1 mutations in hormone receptor-positive advanced breast cancer. Front Oncol 2017;7:26.

[35] Smith NG, Gyanchandani R, Shah OS, et al. Targeted mutation detection in breast cancer using MammaSeq™. Breast Cancer Res 2019;21(1):22.

[36] Nardone A, Weir H, Delpuech O, et al. The oral selective oestrogen receptor degrader (SERD) AZD9496 is comparable to fulvestrant in antagonising ER and circumventing endocrine resistance. Br J Cancer 2019;120(3):331–9.

[37] Cizkova M, Susini A, Vacher S, et al. PIK3CA mutation impact on survival in breast cancer patients and in ERα, PR and ERBB2-based subgroups. Breast Cancer Res 2012,14(1):R28.

[38] André F, Ciruelos E, Rubovszky G, et al. Alpelisib for PIK3CA-mutated, hormone receptor-positive advanced breast cancer. N Engl J Med 2019;380(20):1929–40.

[39] Ribas A, Wolchok JD. Cancer immunotherapy using checkpoint blockade. Science 2018;359(6382):1350–5.

[40] Hellmann MD, Ciuleanu T-E, Pluzanski A, et al. Nivolumab plus Ipilimumab in lung cancer with a high tumor mutational burden. N Engl J Med 2018;378(22): 2093–104.

[41] Goodman AM, Kato S, Bazhenova L, et al. Tumor mutational burden as an independent predictor of response to immunotherapy in diverse cancers. Mol Cancer Ther 2017;16(11):2598–608.

[42] Samstein RM, Lee C-H, Shoushtari AN, et al. Tumor mutational load predicts survival after immunotherapy across multiple cancer types. Nat Genet 2019;51(2): 202–6.

[43] Truesdell J, Miller VA, Fabrizio D. Approach to evaluating tumor mutational burden in routine clinical practice. Transl Lung Cancer Res 2018;7(6):678–81.

[44] Vilar E, Gruber SB. Microsatellite instability in colorectal cancer-the stable evidence. Nat Rev Clin Oncol 2010; 7(3):153–62.

[45] Le DT, Durham JN, Smith KN, et al. Mismatch repair deficiency predicts response of solid tumors to PD-1 blockade. Science 2017;357(6349):409–13.

[46] Vanderwalde A, Spetzler D, Xiao N, et al. Microsatellite instability status determined by next-generation sequencing and compared with PD-L1 and tumor mutational burden in 11,348 patients. Cancer Med 2018;7(3):746–56.

[47] Cree IA, Uttley L, Buckley Woods H, et al. The evidence base for circulating tumour DNA blood-based biomarkers for the early detection of cancer: a systematic mapping review. BMC Cancer 2017;17(1):697.

[48] Zhang J, Chen K, Fan ZH. Circulating tumor cell isolation and analysis. Adv Clin Chem 2016;75:1–31.

[49] Lyu M, Zhou J, Ning K, et al. The diagnostic value of circulating tumor cells and ctDNA for gene mutations in lung cancer. Oncotargets Ther 2019;12:2539–52.

[50] Sharp A, Welti JC, Lambros MBK, et al. Clinical utility of circulating tumour cell androgen receptor splice variant-7 status in metastatic castration-resistant prostate cancer. Eur Urol 2019. https://doi.org/10.1016/j.eururo.2019.04.006.

[51] Lanman RB, Mortimer SA, Zill OA, et al. Analytical and clinical validation of a digital sequencing panel for quantitative, highly accurate evaluation of cell-free circulating tumor DNA. PLoS One 2015;10(10):e0140712.

[52] Clark TA, Chung JH, Kennedy M, et al. Analytical validation of a hybrid capture-based next-generation sequencing clinical assay for genomic profiling of cell-free circulating tumor DNA. J Mol Diagn 2018;20(5): 686–702. https://doi.org/10.1016/j.jmoldx.2018.05.004.

[53] Feynman's Talk. Available at: http://www.zyvex.com/nanotech/feynman.html. Accessed May 30, 2019.

[54] Zhang Y, Liu X, Zhao Y, et al. Single molecule DNA resensing using a two-pore device. Small 2018;14(47): e1801890.

[55] Machacek C, Nabavi M, Tabone J, et al. Sequencing by Expansion-A Novel Technology Enabling Rapid Clinical DNA Sequencing. Presented at the: American Society of Human Genetics. San Diego, CA, October 18, 2018.

[56] Schibel AEP, Ervin EN. Decreasing the limits of detection and analysis time of ion current rectification biosensing measurements via a mechanically applied pressure differential. Anal Chem 2015;87(13):6646–53.

[57] Esfandyarpour H, Parizi KB, Barmi MR, et al. High accuracy DNA sequencing on a small, scalable platform via electrical detection of single base incorporations. Biorxiv 2019;604553. https://doi.org/10.1101/604553.

Advances in Molecular Pathology 2 (2019) 177–185

ADVANCES IN MOLECULAR PATHOLOGY

Evidence Builds for Tumor Mutation Burden as an Immunotherapy Biomarker

Andrea Ferreira-Gonzalez, PhD, HCLD(ABB), CC(ABB), FACB

Department of Pathology, Virginia Commonwealth University, 403 North 13th Street, CSC Building Room 246, Richmond, VA 23298-0248, USA

KEYWORDS

• Immunotherapy • Tumor mutation burden • Cell free tumor DNA • Blood tumor mutation burden

KEY POINTS

- Tumor mutation burden represents a new determinant of clinical benefit for immune therapy.
- Tumor mutation burden is an independent predictor from programmed death ligand-1 expression for response to immune therapy.
- Tumor mutation burden can be assessed using cell free tumor DNA, but new thresholds would need to be evaluated for the stratification of patients.

Discovery of immune checkpoint cytotoxic T lymphocyte–associated antigen 4 (CTLA-4), programmed cell death protein 1 (PD-1), and programmed death ligand-1 (PD-L1) as key regulators of the adaptive immune response motivated the development of immune checkpoint blockade therapeutics targeting pathways for cancer treatment [1]. Immune checkpoint therapies have developed rapidly owing to their high efficacies and low side effects relative to those of chemoradiotherapy in advanced cancers. In contrast to targeting the tumor cell directly, they target molecules involved in activation of T cells in order to enhance the endogenous antitumor immune response (Fig. 1). The CTLA-4 antibody ipilimumab was the first checkpoint inhibitor approved by the Food and Drug Administration (FDA). Soon after, the FDA approved an additional 6 immune checkpoint inhibitors for 3 different targets for more than 10 applications [2–4]. The anti-PD-1 nivolumab and pembrolizumab, and the anti-PD-L1 antibody atezolizumab, have shown remarkable clinical benefits in various solid tumors [5–10]. These immune checkpoint agents bring about durable clinical responses, however, only in a fraction of patients. Despite the marked success of applications of immunotherapy in clinical practice, the efficacy and responsiveness of these agents vary greatly among different tumor types and across individual patients. Furthermore, the combination of checkpoint inhibitors caused severe immune-related side effects, such as dermatitis, enteritis, and hepatitis [11,12]. Therefore, establishment of predictive biomarkers for checkpoint blockades is of the utmost importance to identify which populations are likely to experience a response to immunotherapy.

Disclosure Statement: The author has nothing to disclose.
E-mail address: Andrea.ferreira-gonzalez@vcuhealth.org

https://doi.org/10.1016/j.yamp.2019.07.015
2589-4080/19/

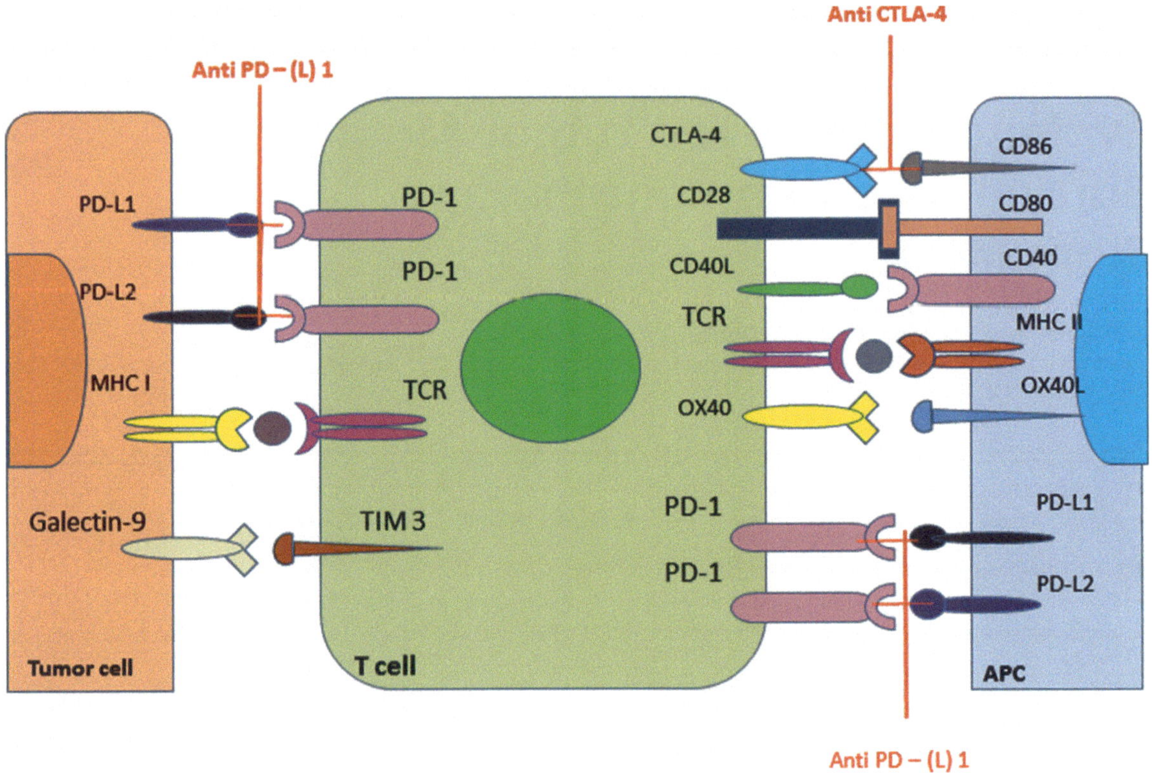

FIG. 1 Cancer immunotherapy through checkpoint blockade.

PREDICTIVE BIOMARKERS IN IMMUNOTHERAPY

PD-L1 Expression

The FDA has approved 5 PD-L1 clinical trials using PD-L1 expression as adjuvant or companion diagnosis for PD-1/PD-L1 inhibitors [1–5]. PD-L1 expression on tumor surfaces can be detected by immunohistochemistry (IHC). Positive cutoff values varied depending on the FDA-approved assay used, from 50% to greater than 1% for the same drug, such as pembrolizumab [13]. The FDA also approved 2 other PD-L1 tests for companion diagnosis and adjuvant diagnosis for atezolizumab and durvalumab [14]. However, the practical use of IHC for detecting the expression level of PD-L1 is still problematic. Although the increase of response rate in PD-1/PD-L1 inhibitor treatments correlate with the upregulation of PD-L1 expression, some patients with negative PD-L1 expression still respond to these treatments, and thus, PD-L1 expression is the only effective biomarker for PD-1/PD-L1 inhibitor efficacy. However, the value is not absolute. Both biological and technical complexities hamper the maturation of PD-L1 expression as a universal predictive biomarker for immunotherapy [15,16].

Genome Instability

In May 2017, the FDA approved the use of pembrolizumab by Merck in the treatment of all Microsatellite Instability High/deficient Mismatched Repair solid tumors. Mutations of tumor cells, especially mutations involved in DNA replication and mismatch repair (MMR), are associated with the effects of tumor immunotherapy [17]. The high-fidelity replication of DNA is performed by DNA polymerase, and the respective exonuclease proofreading domain is encoded by polymerase epsilon (POLE) and Polymerase Delta (POLD). The MMR protein also plays a vital role in ensuring DNA integrity. The probability of an intact DNA polymerase in making a replication error is 10^{-5} to 10^{-4}; however, after the effect of MMR proteins, the probability of error is reduced to 10^{-10} [17]. The presence of microsatellite instability in cancer cells, which indicates mutations in the MMR protein, correlates strongly with the clinical benefit of treatment with immune checkpoint inhibitors [18]. The junction of these mutant phenotypes with the immunotherapeutic responses can be explained by the production of neoantigens. Wang and colleagues [18] showed that MMR-deficient patients with colorectal cancer and other cancers show an improved clinical response to pembrolizumab therapy. Le and colleagues [19] evaluated the effect of using PD-1 inhibitors in 12 different types of cancers with severe MMR deficiency. Approximately 53% of the patients show an objective imaging response; 21% show a complete response and a long-lasting response, and the median progression-free survival is prolonged. Therefore, the clinician can determine whether the patient can benefit from immunotherapy based on the patient's DNA MMR ability.

TUMOR MUTATION BURDEN

Tumor mutation burden (TMB) has newly emerged as a possible independent biomarker to predict patient responses to immunotherapy in different tumor types, including lung cancer [20,21]. TMB measures the number of nonsynonymous somatic mutations within a tumor and thus is defined as the total number of somatic mutations per coding area of a tumor genome. In general, the accumulation of somatic mutations in the cancer genome is a multifactorial process, caused by factors that can be intrinsic, which include deficiencies or alterations in DNA repair genes or genes involved in DNA replication, such as the POLE, and extrinsic, environmental factors, such as smoking status or UV exposure [22]. Most of these mutations are passenger mutations, which can affect the immune editing process and exert selective pressure on the immune system. The presence of high numbers of somatic mutations can lead to modifications of the proteins that are encoded by the mutated genes. The modified proteins are recognized by the immune system as "non-self" and may therefore represent tumor-specific neoantigens capable of activating specific antitumor immune responses. Indeed, the accumulation of somatic mutations and the neoantigen load has been demonstrated to correlate with response to immune therapy also in non–small cell lung cancer (NSCLC) [22]. The clinical response of checkpoint inhibitors is related to the total mutation burden of tumor cells. One study analyzed the correlation between mutational burden and clinical outcomes by sequencing the whole exons (WES) of patients with advanced melanoma treated with ipilimumab. Patients with numerous mutations and nonsynonymous mutations showed long overall survival (OS) rates [23]. Similarly, 2 groups of retrospective studies of pembrolizumab analyzed the mutation burden of patients with advanced NSCLC and found that patients with high nonsynonymous mutation burden show long median progression-free survival. In other words, patients with high mutational burden show a long sustained clinical benefit (>6 months) [22]. The phase 2 clinical trial of atezolizumab in the treatment of patients with advanced bladder cancer shows that the median mutation burden is significantly higher in patients who responded to treatment than in patients who did not [24]. Considering the complexity of the mechanisms that cause the accumulation of somatic mutations, the TMB value can differ among different tumor types and within the same tumor histotype [25]. The Cancer Genome Atlas Project and other studies have used WES to measure TMB across cancer types and found a wide distribution of TMB across 20 to 30 cancer types, documenting the highest levels of TMB in melanoma and NSCLC and other squamous carcinomas, whereas leukemia and pediatric tumors show the lowest levels of TMB. Cancers such as breast, kidney, and ovary display intermediate levels of mutational load. In addition to the variation of tumor load, across tumor types [25], a significant TMB range is also observed within the same cancer type. Within NSCLC, there is a high degree of variation in TMB attributable to smoking status compared with gastric and breast. Mutational signatures characterized by the Stratton group have shed some light on the origins of tumor somatic mutilations [26]. For example, UV light and Tabaco carcinogens are the dominant mutational processes in melanoma and NSCLC, respectively. Later in tumor evolution, mutations present in some cells but not others (called subclonal mutations) occur. Furthermore, in lung cancer, for example, although the level of somatic mutations is generally high, it is significantly reduced in tumors carrying driver mutations (ie, alterations in EGFR, ALK, ROS genes), whereas it seems not affected by the presence of KRAS or BRAF alterations [26]. Because EGFR, ALK, and ROS1 alterations are more frequent among never or light smokers, this correlation further strengthens the connection between smoking and TMB.

However, some patients with high mutation burdens do not respond to immune checkpoint inhibitors, although some with low mutation burdens still respond. Rizvi and colleagues [19] found that in patients responding well to pembrolizumab, the reactivation of neoantigen specific T cells is correspondingly increased, indicating that the specific neoantigen is the main driving force of response to immunotherapy. They also found that response to pembrolizumab is associated with the biomarkers of tobacco carcinogen-related mutations, and patients with high smoking labels show a great likelihood of responding to PD-1 therapy [19]. Immune checkpoint inhibitors exhibit therapeutic effects on other smoking-related malignancies, such as esophageal cancer, head and neck squamous cell carcinoma, and bladder cancer. In addition to the overall mutation burden and the neoantigen burden, low heterogeneity of neoantigen within a tumor is a noticeable factor. McGranahan and colleagues [26] found that NSCLC patients with high mutational burdens and low tumor heterogeneity received continuous benefit from pembrolizumab treatment. The quality of neoantigen rather than its quantity seems to be crucial to the initiation of immune checkpoint inhibitor triggered immune response. This result poses a question about how to link mutation burden to patients' response to immunotherapy. Even though neoantigen load has been correlated with response to immune therapy, no recurrent neoantigens have been found that predict response to date. For all these reasons, the possibility of using TMB measured by means of WES has been used as a proxy to deduce the neoantigen load of the tumors, introducing the rationale for its use as a biomarker for treatment with immunotherapies [20,24].

The use of WES in clinical practice results is difficult, especially in NSCLC, because of required genomic DNA input, minimum coverage needed, and turnaround time. For this reason, using only the genes included in 2 targeted next-generation sequencing (NGS) panels approved by FDA, the Memorial Sloan Kettering-Integrated Mutation Profiling of Actionable Cancer Targets (MSK-IMPACT) and FoundationOne panel, they were able in silico to infer TMB similarly to WES [27,28]. Furthermore, in a study published by Chalmers and collaborators [29], analysis of 100,000 human cancer genomes revealed that measurements of TMB from a comprehensive genomic profiling are strongly correlated with measurements from WES. They showed that TMB calculated using a 1.1-Mb comprehensive genomic profile (CGP) assay agreed well with WES measurements of mutation burden. Rizvi and colleagues [30] used 3 subsequent versions of the MSK-IMPACT NGS gene panel (covering 0.98, 1.06, and 1.22 Mb in the 341-, 410-, and 468-gene panel versions, respectively) to analyze 240 NSCLC patients treated with immuno-therapies (IOs). Using TMB data from the NGS panel to perform clinical correlations, higher TMB (median 8.5 vs 6.6 single nucleotide variants per megabases) was present in patients with durable clinical benefit (DCB), defined as partial response/stable disease for more than 6 months. In addition, MSK-IMPACT was compared with WES in a subgroup of 49 patients, confirming the good correlation between targeted NGS and WES when a minimum area of 1 Mb is sequenced. Pretreatment tumor specimens from 102 first-line and 465 second-line or subsequent NSCLC patients enrolled in the POPLAR, BIRCH, and FIR trials, all evaluating the role of atezolizumab as monotherapy, were analyzed with the FoundationOne panel covering 315 cancer-related genes, corresponding to 1.1 Mb of genomic area. Atezolizumab produced improved outcomes in patients with a TMB value superior to the established cutoffs, defined by the 75th (high) and 50th (median) percentile. Thus, the obtained cutoffs were not univocal. TMB and PD-L1 expression were also independently associated with improved atezolizumab efficacy [31].

Variables Defining Tumor Mutation Burden

Even with the promising results described above, there are several reasons TMB measure faces significant challenges. One of the most critical reasons is availability of tumor material, which might be limited. Large sequencing panels are required for accurate TMB assessment, and these panels necessitate larger amounts of tumor material. Especially in late stages of NSCLC, small biopsies are usually the main source of tumor analysis.

Tumor cell content and sequencing coverage

Tumor content is of extreme importance with some TMB assay requiring not only large amounts of tissue but also at least 20% of tumor content. In this context, the limited amounts of tumor DNA obtained following a conventional biopsy or fine needle biopsy might make the TMB assessment challenging. The ability to detect somatic variants with NGS primarily depends on the variant frequency within the tumor as well as on sequencing depth. Theoretically, a ×50 coverage, 95% of single nucleotide variants, and short insertions or deletions with a variant frequency of 15% or higher can be consistently detected. However, contamination of no tumor cells, tumor heterogeneity, and aneuploidy are additional complexity factors. Therefore, there is a need for deeper sequencing in samples with lower purity or higher heterogeneity. Targeted panels enable deeper sequencing coverage compared with WES, which means that higher sensitivity is achieved when suing these targeted platforms even when tumor cell content of the sample is low (<10%), and especially when the depth of sequencing or coverage increases to ×500 to ×1000.

Preanalytic factors affecting tumor mutation burden measurement

TMB is most commonly measured by assessing the formalin-fixed paraffin-embedded (FFPE) tissue samples using NGS methods. One of the most important preanalytic factors is the tissue processing before TMB testing. In order to preserve morphology, tissues are normally fixed in buffered formaldehyde. It is well known that formaldehyde induces various cross-links (protein-protein, protein-DNA, interstrand DNA cross-links, and so forth) and is a source of sequencing artifacts (apparent sequence changes that are not present in the original sample). The most prevalent alterations in FFPE samples are DNA fragmentation, denaturation, and deamination of cytosine bases. Cytosine deamination is the major cause of baseline noise in NGS, leading to the most prevalent sequence artifacts in FFPE (C:G > T:A). The existence of these artifacts complicates the analysis of NGS results, which makes analyzing low-frequency mutations extremely challenging. The impact of sequence artifacts in FFPE DNA can be minimized through preanalytical assessment to identify tumor-rich areas for macrodissection, de-cross-linking by heat treatment before DNA extraction, or use of specialized nucleic acid extraction procedures to revert these artifacts. High-fidelity polymerase use, sequencing of both strands of DNA, use of molecular bar codes or capture-based sequencing approaches, and frequency and variant filtering could help with artifacts.

Size of the gene-targeted panel and the genes included

It has been shown that as panels become smaller, the zone of uncertainty associated with TMB estimation increases rapidly. In addition, the coefficient of variance increases rapidly when the size of the targeted panels is less than 1 Mb [31,32]. Therefore, the minimum size of the panel for determining the TMB of more than 300 genes or 1 Mb has been calculated [31]. Regarding the selected genes included in these panels, further investigation is needed as to the impact of the mutational study of different genes on TMB calculation.

Bioinformatic pipeline

Although the higher occurrence of synonymous variants may indicate a mutational process that also results in nonsynonymous changes, in general, synonymous and germline variants are discarded in the calculation of TMB, because it is assumed that these variants are not likely to be directly involved in creating neoantigens. In order to filter out germline variants, the ideal situation would be to sequence a matched nontumor sample from each patient. However, in a clinical practice setting, the availability of this matched sample may vary across different institutions, and diverse organizational factors may hamper the feasibility of maintaining short turnaround times and the affordability of the test. In the setting of tumor-only sequencing, germline false positive variants may be filtered out by using large, publicly available germline variant data sets. The use of these germline databases is a critical step in this process, because it is necessary to use germline databases with a sufficiently broad representation of all populations. Otherwise, patients with ethnic backgrounds who are underrepresented in these databases may have elevated rates of germline false positive mutations.

There is a certain degree of variability in the TMB calculation between the different studies, because some of them consider all somatic alterations, including nonsynonymous mutations and copy number alterations, whereas others considered only sequence mutations [32,33]. Similarly, most of the studies removed the variants included in COSMIC in order to avoid bias toward genes with functional mutations in cancer or in order to just exclude alterations likely or known to be bona fide oncogenic drivers and germline polymorphisms.

Cutoffs

Several studies reported a wide range of TMBs across many cancer types, with melanoma and lung tumors representing two of the cancer types with the highest TMB. In the lung, the median TMB across more than 18,000 lung cancer cases was 7.2 mutations per megabases, with approximately 12% of the patients showing more than 20 mutations per megabases. Nevertheless, cutoffs may not be coincident for all tumor types, and clinical cutoffs should be accurately established for each tumor type in order to translate the use of TMB biomarker into clinical practice. The initial WES study from Rizvi and collaborators in advanced NSCLC patients defined 178 nonsynonymous mutations (approximately 5 mutations per megabases if 38 Mb is used as the estimate of the exome size as the cut point that combined maximal sensitivity [100%] with maximal specificity [67%]); this cut point was associated with a likelihood ratio of a DCB of 3.0 [34]. Note that the study of Campesato and collaborators [28] using the same WES data yielded median numbers of nonsynonymous somatic mutations per megabases (calculated by analyzing only the genes contained in the Foundation Medicine panel) of 9 and 5 for tumors from patients with a DCB and with a nondurable clinical benefit, respectively. In the CheckMate 227 phase 3 trial, TMB was evaluated using the FoundationOne CDx panel with a cutoff of 10 mutations per megabases of DNA and was associated with an overall response rate of approximately 44%. Increasing this cutoff to 15 mutations per megabases did not identify patients with a greater likelihood of response, and a lower cutoff was associated with significantly lower response rates [30]. Therefore, in patients with advanced NSCLC whose first-line treatment is the combination immunotherapy (nivolumab-ipilimumab), a tumor mutational burden greater than or equal to 10 mutations per megabases was identified as the optimal cutoff for benefits owing to combination immunotherapy, showing a longer progression-free survival than chemotherapy treatment. Overall, from these different studies, it was observed that the optimal cutoffs to establish a tumor with a high TMB have yet to be defined. Three categories of TMB seem to be emerging, one clearly high (>10 mutations per megabases), one clearly low (<5), and the last "undetermined," for which more studies are needed in order to evaluate the response to immune checkpoint inhibitors [31,33].

Tumor Mutation Burden Liquid Biopsy

Despite improvements in the prediction of responders undergoing immune check-point inhibitors (ICI), many challenges persist. One of the major challenges is availability of sufficient primary tumor sample usually in the form of FFPE, fine needle aspiration biopsy, or cytologic samples, which is considered the standard starting material to perform NGS and TMB assessment. The predictive therapeutic response based on PD-L1 IHC and/or TMB assessment is not always possible to determine because of the lack of available tissue and/or the low percentage of tumor cells in the tissue sample. Because of the relative cost and complexity involved in procuring and sequencing tumor samples, there has been a recent focus on finding noninvasive biomarkers. Liquid biopsy is becoming a common alternative approach to perform molecular analysis, because it is less invasive that tumor biopsy and it is easily repeatable, cost-effective, and rapidly gives information to the physician who guides decision making for therapeutic strategy [34,35]. Cell-free DNA (cfDNA), or more specifically circulating tumor DNA (ctDNA), is the most important source in liquid biopsies and, consequently, efforts have been made to implement cfDNA in the field of immunooncology. Importantly, the methods for extraction of cfDNA from the blood have considerably improved over the last few years, and the analysis for some genomic alterations in cfDNA is now performed in daily practice. Liquid biopsy uses fluids, mostly blood, but also cerebrospinal fluid and urine for biological testing. cfDNA is easily accessible for genetic analysis and, given the promising results of TMB as a novel tissue-based biomarker for cancer immunotherapy, assessment of TMB from cfDNA represents a promising evolution that could expand its use in patients in which the initial material is scarce or of limited quality for proper TMB testing in tissue samples. However, the assessment of blood tumor mutation burden (bTMB) requires a sufficient quantity of high-quality DNA, which might not always be achievable. Moreover, the cutoff for the bTMB and the exact panel of genes may be questionable and may need further validation and standardization [36]. Furthermore, bTMB seems to be independent of tissue TMB, and thus, new thresholds would need to be evaluated for the stratification of patients. Furthermore, the detection of different mutations in cfDNA allows assessment of tumor dynamics [36].

Using a blood-based assay to measure bTMB from plasma ctDNA instead of solid tumor, Gandara and colleagues [37,38] found bTMB to be moderately positively correlated with TMB in the pretreatment of patients with NSCLC; however, the assays detected overlapping but not identical variants in DNA isolated from asynchronous matching plasma and tissue samples. The bTMB score was determined by identifying all base substitutions present at an allele frequency of greater than 0.5% across coding region of 394 genes (1.1 Mb). Having compared bTMB of the 2 clinical cohorts with tissue-based tumor mutation burden (tTMB), they confirmed that tTMB and bTMB were indeed positively correlated as a whole. The researchers selected bTMB $\geq$16 mutations per megabases as the threshold, and in the population with bTMB $\geq$16 mutations per megabases, the median OS of patients receiving atezolizumab immunotherapy was 13.5 months, whereas the median OS of patients receiving docetaxel was 6.8 months, which indicated that bTMB does indeed serve as a potential noninvasive biomarker for atezolizumab immunotherapy. An important limitation of the bTMB assay is that it requires a minimum amount of ctDNA to be present in the blood for optimal assay performance, meaning that tumors must shed DNA into the blood and that this ctDNA must contain mutations with an allele frequency of $\geq$1% for a bTMB score to be valid. In addition, the likelihood of detecting ctDNA also depends on the overall tumor burden. Another limitation of the bTMB assay is that the bTMB calculation is based only on single nucleotide variations (SNVs). Although this did not affect the concordance between bTMB and tTMB in this study, it is conceivable that, in certain rare cases, the assay may miss a patient whose tumor has a large number of indels but relatively few SNVs. Further tissue/blood studies are necessary to establish the conditions of using this test in routine clinical practice, in particular, the cutoff value that should be used.

Harmonization Efforts

As already mentioned, variability in current methods for mutation TMB estimation and reporting is evident, demonstrating a need for standardization and harmonization of TMB assessment methodology across different assays and different testing facilities. The increase in TMB assessment by various methods has brought with it a confusing array of information that documents how TMB has been determined and reported. There are 3 harmonization efforts: Friends of Cancer Research, Quality Assurance Initiative Pathology (QuIP), and European Society of Pathology in collaboration with the International Quality Network for Pathology. Friends of Cancer Research proposed an in silico assessment of the variation in TMB quantitation across diagnostic platforms by identifying sources of variability between TMB calculated using WES and 11 different targeted panels across 32 different tumor types. In general, the in silico analysis demonstrated that there is a strong correlation between panel-derived TMB and WES-derived TMB and that the methods to calculate TMB can impact this correlation. Phase 2 consists of empirical analysis of 14 matched tumor/normal cancer cell lines that harbor a range to TMB values to be able to define a universal reference standard. The reference standard will be used as an alignment tool to make TMB values calculated using different gene panels comparable to one another. Phase 3 will accomplish clinical validation by using clinical samples to propose standards for defining clinical application of TMB. Similarly, QuIP has implemented a complementary clinical approach to the one described above with an in silico analysis using publicly available data from The Cancer Genome Atlas to compare TMB values derived from WES and panels. The second phase will determine a comparison of TMB estimates from selected tissue (NSCLC and squamous cell carcinoma of the head and neck), using a WES analysis-derived reference standard, with commercial and laboratory-developed targeted gene panels to evaluate the interlaboratory and the interassay variability. All these efforts will provide a framework for harmonization and standardization as well as additional aspects of TMB measurement to ensure consistency between assays and laboratories, based on the expectation that many laboratories may develop their own tests for TMB assessment.

Future Biomarkers of Immunotherapy Response

Several additional emerging biomarkers, such as tumor infiltrating lymphocyte (TIL), specific immune gene signatures, T-cell receptor clonality, monitoring of peripheral T-cell lymphocytes, and imagining biomarkers, hold promise in selecting patients for treatment with checkpoint inhibitors. Among the factors in tumor microenvironment, TIL may be of greatest value for the prediction of prognosis and response to therapy for many solid tumors and cancers. Patients with tumors infiltrated by TILs are more susceptible to immunotherapies [39]. In recent years, an increasing number of studies have pointed out the connection between the gut microbiome and efficiencies of checkpoint inhibitor immunotherapies. The effect of intratumor heterogeneity (ITH) on the neoantigen landscape offers an additional explanation for the variability in immunotherapy responses. McGranahan and colleagues [39] found increased sensitivity to both PD-1 and CTLA-4 blockade, and improved OS, among NSCLC and melanoma patients with tumors harboring low ITH and high clonal neoantigen burden. Confirming the intricate relationship between immune response and tumor progression, alterations in several canonical oncogenes and tumor suppressors have also recently been associated with response to immunotherapy. Most of these genes function in the MAPK, PI3K-AKT-mTOR, and WNT-β-catenin pathways, all of which are firmly established as oncogenic signaling pathways with longstanding biological evidence for relevance to tumor formation and evolution. In addition, various gene expression profiles (GEPs) are also being explored as possible predictors for immune therapy response. Ayers and colleagues [40] proposed using one such GEP for a set of immune-related genes to predict anti-PD-1 therapy response in multiple cancer types. More research is needed to assess the stability and transferability of such biomarkers across cancer types and under different treatments.

REFERENCES

[1] Klaus WCM, Fenchel D, Dale P, et al. Second- and third-generation drugs for immuno-oncology treatment—the more the better? Eur J Cancer 2017;74:55–72.

[2] Asmar R, Rizvi NA. Immunotherapy for advanced lung cancer. Cancer J 2015;21(5):383–91.

[3] Bellmunt J, Powles T, Vogelzang NJ. A review on the evolution of PD-1/PD-L1 immunotherapy for bladder cancer: the future is now. Cancer Treat Rev 2017;54:58–67.

[4] Gubens MA, Davies M. NCCN guidelines updates: new immunotherapy strategies for improving outcomes in non-small cell lung cancer. J Natl Compr Canc Netw 2019;17(5.5):574–8.

[5] Rizvi NA, Peters S. Immunotherapy for unresectable stage III non-small-cell lung cancer. N Engl J Med 2017;377(20):1986–8.

[6] Ribas A, Hamid O, Daud A, et al. Association of pembrolizumab with tumor response and survival among patients with advanced melanoma. JAMA 2016;315(15):1600–9.
[7] Rizvi NA, Hellmann MD, Brahmer JR, et al. Nivolumab in combination with platinum-based doublet chemotherapy for first-line treatment of advanced non-small-cell lung cancer. Clin Oncol 2016;34(25):2969–79.
[8] Rizvi NA. The use of immunotherapy in the first-line treatment of lung cancer. Clin Adv Hematol Oncol 2017;15(3):190–2.
[9] Remon J, Hendriks LE, Cabrera C, et al. Immunotherapy for oncogenic-driven advanced non-small cell lung cancers: is the time ripe for a change? Cancer Treat Rev 2018;71:47–58.
[10] Hendriks LEL, Henon C, Auclin E, et al. Outcome of patients with non-small cell lung cancer and brain metastases treated with checkpoint inhibitors. J Thorac Oncol 2019;14(7):1244–54.
[11] Phillips GS, Wu J, Hellmann MD, et al. Treatment outcomes of immune-related cutaneous adverse events. J Clin Oncol 2019;JCO1802141.
[12] Antonia S, Goldberg SB, Balmanoukian A, et al. Safety and antitumour activity of durvalumab plus tremelimumab in non-small cell lung cancer: a multicentre, phase 1b study. Lancet Oncol 2016;17(3):299–308.
[13] Hui R, Garon EB, Goldman JW, et al. Pembrolizumab as first-line therapy for patients with PD-L1-positive advanced non-small cell lung cancer: a phase 1 trial. Ann Oncol 2017;28(4):874–81.
[14] Boothman AM, Scott M, Ratcliffe M, et al. Impact of patient characteristics, prior therapy, and sample type on tumor cell programmed cell death ligand 1 expression in patients with advanced NSCLC screened for the ATLANTIC study. J Thorac Oncol 2019;14(8):1390–9.
[15] Heymann JJ, Bulman WA, Swinarski D, et al. A. PD-L1 expression in non-small cell lung carcinoma: comparison among cytology, small biopsy, and surgical resection specimens. Cancer Cytopathol 2017;125(12):896–907.
[16] Grigg C, Rizvi NA. PD-L1 biomarker testing for non-small cell lung cancer: truth or fiction? J Immunother Cancer 2016;4:48.
[17] Conway JR, Kofman E, Mo SS, et al. Genomics of response to immune checkpoint therapies for cancer: implications for precision medicine. Genome Med 2018;10(1):93.
[18] Wang T, Lee LH, Vyas M, et al. Colorectal carcinoma with double somatic mismatch repair gene inactivation: clinical and pathological characteristics and response to immune checkpoint blockade. Mod Pathol 2019. https://doi.org/10.1038/s41379-019-0289-6.
[19] Rizvi NA, Hellmann MD, Snyder A, et al. Cancer immunology. Mutational landscape determines sensitivity to PD-1 blockade in non-small cell lung cancer. Science 2015;348(6230):124–8.
[20] Chowell D, Morris LGT, Grigg CM, et al. Patient HLA class I genotype influences cancer response to checkpoint blockade immunotherapy. Science 2018;359(6375):582–7.
[21] Endris V, Buchhalter I, Allgäuer M, et al. Measurement of tumor mutational burden (TMB) in routine molecular diagnostics: in silico and real-life analysis of three larger gene panels. Int J Cancer 2019;144(9):2303–12.
[22] Blons H, Garinet S, Laurent-Puig P, et al. Molecular markers and prediction of response to immunotherapy in non-small cell lung cancer, an update. J Thorac Dis 2019;11(Suppl 1):S25–36.
[23] Hellmann MD, Callahan MK, Awad MM, et al. Tumor mutational burden and efficacy of nivolumab monotherapy and in combination with ipilimumab in small-cell lung cancer. Cancer Cell 2019;35(2):329.
[24] Necchi A, Joseph RW, Loriot Y, et al. Atezolizumab in platinum-treated locally advanced or metastatic urothelial carcinoma: post-progression outcomes from the phase II IMvigor210 study. Ann Oncol 2017;28(12):3044–50.
[25] Samstein RM, Lee CH, Shoushtari AN, et al. Tumor mutational load predicts survival after immunotherapy across multiple cancer types. Nat Genet 2019;51(2):202–6.
[26] Alexandrov LB, Nik-Zainal S, Wedge DC, et al. Signatures of mutational processes in human cancer. Nature 2013;500(7463):415–21.
[27] Drilon A, Wang L, Arcila ME, et al. Broad, hybrid capture-based next-generation sequencing identifies actionable genomic alterations in lung adenocarcinomas otherwise negative for such alterations by other genomic testing approaches. Clin Cancer Res 2015;21(16):3631–9.
[28] Campesato LF, Barroso-Sousa R, Jimenez L, et al. Comprehensive cancer-gene panels can be used to estimate mutational load and predict clinical benefit to PD-1 blockade in clinical practice. Oncotarget 2015;6(33):34221–7.
[29] Chalmers ZR, Connelly CF, Fabrizio D, et al. Analysis of 100,000 human cancer genomes reveals the landscape of tumor mutational burden. Genome Med 2017;9(1):34.
[30] Rizvi H, Sanchez-Vega F, La K, et al. Molecular determinants of response to anti-programmed cell death (PD)-1 and anti-programmed death-ligand 1 (PD-L1) blockade in patients with non-small-cell lung cancer profiled with targeted next-generation sequencing. J Clin Oncol 2018;36(7):633–41.
[31] Buchhalter I, Rempel E, Endris V, et al. Size matters: dissecting key parameters for panel-based tumor mutational burden analysis. Int J Cancer 2019;144(4):848–58.
[32] Hellmann MD, Rizvi NA, Goldman JW, et al. Nivolumab plus ipilimumab as first-line treatment for advanced non-small-cell lung cancer (CheckMate 012): results of an open-label, phase 1, multicohort study. Lancet Oncol 2017;18(1):31–41.
[33] Hellmann MD, Callahan MK, Awad MM, et al. Tumor mutational burden and efficacy of nivolumab monotherapy and in combination with ipilimumab in small-cell lung cancer. Cancer Cell 2018;33(5):853–61 [Erratum in: Cancer Cell. 2019 Feb 11;35(2):329].
[34] Cai LL, Wang J. Liquid biopsy for lung cancer immunotherapy. Oncol Lett 2019;17(6):4751–60.

[35] Iqbal M, Roberts A, Starr J, et al. Feasibility and clinical value of circulating tumor DNA testing in patients with gastric adenocarcinomas. J Gastrointest Oncol 2019; 10(3):400–6.
[36] Volckmar AL, Sültmann H, Riediger A, et al. A field guide for cancer diagnostics using cell-free DNA: from principles to practice and clinical applications. Genes Chromosomes Cancer 2018;57(3):123–39.
[37] Gandara DR, Paul SM, Kowanetz M, et al. Blood-based tumor mutational burden as a predictor of clinical benefit in non-small-cell lung cancer patients treated with atezolizumab. Nat Med 2018;24(9):1441–8.
[38] Stenzinger A, Allen JD, Maas J, et al. Tumor mutational burden standardization initiatives: recommendations for consistent tumor mutational burden assessment in clinical samples to guide immunotherapy treatment decisions. Genes Chromosomes Cancer 2019;58(8):578–88.
[39] Addeo A, Banna GL, Weiss GJ. Tumor mutation burden-from hopes to doubts. JAMA Oncol 2019. https://doi.org/10.1001/jamaoncol.2019.0626.
[40] Rizvi NA, Chan TA. Immunotherapy and oncogenic pathways: the PTEN connection. Cancer Discov 2016; 6(2):128–9.

Identify/HLA

Advances in Molecular Pathology 2 (2019) 187–199

ADVANCES IN MOLECULAR PATHOLOGY

Human Leukocyte Antigen Typing Using High-Throughput DNA and RNA Sequencing and Application for Cell Line Identification

Sebastian Boegel, PhD[a,*], John C. Castle, PhD[b]

[a]Johannes Gutenberg University, Mainz, Germany; [b]Agenus Inc, 3 Forbes Road, Lexington, MA 02421-7305, USA

KEYWORDS

• Cell line misidentification • Cell line authentication • HLA typing • High-throughput sequencing • Bioinformatics

KEY POINTS

- The HLA type is encoded by a highly variable region of the human genome.
- This review provides an overview of methods using high-throughput sequencing for HLA typing, including wet laboratory protocols and in silico tools.
- Cross-contaminated and misidentified cell lines can confound the results drawn from experiments.
- Using high-throughput sequencing, the HLA type can be used as a fundamental cell line "barcode" to track samples and prevent sample annotation swaps and contamination.

INTRODUCTION

Human cell lines are essential tools for biological and medical research, such as models predicting response to a treatment [1,2], for identification of disease-specific biomarkers [3,4], and for novel cancer immunotherapies [5,6]. However, up to 36% of active cell lines are either cross-contaminated or misidentified [7]. A recent analysis of 13 studies comprising ~3600 cell lines found contamination in 23% of the samples, ranging from 10% to 100% depending on the study [8]. In addition, 32,755 papers were identified that used known misidentified cell lines in their experiments [9]. This issue is a serious one [10], with only 25 published retractions in the literature as of November 2018 [8]. Scientific journals now require cell line authentication before publication [11], and many research funders also require authentication for grant submissions (see National Institutes of Health notices NOT-OD-16-011 [12] and NOT-OD-16-012 [13]).

Short tandem repeats (STRs) and single nucleotide polymorphisms are commonly used to determine the identity of a cell line [14]. In 2001, Giacomini and colleagues [15] proposed the HLA type of a cell line as an ID card to prevent usage of cell lines "sans papiers" (ie, cell lines without a valid identity check). Furthermore, Adams and colleagues [16] provided the HLA class I and II types from the NCI-60 cell lines as a reference catalog, stating "accurate information about the HLA genotype of each cell line may, in addition, help their identification, validation and qualification among

Disclosure: J.C. Castle is employed by Agenus Inc, a company developing immunotherapies. S. Boegel has nothing to disclose.

*Corresponding author, *E-mail address:* seb.boegel@gmail.com

https://doi.org/10.1016/j.yamp.2019.07.013
2589-4080/19/

different laboratories excluding possible errors related to switching of cell lines or culture contamination". With colleagues, the authors' laboratory characterized the HLA types and expression of more than 1000 cancer cell lines and showed how this catalog represents an easy-to-perform solution for cell line identity checking and tracking [17,18].

HLA molecules play a central role in the adaptive immune system. They present self, non-self (eg, neoepitopes arising from mutations), and foreign (eg, pathogenic) peptide antigens that are either derived from intracellular proteins (in the case of HLA class I) or from extracellular proteins (HLA class II) [19] (Fig. 1A). A hallmark of the HLA system is that it is polygenic (Fig. 1B) and highly polymorphic (Fig. 1C) [20–22]. More than 15,000 alleles have been sequenced in the human population for the 3 classical HLA class I genes (HLA-A, -B, and -C) and more than 6000 alleles for the classical HLA class II genes (HLA-DP, -DQ, and -DR) (Fig. 1D) [23]. Deciphering an individual's composition of HLA alleles, HLA typing, is needed for, for example, organ and stem cell transplantation [24] and mutanome-based cancer immunotherapies [25,26]. In addition, the HLA type of a cell line can be used for cell line authentication and tracking.

The standard laboratory-based HLA typing techniques use genomic DNA for selective polymerase chain reaction (PCR) amplification of the target HLA alleles followed by sequence-specific oligonucleotide probe hybridization [27], detection via a sequence-specific primer gel electrophoresis [28], or direct Sanger sequencing [29]. In contrast, high-throughput sequencing (HTS) approaches for HLA typing allow the parallel sequencing of nucleic acids of many

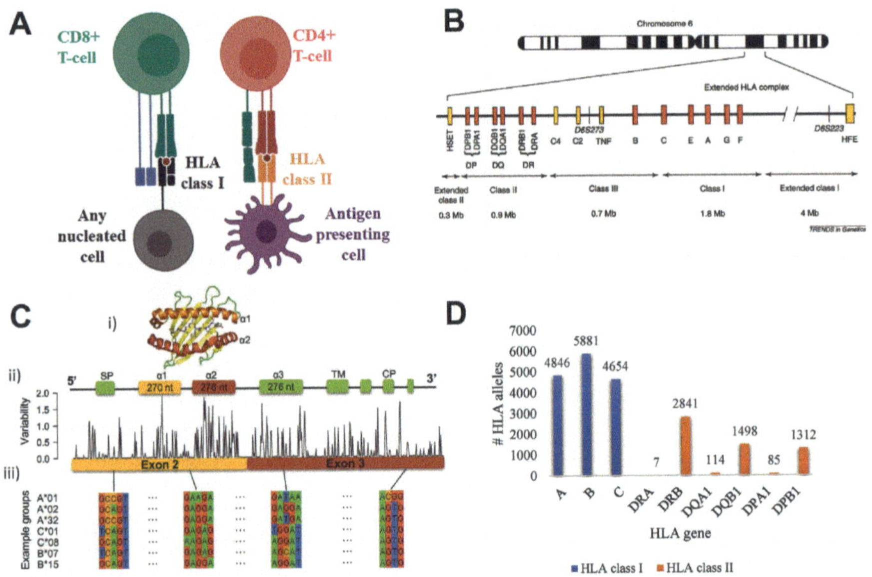

FIG. 1 The HLA system. (**A**) HLA class I and II molecules present self, non-self, and foreign peptide antigens on the cell surface, that are mainly derived from intracellular (HLA class I) or extracellular proteins (HLA class II), where the peptide-HLA complexes can be recognized by CD8$^+$ T cells (HLA class I) or CD4$^+$ T cells (HLA class II). Image made with BioRender (www.biorender.com). (**B**) The HLA complex consists of more than 200 genes (not all shown) located in close proximity on chromosome 6 and is divided into 3 regions, of which class I and class II genes (depicted in *red*) are responsible for antigen presentation. (**C**) The HLA system is highly polymorphic. Depicted is a sequence variability analysis for HLA class I alleles. (i) The helices encoded by exons 2 (α1-chain: *orange*) and 3 (α2-chain: *red*) of HLA class I alleles bind peptides (crystal structure 3OXR from PDB). (ii) The nucleotide variability at each position of a multiple sequence alignment of all HLA class I (A, B, and C) alleles, where 0 and 2 represent minimum and maximum variability, (iii) Example sequences are shown for 4 regions in 7 HLA groups, that is, 2-digit resolution. (**D**) HLA class I and class II allele frequencies, numbers assigned as of April 2016 from [23]. ([*B*] *From* Undlien DE, Lie BA, Thorsby E. HLA complex genes in type 1 diabetes and other autoimmune diseases. Which genes are involved? Trends Genet. 2001;17:94; with permission; and [*C*] *Adapted from* Boegel S, Löwer M, Schäfer M, et al. HLA typing from RNA-Seq sequence reads. Genome Med. 2012;4:102.)

samples, and thus, can be both cost and time-effective. In addition, HTS enables the rapid generation of billions of nucleic acid sequences (ie, "sequencing reads"), enabling determination of the whole HLA locus as compared with only the exons containing the most variations.

Excitingly, raw DNA and RNA sequence data (fastq files) from more than 28,000 human samples have been deposited in the public Sequence Read Archive as of April 2019. Consortia, such as Genotype-Tissue Expression [30], The Cancer Genome Atlas [31], International Cancer Genome Consortium [32], and the Cancer Cell Line Encyclopedia (CCLE) [33], have sequenced the genome and transcriptome of many tumors, normal tissues, and cell lines. Although the experiments did not aim to determine the HLA type of each samples, the raw data are publicly available and can be reanalyzed to determine the HLA type.

In this review, the authors (i) provide an overview of laboratory protocols developed for high-throughput HLA typing, (ii) describe algorithms developed for HLA typing from standard DNA and RNA-sequencing data, and (iii) describe the application of HLA typing for cell line authentication (Fig. 2).

Human Leukocyte Antigen Nomenclature

Each HLA allele has a unique name [34] consisting of the prefix "HLA-", followed by the HLA locus, for example, "A" and the separator "*", followed by numbers that specify the respective allele of this gene. The first field (also called "2-digit resolution") denotes the allele group (eg, "HLA-A*02"); the second field ("4-digit resolution") specifies the specific allele encoding a unique protein (eg, "HLA-A*02:01"); the third field ("6-digit resolution") specifies the allele nucleotide sequence, including synonymous substitutions within the coding region (eg, "HLA-A*02:01:01"), and the fourth field ("8-digit resolution") is used to include noncoding regions (eg, "HLA-A*02:01:01:01").

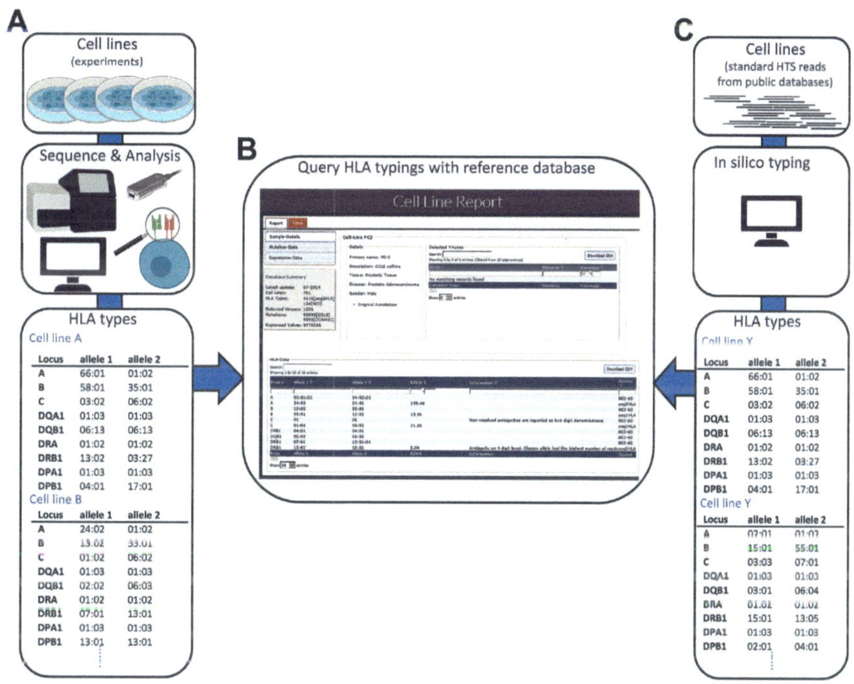

FIG. 2 HLA type as cell line barcode. (A) Established laboratory protocols for second and third generation sequencing platforms enable efficient HLA typing for cell lines in an experiment. (B) A reference database of ground truthed HLA types for cell lines will enable researchers running experiments with cell lines generating HTS data could straightforwardly validate the cell line identity. (C) Consortia and researchers worldwide have sequenced the genomes and transcriptomes of many tumors, normal tissues, and cell lines. The raw data are publicly available and can be reanalyzed. In silico HLA typing tools should be a standard part in HTS processing workflows, thereby providing an easy way for cell line identification and sample tracking. Images made with BioRender (www.biorender.com). TNF, tumor necrosis factor.

SEQUENCING PLATFORMS

Sequencing platforms such as Illumina and Ion Torrent, often called "Next-Generation Sequencing" (NGS) or "second-generation sequencing" platforms [35], are effective, highly parallelized platforms enabling high-resolution HLA genotyping with few ambiguities [36,37] and accuracies greater than 97% for HLA class I and 90% to 99% for HLA class II genes [38]. Tissue typing laboratories are adapting these platforms [39–42].

HLA typing by second-generation sequencing platforms involves the following:

1. Amplification of the target region, which can be the complete HLA region, specific exons, or the full sequence of the HLA genes of interest
2. Library preparation, including, among other steps, ligation of barcodes (ie, indexed adaptors) to the amplicons that allow sequencing of many samples (eg, different donors) in a single run
3. Sequencing
4. Processing of the reads and in silico HLA typing analysis

The core principles of second-generation sequencing (Ion Torrent and Illumina) are clonal amplification of the isolated nucleic acid fragments followed by highly parallelized sequencing, producing billions of short reads (<300 nucleotides [nt]), either single or paired end. Paired-end reads, in which both ends of the DNA fragments are sequenced, are more suitable for reconstructing the allele composition of the highly polymorphic HLA region in a sample. One challenge of the second-generation sequencing platform is aligning the short reads to determine the full sequence of the HLA alleles.

Third-generation sequencing platforms from Pacific Biosciences (PacBio) and Oxford Nanopore produce reads up to 2.3 Mb by sequencing a single DNA molecule without amplification. Despite their higher error rate, it has been shown that accurate genotypes of the HLA loci are possible.

In this later discussion, the different sequencing platforms are introduced and studies are reviewed that developed protocols for high-throughput accurate HLA typing on these platforms.

Illumina

The sequencing technology used by Illumina is based on sequencing by synthesis using DNA fragments attached to the surface of a glass flow cell, hybridization of the DNA fragments in the sample (using specific adapters ligated to these fragments in a step called library preparation), and subsequently, incorporation of differently labeled fluorescent nucleotides, followed by an imaging step to detect the identity of the incorporated base. The result is millions of short reads typically 150 nt long on the HiSeq and NextSeq instruments and 300 nt on the MiSeq. When sequenced in paired-end mode, 150 (300) nt are sequenced from each end of the DNA fragment.

Wittig and colleagues [43] developed a bait-based capturing approach for HLA genotyping (HLA-A, -B, -C, -DRB1, -DQA1, -DQB1, -DPA1, -DPB1) of 96 samples in parallel on a single HiSeq2500 run with an allele call rate of 0.99 (see Ref. [44] for the protocol). Ehrenberg and colleagues [45] developed a 6-locus multilocus individual tagging-NGS approach to sequence full-length HLA class I and class II genes (HLA-A, -B, -C, -DRB1, -DPB1, -DQB1) from 96 individuals in a single MiSeq run, including the identification of novel alleles (see Ref. [46] for the protocol). Yin and colleagues [47] developed an automated workflow of sequencing 5 HLA loci (HLA-A, -B, -C, -DRB1, -DQB1) from buccal swab DNA using multiplex long-range PCR in conjunction with the MiSeq platform and applied it to more than 10,000 National Marrow Donor Program registry donors, resulting in 99.84% accuracy of the successfully amplified and reported typings (see Ref. [48] for the protocol).

Ion Torrent personal genome machine

The sequencing technology used by the Ion Torrent personal genome machine (PGM) is based on sequential addition of the 4 nt to a DNA template nucleotide incorporation by the DNA polymerase and the measurement of hydrogen ion release every time a nucleotide is incorporated [49], generating 0.4 to 5 million sequencing reads with read lengths up to 400 bases in 3 to 7 hours depending on the chip used [50].

Shiina and colleagues [51] developed an approach for high-resolution (8 digits) single-molecule sequencing and typing for HLA class I and class II using PGM (see Ref. [50] for the protocol). Furthermore, the efficacy of the PGM for HLA typing of 285 genomic DNA was shown by Barone and colleagues [52], with concordance rates of more than 99% for HLA-A, -B, -C, -DRB1, -DQB1, and more than 98% for HLA-DPB1. In addition, Guerra and colleagues [53] evaluated HLA class I and class II (HLA-DRB1, -DRB345, -DQB1, -DPB1) typing on the PGM of 362 registry donors from 4 ethnic populations and obtained concordance rates of 91% to 98% compared with PCR-SSO HLA types with a turnaround of 4 days for typing 44 samples.

PacBio single-molecule real time sequencing

The PacBio platform is based on single-molecule real-time sequencing (SMRT) [54], in which a single long DNA fragment together with a DNA polymerase is immobilized in a chamber of an SMRT cell, and the detection of the fluorescent light pulse resulting from the release of phospholinked fluorophores upon incorporation of nucleotides in the DNA strand [55]. Depending on the lifetime of the DNA polymer, the DNA fragment can be sequenced multiple times, thus increasing the accuracy [56]. By sequencing long fragments, this platform generates reads with an average length of up to 14 kb [57].

Gowda and Ambardar [58] used the PacBio platform for large-scale HLA class I and class II (HLA-DRB1, -DQB1) typing of Indian HLA types (see Ref. [59] for the protocol). Suzuki and colleagues [60] used the PGM and PacBio SMRT platforms to perform full-length HLA allele sequencing to provide polymorphic gene reference sequences at genomic allelic resolution that serves as a foundation in precision medicine.

MinION nanopore

MinION by Oxford Nanopore is a portable real-time device the size of a memory stick, which is connected to a computer via a USB port. Using an enzyme motor, a single DNA or RNA fragment passes through a nanoscale hole base by base while the fluctuations in current identify the passing nucleotide [61]. Protocols have been developed that generate average read lengths greater than 100 kb [62] with individual reads up to 2.3 Mb [63]. Despite the relatively high per-read error rate [64,65], Ton and colleagues [66] accurately typed HLA-B in Māori and Polynesian populations, Liu and colleagues [67] demonstrated 100% accuracy for HLA class I alleles, and Lang and colleagues [68] published a protocol to characterize HLA class I genotypes from genomic DNA using the MinION Nanopore.

Human Leukocyte Antigen–Determining Algorithms

Because there is a high level of homology between the HLA alleles (see Fig. 1B), it is challenging to determine the HLA type from short sequencing reads. Furthermore, the human reference genome, the standard reference used in bioinformatic workflows for reconstructing the genome and transcriptome of the sample from a sequencing experiment, does not reflect the diversity of the HLA alleles in the human population, confounding read alignment and HLA determination. Last, distinguishing between homozygous (eg, HLA-A*02:01/HLA-A*02:01) and heterozygous loci (eg, HLA-A*02:01/HLA-A*24:01) using short reads is difficult, especially from RNA-Seq data.

In the last decade, there has been a tremendous evolution of bioinformatic tools for HLA typing from HTS data (Table 1). These tools use a variety of algorithms for input from different HTS assays: whole-genome sequencing (WGS), whole-exome sequencing (WXS), targeted (amplicon) sequencing, or transcriptome sequencing (RNA-Seq), allowing either standard HTS sequencing reads (in fastq format) or processed alignment files (in bam format). The software tools also differ in the output, for example, HLA class I only or also HLA class II, the typing depth (2-field, 3-field, or 4-field), additional information, such as confidence score, expression, or ambiguities. All methods determine the HLA type in at least 4-digit resolution (2-field), which denotes the actual protein sequence of the HLA allele.

A subset of the tools has been benchmarked. Optitype [69,70] showed the highest accuracy of HLA class I for WXS [71–73] and RNA-Seq data [72]. In addition, seq2HLA [74] and PHLAT [75] showed the highest combined accuracy for HLA class I and class II calls. Seq2HLA had the shortest runtime [72]. Furthermore, Liu and Yang [76] found ATHLATES [76] to be as accurate as Optitype for WXS HLA class I and HLAreporter [77] to have the best accuracy for WXS HLA class II. An ensemble approach combining different HLA callers further increased the accuracy to 100% accuracy for class I and 99% for class II [78]. Some HLA calling tools report accuracies greater than 99% for WGS, for example, Kourami [79], WXS, for example, HLA-HD [80], and HLAscan [81], or RNA-Seq assays, such as HLAprofiles [82] and arcasHLA [83].

Of note, Bauer and colleagues [72] were not able to run 4 of the 9 HLA typing tools included in their benchmark study, despite seeking advice from the developers. Software installation surprisingly remains a general issue in the deployment of biomedical software [84–86]; the authors therefore published methods for HLA typing [87] that provided protocols and manuals for several of the tools in Table 1, thereby facilitating reuse and reproducibility.

Taken together, the plethora of tools and their high accuracies suggest that the issue of 4-digit HLA class I and class II typing (2 fields), which is sufficient for most applications, from standard HTS data using second generation is solved and should therefore be a standard part in HTS

TABLE 1
Bioinformatic Tools for Human Leukocyte Antigen Typing from High-Throughput Sequencing Data

Name	Designed for	Description	Source Code
HLApers [88]	RNA-Seq	Mapping, allele-specific expression estimation, eQTL mapping	https://github.com/genevol-usp/HLApers
Phlat [75,89]	RNA-Seq, WXS, targeted amplicon seq	Alignment-based	https://sites.google.com/site/phlatfortype/
Seq2HLA [21,74]	RNA-Seq	Alignment-based, HLA class I (classical and nonclassical), HLA class II, locus-specific expression estimation, 4-digit resolution	https://github.com/TRON-Bioinformatics/seq2HLA
HLAProfiler [82]	RNA-Seq	k-mer profile-based method, competitive alignment, rare alleles	https://github.com/ExpressionAnalysis/HLAProfiler
HLA*PRG:LA [90]	WGS, WXS, long-read Oxoford Nanopore & PacBio (WGS & targeted), genome assemblies	Alignment-based representing reference database as graphs	https://github.com/DiltheyLab/HLA-PRG-LA
ALPHLARD-NT [91]	WGS	Bayesian method, detection of rare germline variants, and somatic mutation in HLA genes	n.a.
HLAreporter [77]	WXS	Assembly and alignment-based	http://paed.hku.hk/genome/software.html
HLAforest [92]	RNA-Seq	Alignment-based, hierarchical read weighting	https://code.google.com/archive/p/hlaforest/
Kourami [79,93]	WGS	Graph-guided assembly, novel HLA allele discovery	https://github.com/Kingsford-Group/kourami
HLA-VBSeq [94]	WGS	Variational Bayesian inference, full resolution	http://nagasakilab.csml.org/hla/
Optitype [69,70]	RNA-Seq, WXS	Alignment-based, optimization problem using integer linear programming, no HLA class II	https://github.com/FRED-2/OptiType
xHLA [95]	WGS, WXS	Integer linear programming, protein-level alignment of exons, 4-digit resolution, ~3 min to process a 30× WGS BAM file on a desktop computer	https://github.com/humanlongevity/HLA
Prohlatype [96]	DNA and RNA	Bayesian inference of HLA types, Profile Hidden Markov Models, alignment-based	https://github.com/hammerlab/prohlatype

(continued on next page)

TABLE 1
(continued)

Name	Designed for	Description	Source Code
HLAminer [97]	WGS, Exon capture, RNA-Seq, long read seq (eg, Oxford Nanopore)	Assembly and alignment-based, v1.4 supports HLA prediction from raw uncorrected shotgun nanopore long reads (such as those from Oxford Nanopore)	https://github.com/warrenlr/HLAminer
BayesTyping1 [98]	long read seq (PacificBiosciences)	Circular consensus sequencing reads, using Bayes' theorem	n.a.
HLAscan [81]	WGS, WXS, targeted amplicon seq	Analysis of genomic reads from Illumina X-Ten	http://www.genomekorea.com/display/tools/HLAscan
AmpliHLA/AmpliSAS [99,100]	RNA-Seq, WXS, amplicon	Web server, implementation of seq2HLA for RNA-Seq and WXS, MHC prediction also for nonmodel species	http://evobiolab.biol.amu.edu.pl/amplisat/index.php?amplihla
HLA-HD [80,101]	WXS	Alignment-based, 6-digit-resolution	https://www.genome.med.kyoto-u.ac.jp/HLA-HD/
ATHLATES [76,102]	WXS, (WGS, RNA-Seq)	Alignment-based, contig assembly	https://www.broadinstitute.org/viral-genomics/athlates
Polysolver [103]	WXS	Alignment-based Bayesian probabilistic model to reassign reads that did not map to reference, no HLA class II, somatic mutation detection in HLA class I alleles	https://software.broadinstitute.org/cancer/cga/polysolver
Hla-mapper [104]	WGS, WXS, targeted	No HLA typing, optimizing the mapping of HLA sequences, possibly a useful preprocessing step	http://www.castelli-lab.net/apps/hla-mapper/
arcasHLA [83]	RNA-Seq	Accepts prealigned BAM files or standard fastq files as input, 3-field resolution for HLA class I and class II in <2 min	https://github.com/RabadanLab/arcasHLA

Abbreviation: n.a., not applicable from the publication.

processing workflows. Technical advancements of third-generation sequencing platforms will also lead to the development of many more bioinformatic HLA typing tools for these instruments, resulting in higher resolutions.

HUMAN LEUKOCYTE ANTIGEN TYPE FOR CELL LINE IDENTIFICATION

Here, the authors provide examples how the HLA type can be used for quality control throughout experiments with cell lines. They are the standard workhorses in biomedical research; the advent of HTS platforms has enabled characterization of these cell lines on genomic and transcriptomic levels. Indeed, many cell lines have been subject to HTS experiments: COSMIC Cell Lines Project [105] has curated comprehensive data on somatic mutations in a broad range of human cell lines; the Broad-Novartis CCLE [33] has determined genetic alterations and gene expression profiles in more than 1000 cell lines; and the transcriptome of 675 cell lines has been analyzed [106]. Less attention has been given to the characterization of the HLA types but, excitingly, the raw data files from these studies are available for reanalysis [16,107–109].

The authors' team reanalyzed raw RNA-Seq data from more than 1000 human cancer cell lines, using seq2HLA to determine the HLA class I and II type and HLA expression, and placed the results in a public Web server [17,18]. The authors examined possible annotation discrepancies between related cell lines. As an example, the transcriptome of ovarian cancer cell lines PEO1, PEO4, PEO14, and PEO23 was sequenced by Ng and colleagues [110] to examine structural variations in high-grade serous ovarian cancers. Cell lines PEO1 (Cellosaurus [109] identifier: CVCL_2686) and PEO4 (CVCL_2690) are derived from the same patient, whereas PEO14 (CVCL_2687) and PEO23 (CVCL_2689) came from different patients [111]. As expected, the determined HLA type between the pairs from the same individual matched. Similarly, different samples of the breast cancer cell lines 21NT (CVCL_7933) and 21PT (CVCL_7934), which are from primary tumors, and 21MT1 (CVCL_7931) and 21MT2 (CVCL_7932), which are from metastasis of the original tumor, were sequenced by Daemen and colleagues [112]. These lines were originally derived from the same individual [113], and, indeed, the same HLA type is found in all samples. Furthermore, the same study provided RNA-Seq data from the breast carcinoma cell line HCC-1937 (CVCL_0290) and the matched lymphocyte cell line HCC-1937 (CVCL_3281; mistakenly called HCC-2337 in some publications), and again, the authors obtained the same HLA type for these samples. However, they also identified 2 studies using the breast cancer cell line SUM149PT (CVCL_3422) that, when the authors analyzed the HLA types, showed discrepant HLA types [18], suggesting a possible sample annotation or authentication issue.

Often cancer research studies sequence both transcriptomes and exomes of tumor and normal samples from the same individual, and such isogenic samples should have the same HLA type. HLA typing tools applied to these data provide a fast and easy quality control method to validate annotation and to identify inconsistencies without additional laboratory work.

DISCUSSION

Cross-contaminated and misidentified cell lines can confound the results drawn from experiments. Fortunately, the HLA type can be used as a fundamental cell line "barcode" to track samples and prevent sample annotation swaps and contamination. The HLA type itself can now be readily "read" using HTS data.

When the HLA type of a cell line is known [16,107–109], the authors were able to compare the locally determined HLA type with the published one for identification. For a given cell line, a limitation of the approach is the lack of a curated searchable reference catalog of cell line HLA types, that is, ground truth of HLA class I and class II typings. One solution is the creation of a curated cell line database integrating cell line HLA class I and class II types with additional characterizations important for authentication (eg, STR genotypes) or biological function (eg, mutation profiles). Having this reference database in place, researchers running experiments with cell lines generating HTS data could straightforwardly validate the cell line identity. As part of this solution, the authors generated the TRON cell line portal (http://celllines.tron-mainz.de), integrating HLA type and expression with genomic data, as well as immunomic information, such as determined from RNA-Seq data and public resources, for 1082 widely used cancer cell lines. The portal provides an interactive user interface and advanced search capabilities, such that researchers can effectively search for cell lines that fit the requirements of their experiments.

A drawback of the information in this portal is that no established gold-standard HLA types exist for most of the cell lines, and thus, the authors need to rely on the validity of the cell line samples used for sequencing and the integrity of the datasets (eg, correct sample annotation). Projects, such as "NGS in Reference cell lines," from the International HLA and Immunogenetics Workshop [114] and efforts by cell line distributors to determine the HLA class I and class II type cell lines help generate curated references, which could be integrated in resources, such as the Cellosaurus database (https://web.expasy.org/cellosaurus/ [109]). Cellosaurus is an excellent, curated resource of information, aggregating available characteristics of more than 80,000 human cell lines, including STR genotypes, mutation data, and HLA typings.

Primary tumor tissues evolve, eventually leading to mutations in the HLA gene locus [103] and loss of heterozygosity in HLAs [115]. Similarly, cell lines evolve over time, and passage, for example, during cultivation leading to changes in the genomic and transcriptomic profile [116–118], potentially hamper authentication of overpassaged cell lines [7]. Nevertheless, even in the cases when no curated information about the HLA type of a cell line or tumor sample is available, the HLA type barcode provides an excellent tracking barcode for samples and datasets within an experiment that are derived from the sample donor material, such as tumor/normal pairs.

Using HTS for HLA typing, groups have identified novel alleles, which are available in the IPD-IMGT/HLA database [119,120]. With nucleic acid sequences of more than 21,000 HLA alleles, this database is a key resource in the development of HLA typing methods of both laboratory protocols and bioinformatic tools. Indeed, although the reference human genome lacks genetic variation at the HLA locus, tools such as vg [121] provide the possibility to build nonlinear variation graphs of DNA sequences representing genetic variation across a population, which could directly integrate the genetic HLA variability [122].

Obtaining the HLA type of cell lines using HTS is feasible, and the HLA type can be used as a sample barcode. The cited laboratory protocols for second- and third-generation sequencing platforms enable efficient HLA typing. The bioinformatic software tools for HLA typing from standard HTS data can be straightforwardly integrated into HTS processing workflows, thereby providing an easy way for cell line identification and sample tracking.

ACKNOWLEDGMENTS

The authors would like to acknowledge the former colleagues at TRON, who codeveloped seq2HLA [21] as well as TCLP [17], and all the researchers who contributed to the development of protocols and bioinformatic tools to make HLA typing from HTS data possible. They would also like to thank Dr Christopher Korch for fruitful discussion and excellent comments that enhanced this review.

REFERENCES

[1] Domcke S, Sinha R, Levine DA, et al. Evaluating cell lines as tumour models by comparison of genomic profiles. Nat Commun 2013;4:2126.

[2] Niu N, Wang L. In vitro human cell line models to predict clinical response to anticancer drugs. Pharmacogenomics 2015;16:273–85.

[3] Huang Y-H, Vakoc CR. A biomarker harvest from one thousand cancer cell lines. Cell 2016;166:536–7.

[4] Dowling P, Clynes M. Conditioned media from cell lines: a complementary model to clinical specimens for the discovery of disease-specific biomarkers. Proteomics 2011;11:794–804.

[5] Castle JC, Kreiter S, Diekmann J, et al. Exploiting the mutanome for tumor vaccination. Cancer Res 2012;72:1081–91.

[6] Kreiter S, Vormehr M, van de Roemer N, et al. Mutant MHC class II epitopes drive therapeutic immune responses to cancer. Nature 2015;520:692–6.

[7] Hughes P, Marshall D, Reid Y, et al. The costs of using unauthenticated, over-passaged cell lines: how much more data do we need? Biotechniques 2007;43:575, 577–8, 581–2 passim.

[8] Korch C, Varella-Garcia M. Tackling the human cell line and tissue misidentification problem is needed for reproducible biomedical research. Adv Mol Pathol 2018;209–28.e6.

[9] Horbach SPJ, Halffman W. The ghosts of HeLa: how cell line misidentification contaminates the scientific literature. PLoS One 2017;12:e0186281.

[10] Vaughan L, Glänzel W, Korch C, et al. Widespread use of misidentified cell line KB (HeLa): incorrect attribution and its impact revealed through mining the scientific literature. Cancer Res 2017;77:2784–8.

[11] Fusenig NE, Capes-Davis A, Bianchini F, et al. The need for a worldwide consensus for cell line authentication: experience implementing a mandatory requirement at the International Journal of Cancer. PLoS Biol 2017;15:e2001438.

[12] NOT-OD-16-011: implementing rigor and transparency in NIH & AHRQ Research Grant Applications. Available at: https://grants.nih.gov/grants/guide/notice-files/NOT-OD-16-011.html. Accessed April 11, 2019.

[13] NOT-OD-16-012: implementing rigor and transparency in NIH & AHRQ Career Development Award Applications. Available at: https://grants.nih.gov/grants/guide/notice-files/NOT-OD-16-012.html. Accessed April 11, 2019.

[14] Almeida JL, Cole KD, Plant AL. Standards for cell line authentication and beyond. PLoS Biol 2016;14:e1002476.

[15] Giacomini P, Giorda E, Pera C, et al. An ID card for tumour cell lines: HLA typing can help. Lancet Oncol 2001;2:658.

[16] Adams S, Robbins F-M, Chen D, et al. HLA class I and II genotype of the NCI-60 cell lines. J Transl Med 2005;3:11.

[17] Scholtalbers J, Boegel S, Bukur T, et al. TCLP: an online cancer cell line catalogue integrating HLA type, predicted neo-epitopes, virus and gene expression. Genome Med 2015;7:118.

[18] Boegel S, Löwer M, Bukur T, et al. A catalog of HLA type, HLA expression, and neo-epitope candidates in human cancer cell lines. Oncoimmunology 2014;3: e954893.

[19] Rock KL, Reits E, Neefjes J. Present yourself! By MHC class I and MHC class II molecules. Trends Immunol 2016;37:724–37.

[20] Undlien DE, Lie BA, Thorsby E. HLA complex genes in type 1 diabetes and other autoimmune diseases. Which genes are involved? Trends Genet 2001;17:93–100.

[21] Boegel S, Löwer M, Schäfer M, et al. HLA typing from RNA-Seq sequence reads. Genome Med 2012;4:102.

[22] Frenet EM, Scaradavou A. Human leukocyte antigens. Transfusion medicine and hemostasis. Elsevier; 2019. p. 191–7.

[23] HLA Nomenclature @ hla.alleles.org. Available at: http://hla.alleles.org/nomenclature/stats.html. Accessed April 13, 2019.

[24] Petersdorf EW. HLA mismatching in transplantation. Blood 2015;125:1058–9.

[25] Vormehr M, Diken M, Boegel S, et al. Mutanome directed cancer immunotherapy. Curr Opin Immunol 2016;39:14–22.

[26] Vormehr M, Türeci Ö, Sahin U. Harnessing tumor mutations for truly individualized cancer vaccines. Annu Rev Med 2019;70:395–407.

[27] Cao K, Chopek M, Fernández-Viña MA. High and intermediate resolution DNA typing systems for class I HLA-A, B, C genes by hybridization with sequence-specific oligonucleotide probes (SSOP). Rev Immunogenet 1999;1:177–208.

[28] Olerup O, Zetterquist H. HLA-DR typing by PCR amplification with sequence-specific primers (PCR-SSP) in 2 hours: an alternative to serological DR typing in clinical practice including donor-recipient matching in cadaveric transplantation. Tissue Antigens 1992;39:225–35.

[29] Santamaria P, Boyce-Jacino MT, Lindstrom AL, et al. HLA class II "typing": direct sequencing of DRB, DQB, and DQA genes. Hum Immunol 1992;33:69–81.

[30] Gamazon ER, Segrè AV, van de Bunt M, et al. Using an atlas of gene regulation across 44 human tissues to inform complex disease- and trait-associated variation. Nat Genet 2018;50:956–67.

[31] Blum A, Wang P, Zenklusen JC. SnapShot: TCGA-analyzed tumors. Cell 2018;173:530.

[32] Zhang J, Baran J, Cros A, et al. International cancer genome consortium data portal–a one-stop shop for cancer genomics data. Database 2011;2011: bar026.

[33] Barretina J, Caponigro G, Stransky N, et al. The cancer cell line encyclopedia enables predictive modelling of anticancer drug sensitivity. Nature 2012;483:603–7.

[34] Marsh SGE. WHO Nomenclature Committee for factors of the HLA system. Nomenclature for factors of the HLA system, update October, November, and December 2018. Hladnikia (Ljubl) 2019;93:140–81.

[35] Heather JM, Chain B. The sequence of sequencers: the history of sequencing DNA. Genomics 2016;107:1–8.

[36] Weimer ET, Montgomery M, Petraroia R, et al. Performance characteristics and validation of next-generation sequencing for human leucocyte antigen typing. J Mol Diagn 2016;18:668–75.

[37] Profaizer T, Lázár-Molnár E, Pole A, et al. HLA genotyping using the Illumina HLA TruSight next-generation sequencing kits: a comparison. Int J Immunogenet 2017;44:164–8.

[38] Osoegawa K, Vayntrub TA, Wenda S, et al. Quality control project of NGS HLA genotyping for the 17th International HLA and Immunogenetics Workshop. Hum Immunol 2019;80:228–36.

[39] Schöfl G, Lang K, Quenzel P, et al. 2.7 million samples genotyped for HLA by next generation sequencing: lessons learned. BMC Genomics 2017;18:161.

[40] Weimer ET. Clinical validation of NGS technology for HLA: an early adopter's perspective. Hum Immunol 2016;77:820–3.

[41] Edgerly CH, Weimer ET. The past, present, and future of HLA typing in transplantation. Methods Mol Biol 2018; 1802:1–10.

[42] Baier DM, Hofmann JA, Fischer H, et al. Very low error rates of NGS-based HLA typing at stem cell donor recruitment question the need for a standard confirmatory typing step before donor work-up. Bone Marrow Transplant 2018. https://doi.org/10.1038/s41409-018-0411-2.

[43] Wittig M, Anmarkrud JA, Kässens JC, et al. Development of a high-resolution NGS-based HLA-typing and analysis pipeline. Nucleic Acids Res 2015;43:e70.

[44] Wittig M, Juzenas S, Vollstedt M, et al. High-resolution HLA-typing by next-generation sequencing of randomly fragmented target DNA. Methods Mol Biol 2018;1802: 63–88.

[45] Ehrenberg PK, Geretz A, Sindhu RK, et al. High-throughput next-generation sequencing to genotype six classical HLA loci from 96 donors in a single MiSeq run. Hladnikia (Ljubl) 2017;90:284–91.

[46] Ehrenberg PK, Geretz A, Thomas R. High-throughput contiguous full-length next-generation sequencing of HLA class I and II genes from 96 donors in a single MiSeq run. Methods Mol Biol 2018;1802:89–100.

[47] Yin Y, Lan JH, Nguyen D, et al. Application of high-throughput next-generation sequencing for HLA typing on buccal extracted DNA: results from over 10,000 donor recruitment samples. PLoS One 2016;11. e0165810.

[48] Yin Y, Lan J, Zhang Q. Application of high-throughput next-generation sequencing for HLA typing on buccal extracted DNA. Methods Mol Biol 2018;1802:101–13.

[49] Ambardar S, Gupta R, Trakroo D, et al. High throughput sequencing: an overview of sequencing chemistry. Indian J Microbiol 2016;56:394–404.

[50] Shiina T, Suzuki S, Kulski JK, et al. Super high resolution for single molecule-sequence-based typing of

classical HLA loci using Ion Torrent PGM. Methods Mol Biol 2018;1802:115–33.
[51] Shiina T, Suzuki S, Ozaki Y, et al. Super high resolution for single molecule-sequence-based typing of classical HLA loci at the 8-digit level using next generation sequencers. Tissue Antigens 2012;80: 305–16.
[52] Barone JC, Saito K, Beutner K, et al. HLA-genotyping of clinical specimens using Ion Torrent-based NGS. Hum Immunol 2015;76:903–9.
[53] Guerra SG, Chong W, Brown CJ, et al. Evaluation of Ion Torrent sequencing technology for rapid clinical human leucocyte antigen typing. Int J Immunogenet 2018;45: 230–5.
[54] Clarke J, Wu H-C, Jayasinghe L, et al. Continuous base identification for single-molecule nanopore DNA sequencing. Nat Nanotechnol 2009;4:265–70.
[55] Eid J, Fehr A, Gray J, et al. Real-time DNA sequencing from single polymerase molecules. Science 2009;323: 133–8.
[56] Rhoads A, Au KF. PacBio sequencing and its applications. Genomics Proteomics Bioinformatics 2015;13: 278–89.
[57] Ardui S, Ameur A, Vermeesch JR, et al. Single molecule real-time (SMRT) sequencing comes of age: applications and utilities for medical diagnostics. Nucleic Acids Res 2018;46:2159–68.
[58] Gowda M, Ambardar S. Comparative analyses of low, medium and high-resolution HLA typing technologies for human populations. J Clin Cell Immunol 2016;07. https://doi.org/10.4172/2155-9899.1000399.
[59] Ambardar S, Gowda M. High-resolution full-length HLA typing method using third generation (Pac-Bio SMRT) sequencing technology. Methods Mol Biol 2018;1802:135–53.
[60] Suzuki S, Ranade S, Osaki K, et al. Reference grade characterization of polymorphisms in full-length HLA class I and II genes with short-read sequencing on the ION PGM system and long-reads generated by single molecule, real-time sequencing on the PacBio platform. Front Immunol 2018;9:2294.
[61] Wang Y, Yang Q, Wang Z. The evolution of nanopore sequencing. Front Genet 2015;5. https://doi.org/10.3389/fgene.2014.00449.
[62] Jain M, Koren S, Miga KH, et al. Nanopore sequencing and assembly of a human genome with ultra-long reads. Nat Biotechnol 2018;36:338–45.
[63] Payne A, Holmes N, Rakyan V, et al. BulkVis: a graphical viewer for Oxford nanopore bulk FAST5 files. Bioinformatics 2018. https://doi.org/10.1093/bioinformatics/bty841
[64] Laver T, Harrison J, O'Neill PA, et al. Assessing the performance of the Oxford nanopore technologies MinION. Biomol Detect Quantif 2015;3:1–8.
[65] Ip CLC, Loose M, Tyson JR, et al. MinION analysis and reference consortium: phase 1 data release and analysis. F1000Res 2015;4. https://doi.org/10.12688/f1000research.7201.1.
[66] Ton KNT, Cree SL, Gronert-Sum SJ, et al. Multiplexed nanopore sequencing of HLA-B locus in Māori and Pacific Island samples. Front Genet 2018;9:152.
[67] Liu C, Xiao F, Hoisington-Lopez J, et al. Accurate typing of human leukocyte antigen class i genes by Oxford nanopore sequencing. J Mol Diagn 2018;20: 428–35.
[68] Lang K, Surendranath V, Quenzel P, et al. Full-length HLA class I genotyping with the MinION nanopore sequencer. Methods Mol Biol 2018;1802:155–62.
[69] Szolek A, Schubert B, Mohr C, et al. OptiType: precision HLA typing from next-generation sequencing data. Bioinformatics 2014;30:3310–6.
[70] Szolek A. HLA typing from short-read sequencing data with OptiType. Methods Mol Biol 2018;1802:215–23.
[71] Kiyotani K, Mai TH, Nakamura Y. Comparison of exome-based HLA class I genotyping tools: identification of platform-specific genotyping errors. J Hum Genet 2017;62:397–405.
[72] Bauer DC, Zadoorian A, Wilson LOW, et al. Evaluation of computational programs to predict HLA genotypes from genomic sequencing data. Brief Bioinform 2018; 19:179–87.
[73] Matey-Hernandez ML, Danish Pan Genome Consortium, Brunak S, et al. Benchmarking the HLA typing performance of Polysolver and Optitype in 50 Danish parental trios. BMC Bioinformatics 2018;19:239.
[74] Boegel S, Bukur T, Castle JC, et al. In silico typing of classical and non-classical HLA alleles from standard RNA-Seq reads. Methods Mol Biol 2018;1802: 177–91.
[75] Bai Y, Wang D, Fury W. PHLAT: inference of high-resolution HLA types from RNA and whole exome sequencing. Methods Mol Biol 2018;1802: 193–201.
[76] Liu C, Yang X. Using exome and amplicon-based sequencing data for high-resolution HLA typing with ATHLATES. Methods Mol Biol 2018;1802: 203–13.
[77] Huang Y, Yang J, Ying D, et al. HLAreporter: a tool for HLA typing from next generation sequencing data. Genome Med 2015;7:25.
[78] Larjo A, Eveleigh R, Kilpeläinen E, et al. Accuracy of programs for the determination of human leukocyte antigen alleles from next-generation sequencing data. Front Immunol 2017;8. https://doi.org/10.3389/fimmu.2017.01815.
[79] Lee H, Kingsford C. Accurate assembly and typing of HLA using a graph-guided assembler Kourami. Methods Mol Biol 2018;1802:235–47.
[80] Kawaguchi S, Higasa K, Yamada R, et al. Comprehensive HLA typing from a current allele database using next-generation sequencing data. Methods Mol Biol 2018;1802:225–33.

[81] Ka S, Lee S, Hong J, et al. HLAscan: genotyping of the HLA region using next-generation sequencing data. BMC Bioinformatics 2017;18:258.
[82] Buchkovich ML, Brown CC, Robasky K, et al. HLAProfiler utilizes k-mer profiles to improve HLA calling accuracy for rare and common alleles in RNA-seq data. Genome Med 2017;9:86.
[83] Orenbuch R, Filip I, Comito D, et al. ArcasHLA: high resolution HLA typing from RNA seq [Internet]. bioRxiv 2018;479824. https://doi.org/10.1101/479824.
[84] Wilson G, Aruliah DA, Brown CT, et al. Best practices for scientific computing. PLoS Biol 2014;12:e1001745.
[85] Joppa LN, McInerny G, Harper R, et al. Computational science. Troubling trends in scientific software use. Science 2013;340:814–5.
[86] Silva LB, Jimenez RC, Blomberg N, et al. General guidelines for biomedical software development. F1000Res 2017;6. https://doi.org/10.12688/f1000research.10750.2.
[87] Boegel S, editor. HLA typing. New York: Springer New York; 2018.
[88] Aguiar VRC, Cesar JE, Delaneau O, et al. Expression estimation and eQTL mapping for HLA genes with a personalized pipeline. bioRxiv 2018;365957. https://doi.org/10.1101/365957.
[89] Bai Y, Ni M, Cooper B, et al. Inference of high resolution HLA types using genome-wide RNA or DNA sequencing reads. BMC Genomics 2014;15:325.
[90] Dilthey AT, Mentzer AJ, Carapito R, et al. HLA*PRG:LA - HLA typing from linearly projected graph alignments. bioRxiv 2018;453555. https://doi.org/10.1101/453555.
[91] Hayashi S, Moriyama T, Yamaguchi R, et al. ALPHLARD-NT: Bayesian method for human leukocyte antigen genotyping and mutation calling through simultaneous analysis of normal and tumor whole-genome sequence data. J Comput Biol 2019. https://doi.org/10.1089/cmb.2018.0224.
[92] Kim HJ, Pourmand N. HLA typing from RNA-seq data using hierarchical read weighting [corrected]. PLoS One 2013;8:e67885.
[93] Lee H, Kingsford C. Kourami: graph-guided assembly for novel human leukocyte antigen allele discovery. Genome Biol 2018;19:16.
[94] Nariai N, Kojima K, Saito S, et al. HLA-VBSeq: accurate HLA typing at full resolution from whole-genome sequencing data. BMC Genomics 2015; 16(Suppl 2):S7.
[95] Xie C, Yeo ZX, Wong M, et al. Fast and accurate HLA typing from short-read next-generation sequence data with xHLA. Proc Natl Acad Sci U S A 2017;114: 8059–64.
[96] Rozenberg L, Hammerbacher J. Prohlatype: a probabilistic framework for HLA typing. bioRxiv 2018; 244962. https://doi.org/10.1101/244962.
[97] Warren RL, Choe G, Freeman DJ, et al. Derivation of HLA types from shotgun sequence datasets. Genome Med 2012;4:95.
[98] Chang C-J, Chen P-L, Yang W-S, et al. A fault-tolerant method for HLA typing with PacBio data. BMC Bioinformatics 2014;15:296.
[99] Sebastian A, Herdegen M, Migalska M, et al. AMPLISAS: a web server for multilocus genotyping using next-generation amplicon sequencing data. Mol Ecol Resour 2016;16:498–510.
[100] Sebastian A, Migalska M, Biedrzycka A. AmpliSAS and AmpliHLA: web server tools for MHC typing of non-model species and human using NGS data. Methods Mol Biol 2018;1802:249–73.
[101] Kawaguchi S, Higasa K, Shimizu M, et al. HLA-HD: an accurate HLA typing algorithm for next-generation sequencing data. Hum Mutat 2017;38:788–97.
[102] Liu C, Yang X, Duffy B, et al. ATHLATES: accurate typing of human leukocyte antigen through exome sequencing. Nucleic Acids Res 2013;41:e142.
[103] Shukla SA, Rooney MS, Rajasagi M, et al. Comprehensive analysis of cancer-associated somatic mutations in class I HLA genes. Nat Biotechnol 2015;33: 1152–8.
[104] Castelli EC, Paz MA, Souza AS, et al. HLA-mapper: an application to optimize the mapping of HLA sequences produced by massively parallel sequencing procedures. Hum Immunol 2018;79:678–84.
[105] Forbes SA, Bindal N, Bamford S, et al. COSMIC: mining complete cancer genomes in the catalogue of somatic mutations in cancer. Nucleic Acids Res 2011;39: D945–50.
[106] Klijn C, Durinck S, Stawiski EW, et al. A comprehensive transcriptional portrait of human cancer cell lines. Nat Biotechnol 2015;33:306–12.
[107] HLA typed browse. Culture collections. Available at: https://www.phe-culturecollections.org.uk/products/celllines/hlatyped/browse.jsp. Accessed April 11, 2019.
[108] Robinson J, Halliwell JA, McWilliam H, et al. The IMGT/HLA database. Nucleic Acids Res 2013;41: D1222–7.
[109] Bairoch A. The cellosaurus, a cell-line knowledge resource. J Biomol Tech 2018;29:25–38.
[110] Ng CKY, Cooke SL, Howe K, et al. The role of tandem duplicator phenotype in tumour evolution in high-grade serous ovarian cancer. J Pathol 2012;226: 703–12.
[111] Langdon SP, Lawrie SS, Hay FG, et al. Characterization and properties of nine human ovarian adenocarcinoma cell lines. Cancer Res 1988;48:6166–72.
[112] Daemen A, Griffith OL, Heiser LM, et al. Modeling precision treatment of breast cancer. Genome Biol 2013; 14:R110.
[113] Band V, Zajchowski D, Swisshelm K, et al. Tumor progression in four mammary epithelial cell lines derived from the same patient. Cancer Res 1990;50: 7351–7.
[114] Project: NGS on Reference cell lines > 18th International HLA & Immunogenetics Workshop. In: 18th International HLA & Immunogenetics Workshop

[Internet]. Available at: https://www.ihiw18.org/component-ngs-for-hla/reference-cell-lines/. Accessed April 12, 2019.

[115] McGranahan N, Rosenthal R, Hiley CT, et al. Allele-specific HLA loss and immune escape in lung cancer evolution. Cell 2017;171:1259–71.e11.

[116] Landry JJM, Pyl PT, Rausch T, et al. The genomic and transcriptomic landscape of a HeLa cell line. G3 (Bethesda) 2013;3:1213–24.

[117] Frattini A, Fabbri M, Valli R, et al. High variability of genomic instability and gene expression profiling in different HeLa clones. Sci Rep 2015;5:15377.

[118] Kim M, Rhee J-K, Choi H, et al. Passage-dependent accumulation of somatic mutations in mesenchymal stromal cells during in vitro culture revealed by whole genome sequencing. Sci Rep 2017;7:14508.

[119] Robinson J, Halliwell JA, Hayhurst JD, et al. The IPD and IMGT/HLA database: allele variant databases. Nucleic Acids Res 2015;43:D423–31.

[120] Abraham JP, Barker DJ, Robinson J, et al. The IPD databases: cataloguing and understanding allele variants. Methods Mol Biol 2018;1802:31–48.

[121] Garrison E, Sirén J, Novak AM, et al. Variation graph toolkit improves read mapping by representing genetic variation in the reference. Nat Biotechnol 2018;36:875–9.

[122] Church DM. Genomes for all. Nat Biotechnol 2018;36:815–6.

Advances in Molecular Pathology 2 (2019) 201–213
ADVANCES IN MOLECULAR PATHOLOGY

Expanding the Connectivity Map Concept as the Functional Look-Up Table for Systems Biology

Bernard Kok Bang Lee, PhD[a,b,c], **Sok Ching Cheong, PhD**[b,c], **Aik Choon Tan, PhD**[a,d,*]

[a]Division of Medical Oncology, Department of Medicine, University of Colorado Anschutz Medical Campus, Aurora, CO 80045, USA; [b]Head and Neck Cancer Research Team, Cancer Research Malaysia, Subang Jaya Medical Centre, 2nd Floor, Outpatient Centre, Subang Jaya, Selangor 47500, Malaysia; [c]Department of Oral and Maxillofacial Clinical Sciences, Faculty of Dentistry, University of Malaya, Kuala Lumpur, Malaysia; [d]Department of Biostatistics and Bioinformatics, Moffitt Cancer Center, 12902 Magnolia Drive, Tampa, FL 33612, USA

KEYWORDS

• Connectivity map • Bioinformatics • Systems biology • Drug • Diseases

KEY POINTS

- The "Connectivity Map" (CMap) concept uses gene expression as a "universal language" to connect between biological systems, genes, and drugs.
- The ultimate goal of the CMap concept is to develop a functional look-up table for systems biology, which is similar to the periodic table in chemistry.
- Applications of the CMap concept include identifying disease mechanisms, defining mechanisms of actions of novel compounds, and drug repurposing and repositioning.

INTRODUCTION

The ever-increasing large-scale open-access collections of transcriptional responses to small molecules have had a significant impact on systems biology, facilitated mainly by computational approaches that could digest the enormous amounts of data. Although still challenging, the mining of these datasets promises excellent computational research opportunities for a systemic understanding of how drug perturbations affect the molecular and physiologic processes down to the systemic level, which could lead to more efficient drug discovery. An essential advancement in transcriptional data analysis is the development of the Connectivity Map (CMap) [1]. The CMap concept is based on the following key observations: (1) gene expression can be measured accurately and has shown promise as a "universal language" in disease characterization and prognostication; (2) gene expression can be used to connect different biological states and systems; and (3) biological pathways drive disease phenotypes and, therefore, can be used as connectable traits.

Disclosure Statement: The authors have nothing to disclose.
Funding: B.K.B. Lee gratefully acknowledges PhD funding from the Ong Hin Tiang and Ong Sek Pek Foundation. Cancer Research Malaysia is a nonprofit research organization that is committed to the understanding of cancer prevention, diagnosis, and treatment through fundamental research programs. The authors declare no potential conflicts of interest concerning the authorship and/or publication of this article.

*Corresponding author. Department of Biostatistics and Bioinformatics, Moffitt Cancer Center, 12902 Magnolia Drive, Tampa, FL 33612, USA. *E-mail address:* aikchoon.tan@moffitt.org

https://doi.org/10.1016/j.yamp.2019.07.014
2589-4080/19/

Generally, the computational approach that uses the CMap concept as the functional look-up table consists of 3 main components, that is, a perturbagen-induced reference gene expression database, a set of gene signatures defined by users, and last, a pattern-matching algorithm that correlates these gene signatures to the perturbagen-induced gene expression in the reference database. The output of connectivity mapping is a ranked list of perturbagens, with connectivity scores (CS) that are either positive value (indicating similar gene expression profile) or negative value (indicating negative correlation). Fig. 1 illustrates the principal workflow of CMap.

The purpose of this article is therefore to provide a state-of-the-art survey of the recent advances in computational research using the CMap concept, with the main focus on the application of CMap in the pathology setting, as well as to review the computational tools that apply the CMap concept in the field. The authors also discuss the variety of public databases that use the concept of CMap to answer or gauge different questions in their respective areas.

CONNECTIVITY MAP DATABASES

Connectivity Map

The CMap was set up to answer the questions of how best to streamline the drug discovery and development process. Its most important application lies in the efforts of providing an alternative to running rigorous genetic or chemical screens to connect human disease with the genes that underlie them and the drugs that could treat them. The CMap was initially developed in 2006 [1] as a collection of genome-wide gene expression data derived from cultured human cells that were treated with a compendium of small bioactive molecules. Its goal is to create an extensive public database that collects as many genomics and drugs signatures as possible, to which one can then apply pattern-matching algorithms to detect similarities among these signatures to their genes of interest. Embracing the shift to the systems biology paradigm, the research community generally accepted that biological elements have several interdependencies and are effectively interconnected. Recently, multiple success stories reported on how the CMap was used to identify new candidate drugs to be repurposed on human diseases that would otherwise have no alternative treatment options.

Library of Integrated Cellular Signatures L1000

Based on the promising results of CMap, the National Institutes of Health initiated and funded the Library of Integrated Cellular Signatures (LINCS) program to generate different gene signatures across multiple tissue types as a functional look-up table to study various cellular processes. The LINCS L1000 is the next-generation of CMap, which comprises more than 7494 genetic perturbations (eg, single-gene knockdown or overexpression assays) and more than 19,811 perturbations induced by small molecules (eg, drugs) [2,3]. In addition, more than 1.3 million gene expression responses have been determined and collected using the L1000 technologies [4]. The L1000 platform, developed at the Broad Institute, facilitates rapid, flexible, and high-throughput gene expression profiling at lower costs. Specifically, the L1000 technology measures the expression of only 978 genes (hence termed the "L1000 landmark genes") [2], and the expression values for the remaining transcriptome, approximately 22,000 genes, are estimated by a computational model using additional data from the Gene Expression Omnibus (GEO) [5]. The rationale for using this computational model is that gene expression data contain a high degree of statistical dependencies between measured variables (messenger RNAs [mRNAs]) and the selected 978 landmark genes that would capture most of the information contained within the entire transcriptome [5]. All the LINCS data and computational tools are available at the CLUE Web site (https://clue.io).

Connectivity Map for Anticancer Compounds

To cater to the need of a dedicated gene expression database that specializes in cancer research, Ushijima and colleagues [6] developed a public gene expression database consisting of 83 anticancer compounds tested on 5 human cancer cell lines. Interestingly, some of the anticancer compounds, such as the chemotherapy drugs cisplatin, mitomycin, and docetaxel that were not in the original CMap, were also included in this database, enabling a more robust analysis to be carried out and thus identifying more promising anticancer lead compounds.

PATTERN-MATCHING ALGORITHMS

To date, several pattern-matching algorithms have been developed to connect a query signature to the drug-specific CMap gene expression profile database. Here, the authors highlight a few algorithms that have been widely adopted by the research community. Among others, these are the Kolmogorov-Smirnov (KS) test [1], Weighted Connectivity Score (WTCS) [2], statistically significant Connections Map (ssCMap) [7], eXtreme Sum (XSum) [8], and eXtreme Cosine (XCos)

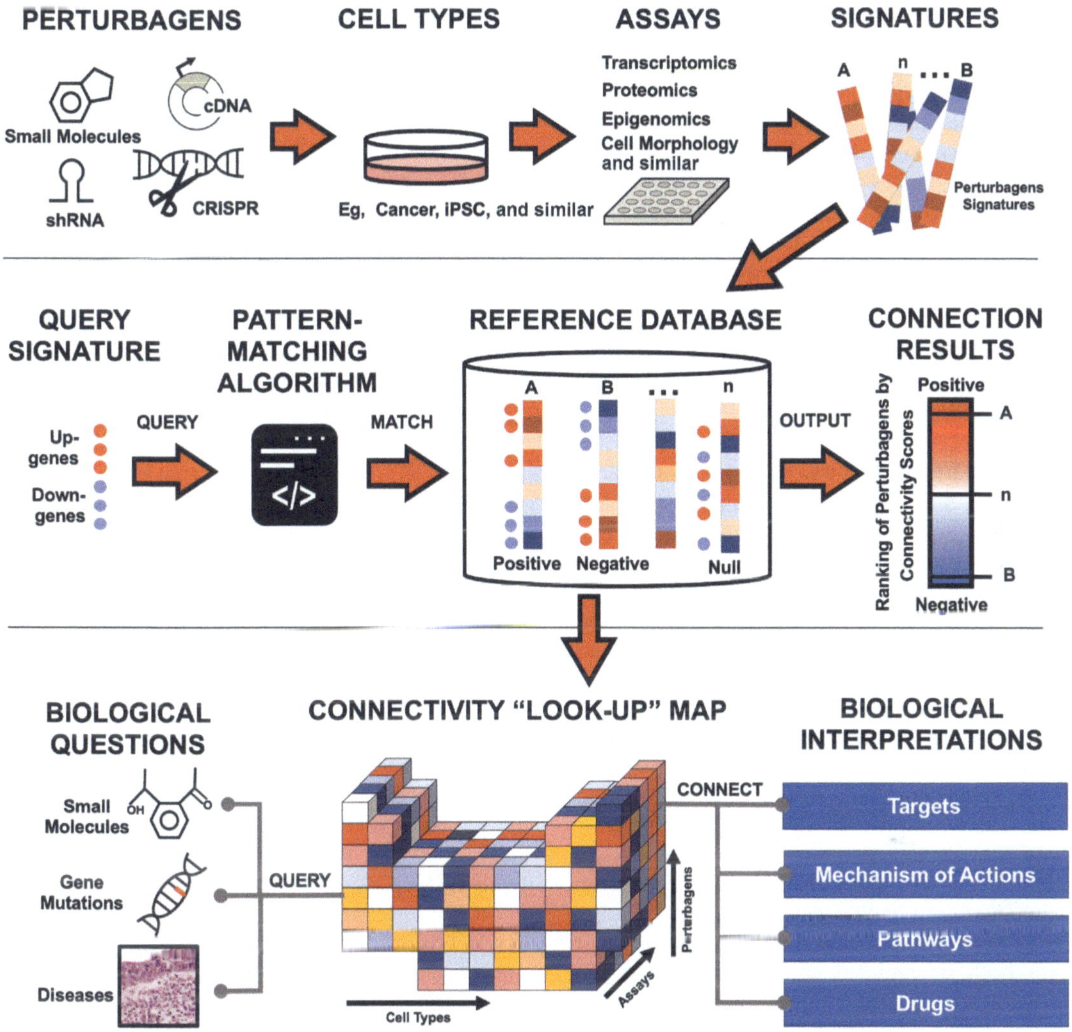

FIG. 1 Overview of the working principle of the CMap. The top panel illustrates the technologies and assays in generating various types of perturbagen-induced signatures. The perturbagens could be small molecules, overexpression by complementary DNA (cDNA), gene knockdown by short hairpin RNA (shRNA), or gene knockout by CRISPR. Depending on the cell types (eg, cancer cell lines or induced pluripotent stem cells [iPSC] or other cell types), the perturbagen-induced signatures could be generated by a wide range of assays (eg, transcriptomics by gene expression microarray, RNA-seq, or L1000 technologies). The middle panel shows the steps of connecting a query gene signature against the reference perturbagen-induced signatures (reference database). A query signature is provided as the input to the CMap (red and blue colors indicate upregulated and downregulated genes), and the pattern-matching algorithm will match the query signature against the reference database. A CS will be assigned to each of the perturbagen-induced signatures in the reference database (eg, from +1 to −1 represents positive and negative connectivity). The CMap system will return the perturbagen-induced signatures ranked by the CS as the output. The bottom panel illustrates the ultimate utility of the CMap as a functional "look-up" table for systems biology. Perturbagen-derived signatures assayed by multi-omics assays across various cell types could be integrated as a connectivity "look-up" map. This resource could be used to "look-up" functional interpretations for different biological questions (eg, querying a new small molecule for MoA, defining the targets and pathways of gene mutations, linking diseases with drugs), which is analogous to the periodic table in chemistry.

[9]. How these algorithms work, their advantages, as well as technical limitations of each algorithm are briefly discussed. Table 1 shows a summary of the similarities and differences between these algorithms. This list is not a comprehensive list of pattern-matching algorithms for CMap analysis, but rather a few algorithms that the authors thought are user-friendly. There are, of course, other algorithms that are being developed, such as the Reverse Gene Expression Score (RGES) developed by Chen and colleagues [10], that evaluates the reverse relationship between disease and drug-gene expression profiles, with lower RGES of a drug indicating higher potency to reverse a disease-specific gene expression, as well as a few other algorithms highlighted by Musa and colleagues [11].

Kolmogorov-Smirnov Test

The KS test is a nonparametric, rank-based pattern-matching algorithm to associate user query gene signatures with the CMap reference expression profiles [1]. A CS ranging from −1 to +1 as a result of querying a gene signature against the signatures in the CMap reference database will reflect the relationship between a query gene signature and a perturbagen. A high-positive CS approaching +1 indicates that the corresponding compound in the CMap database induces expression of the query signature; conversely, a high-negative CS suggests that the corresponding drug may counteract the query signature. Thus, compounds with high-negative scores may have therapeutic potential.

To use the KS test, one must ensure that the query gene signatures are rank-ordered, that is, the most differentially expressed gene is ranked first, and vice versa for both upregulated and downregulated gene lists. In other words, the KS algorithm is susceptible to the ranking of the query gene signatures. Any changes to the ranking of the query genes, such as swapping of a single gene ranking position, will cause a considerable difference to the outcome of the CS. The second limitation of the KS algorithm is that the CS is set to zero if the enrichment scores (ES) of upregulated and downregulated genes have the same algebraic sign, rendering many of the drugs to have CS values of zero.

Weighted Connectivity Score

The WTCS [2] is another nonparametric similarity algorithm based on the weighted KS ES described previously [12]. WTCS is a composite, bidirectional version of ES. The ES values for upregulated and downregulated genes would be computed separately for a given set of query gene pairs. Similar to the KS statistic, WTCS also ranges between −1 and + 1. Signatures that are positively correlated will have positive WTCS, whereas will have negative WTCS for those that are inversely correlated, and near zero for signatures that are unrelated. A null WTCS is assigned for cases where both ES for upregulated and downregulated genes have the same algebraic sign.

WTCS mitigates the limitation of KS in terms of rank-ordered gene signatures by evaluating the ES of the upregulated and downregulated genes that are overlapping with the genes in the reference profile, that is, the running sum of the gene's fold-change value, if the query gene is encountered in the CMap reference profile for upregulated and downregulated genes. With this new intervention, WTCS is no longer dependent on the ranked-order of the query gene signatures. However, the WTCS still has the zero value prediction issue, by which the CS is set to zero if ES of the upregulated and downregulated genes have the same algebraic sign, rendering many of the drugs to have CS values of zero. The developers of KS and WTCS tried to mitigate this limitation by reranking the instances of zero values in descending order of ES for upregulated genes. However, the approach of sorting instances with zero values using ES of upregulated genes might not be optimal, especially in the case where one might argue that downregulated genes might have a more significant biological effect, and therefore, ES of downregulated genes should be used instead.

Statistically Significant Connections Map

The ssCMap algorithm developed by Zhang and Gant [7] orders genes based on their absolute value of differential expression. A query gene signature can be an ordered gene list or just a collection of genes without specific ordering, which will be referred to as *ordered* and *unordered* gene signature, respectively. Based on the ranking, the importance of a gene is determined by the absolute value of its rank rather than its differential expression value. The direction of regulation is maintained by additionally allocating importance with the sign of its rank. Based on the reassigned query gene signature and reference expression profile, the connection strength between them is calculated.

ssCMap ordered analysis overcomes the bias emphasized on ordering prediction results in descending order of ES of upregulated genes in the events of zero values, as in the case for KS and WTCS by treating upregulated and downregulated genes equally in a unified manner, which means that genes that showed a higher differential expression have more weight, regardless of the regulation direction. Thus, a 2-fold downregulated gene is considered equally as important as a 2-fold upregulated

TABLE 1
The Similarities and Differences of Pattern-Matching Algorithms Used in Connectivity Map Analysis

Pattern-Matching Algorithms	Query Signature	Descriptions	Technical Limitations	References
KS test	• Upregulated gene symbols • Downregulated gene symbols	• Nonparametric • Genes are converted to rank	• Query gene signatures must be rank-ordered • The CS is set to zero if ES for the upregulated and downregulated genes have the same algebraic sign	Lamb et al [1], 2006
WTCS	• Upregulated gene symbols • Downregulated gene symbols	• Nonparametric • Genes are converted to rank	The CS is set to zero if ES for the upregulated and downregulated genes have the same algebraic sign	Subramanian et al [2], 2017
ssCMap ordered	• Upregulated gene symbols • Downregulated gene symbols • Fold change values	Genes are ordered using the absolute value of their fold change values	Fold change value of the query genes are required	Zhang and Gant [7], 2008
ssCMap unordered	• Upregulated gene symbols • Downregulated gene symbols	No particular ordering of the genes; +1 for upregulated genes and −1 for downregulated genes	The significance of which genes are more important could not be determined because all genes take on the value of either +1 (upregulated) or −1 (downregulated)	Zhang and Gant [7], 2008
XSum	• Upregulated gene symbols • Downregulated gene symbols	Limited to the top *N* and bottom *N* of the genes in reference profile	Execution of XSum will collapse if there are no overlapping query gene signatures with the genes in the reference profile	Cheng et al [8], 2014
XCos	• Upregulated gene symbols • Downregulated gene symbols • Fold change values	Limited to the top *N* and bottom *N* of the genes in reference profile	• Fold change value of the query genes is a prerequisite for XCos execution • Execution of XCos will collapse if there are nonoverlapping query gene signatures with the genes in the reference profile • Must have at least 2 query genes overlapping with the genes in the reference profile	Cheng et al [9], 2013

gene. In general, the *i*th gene in the list of *N* number of genes will be ranked with $(N - i + 1)$ for upregulation or $-(N - i + 1)$ for downregulation. By doing this, the importance of a gene is reflected by the absolute value of its rank, whereas the sign of its rank indicates its regulation status. However, the use of fold change values has its problems, specifically, in the case wherein users do not have fold-change values for their differential genes of interests, rendering the ssCMap ordered scoring not useable.

To deal with query gene signatures that do not have fold change values, the same group of researchers who developed ssCMap ordered scoring have since developed ssCMap unordered scoring, whereby all the genes in the list have equal weight, with upregulated genes being assigned ranks of +1 and downregulated genes being assigned ranks of −1. However, because there is no particular ordering among the genes, one would not be able to tell which genes are more important than the others. This unique feature, which ignored the ranking of the query genes, was also implemented in WTCS.

eXtreme Sum and eXtreme Cosine

XSum [8] and XCos [9] are pattern-matching algorithms that have similarities with the KS and WTCS methods, as differentially expressed genes (upregulated and downregulated genes) are used to query the reference database and to measure the difference between the 2 corresponding scores for genes that overlap with the reference database. In contrast to KS and WTCS, which evaluate the queried genes that span across the reference profile, XSum and XCos are calculated by retaining only the extreme genes for each drug instance in CMap, that is, only keeping the top *N* and bottom *N* genes. By default, *N* is set at 500. For each drug instance, XSum then sums up the gene expression values of the reference profile that overlaps with the corresponding upregulated and downregulated genes, whereas XCos calculates the dot product of the 2 vectors.

XSum and XCos have different sets of technical limitations, especially in the case wherein there are few query gene signatures (upregulated and downregulated genes). XSum works by summing the gene fold change values of the instance that matches with the query signatures, whereas XCos calculates the sum of the product of the fold change values between the query genes and the reference profile. Because of the need to have overlapping query gene signatures with the top *N* upregulated and bottom *N* downregulated genes for each instance in the reference profile (*N* takes on the value of 500), in the event that there is no match between the query gene signatures with the genes in the reference profile, both XSum and XCos cannot be calculated. In addition, XCos has another additional limitation, in that this algorithm requires there must be at least 2 overlapping gene signatures with the top *N* upregulated and bottom *N* downregulated genes in the reference profile. Instances that yield values of 1 in cases wherein there is only 1 overlapping query gene with the top *N* upregulated and with the bottom *N* downregulated genes in the reference profile would cause the execution of XCos algorithm to collapse.

APPLICATIONS OF CONNECTIVITY MAP IN SYSTEMS BIOLOGY

CMap is an advanced bioinformatics technique that can be used to identify medications that mimic or reverse the gene expression profiles induced by disease. To date, connectivity mapping has been used to identify medications not only in cancers [13–15] but also in rare [16,17] and chronic diseases [18–20]. Furthermore, it has been used to determine the unknown mechanism of actions of herbal extracts [21,22]. In later discussion, the authors highlight some of the applications of the CMap approaches in different systems biology areas. The pattern-matching algorithms used in the studies cited in later discussion have varied strength and advantages, and the reader should evaluate how successful these algorithms were in the context of their limitations described in the above section.

Connecting Diseases with New Therapies

Large-scale integration of expression signatures of human diseases from public databases with drug effect signatures has the potential to confirm already-known therapeutic uses for drugs and to uncover new applications for the Food and Drug Administration (FDA)-approved drugs. For example, Jahchan and colleagues [13] used the bioinformatics approach to query CMap and identified tricyclic antidepressants (TCA) inhibitors as potent inducers of cell death in small cell lung cancer (SCLC) cells. They showed that treatment with 2 such TCA inhibitors, imipramine and promethazine, disrupted the autocrine survival signals involving neurotransmitters and their G protein–coupled receptors. The potential of repurposing TCA inhibitors, as seen for treating SCLC, was also observed in other neuroendocrine tumors, such as Merkel cell carcinoma, midgut carcinoid tumors, pheochromocytoma, and neuroblastoma tumor cells, thus highlighting the importance of autocrine mechanisms in promoting the growth of neuroendocrine tumor cells. Their findings led to the initiation of a phase 2A clinical trial, assessing the efficacy of the TCA inhibitor desipramine in SCLC and other high-grade neuroendocrine tumors (ClinicalTrials.gov Identifier: NCT01719861).

In combating epithelial ovarian cancer (EOC) through the identification of novel therapeutics, Raghavan and colleagues [15] used the EOC gene expression signatures derived from The Cancer Genome Atlas and Mayo Clinic to query CMap and identified 11 drugs to have potential efficacy on EOC. Notably, 5 of those drugs were known a priori to be cytotoxic to the EOC cells. Therefore, it will be interesting to know how the remaining short-listed 6 drugs would fare when tested in vitro; it is hoped promising results will be reported soon.

Treatment of chronic diseases has also benefited from connectivity mapping methods. Dudley and colleagues [18] used the inflammatory bowel disease (IBD) gene expression signatures they obtained from the National Center for Biotechnology Information GEO database to query the CMap. They found that topiramate, an anticonvulsant drug not previously described to have efficacy for IBD, might serve as a therapeutic option for IBD. They tested topiramate efficacy in a trinitrobenzenesulfonic acid–induced rodent model of IBD and observed a significant reduction of gross pathologic signs and microscopic damage in colon tissues of the rodent. Using the same strategy of extracting disease gene expression signatures from public databases and querying the CMap, Sirota and colleagues [14] identified and confirmed the efficacy of cimetidine, an antiulcer drug to be effective against lung adenocarcinoma in vitro and in the mouse model.

Because of advancing genomics techniques, cancer research has made remarkable progress, resulting in many new anticancer drugs approved by the FDA. However, the same does not apply to rare diseases owing to, among other reasons, the insufficient number of patients to conduct clinical trials. One of the key applications of CMap is to identify new therapeutics for rare diseases. For example, Hirschsprung disease (HD) is a congenital intestinal anomaly resulting from a failure to form enteric ganglia nerves in the lower bowel. Several gene expression profiling studies of gut samples from animal models of HD or patients of HD have been done; however, efforts that leverage on the gene expression signatures to find new interventional therapeutics strategies, such as targeted therapies using small molecule inhibitors, have been minimal. Xiao and colleagues [17] used a gene signature consisting of 253 differentially expressed genes that was derived from 8 paired ganglionic and aganglionic samples to query the CMap. In the process, 10 compounds with low CS were suggested to be able to counteract the gene expression observed in HD and thus could be potential novel therapies. Further in vitro and in vivo experiments should be carried out to shed light on the potential uses of these small molecule inhibitors on HD patients.

Identifying Therapeutic Targets in Diseases

By using the CMap, Brum and colleagues [19] identified 3 compounds, withaferin A, calcium folinate, and amylocaine, to have potential in stimulating osteoblast differentiation and mineralization in human mesenchymal stromal cells. A further differential gene analysis revealed that 2 genes, *HMOX1* and *STC1*, as essential factors for human osteogenesis, and thus could potentially be novel targets for bone anabolic therapy.

To overcome cystic fibrosis (CF) lung disease, which is typically categorized by the reduced expression of the NF-κ B downregulator *TNFAIP3*, Malcomson and colleagues [20] used the CMap to identify drugs, such as ikarugamycin and quercetin, that can induce *TNFAIP3* mRNA and protein expression and thus reduce inflammation. However, more work, such as using suitable in vivo model systems to optimize treatments, needs to be done to shed light on the role of the short-listed drugs on CF lung disease.

Deciphering Drug Actions

Besides identifying potential candidate drugs to be treated on a particular disease, connectivity mapping could also be used to infer the possible pharmacologic effects of drugs, especially drugs that are derived from herbal extracts. Kim and colleagues [21] applied the connectivity mapping method and discovered that HepG2 cells treated with extracts from the flowering plant *Scutellaria baicalensis* (commonly called Baikal skullcap or Chinese skullcap) showed top-ranked drug ES that are inversely correlated with those found in type 2 diabetic db/db mouse liver cells. This observation provided clues to the potential use of *S baicalensis* extracts in treating diabetic liver disease in humans, although much work remains to be done to confirm this observation.

Because of their massive gene expression profiles spanning approximately 20,000 drugs, perhaps the most useful application of the L1000 platform would be to decipher the potential new mechanisms of action (MoA) for novel compounds that elicit similar gene expression changes. The application of L1000 technology is especially practical in the case of trying to identify MoA for herbal extracts, such as the traditional Chinese medicine (TCM), owing to their "multicomponent, multitarget" nature that makes them poorly appreciated by the research community. Yoo and colleagues [22] tried to solve this issue by reanalyzing the microarray profiles generated from 102 TCM compounds [23] and performed a more systematic analysis of the MoA of these TCM components. They used the L1000 platform to interrogate the MoA of these 102 TCM components. In the process, they managed to cluster these 102 TCM components into 4 significant clusters based on 7 groups of MoAs. This systematic analysis provides an opportunity for repurposing and positioning some of the TCM components in treating different diseases and symptoms. A Web application called TCM Hub, which allows users to explore and query the 102 TCM components, is freely accessible at http://tanlab.ucdenver.edu/TCMHub/.

INTEGRATING TRANSCRIPTOMIC DATA WITH OTHER DATA TYPES FOR CONNECTIVITY MAP

Beyond the typical usage of gene expression data for CMap analysis, De Bastiani and colleagues [24] explored the inclusion of coexpression networks targeted by transcription factors in a search to identify drugs that could revert the gene expression profiles of pathologic phenotypes. They investigated this idea in bipolar disorder and successfully retrieved several antipsychotics, antidepressive, anti-inflammatory, and antioxidant agents, some of which, such as haloperidol and chlorpromazine, are current clinical therapies for bipolar disorder. These results indicate that the other identified candidate drugs warrant further investigations.

De Wolf and colleagues [25] explored the possibility of increasing the accuracy of compound activity prediction by adding additional biological information of a compound, on top of its existing chemical properties and desired on-target effects. This desirable effort has seen significant steps in the drug discovery and development process. De Wolf and colleagues reported finding that the compound hit rate increased by a factor of 300, as fewer, but more specific chemistry could be screened, based on the upfront computed activity predictions.

The correct interpretation of the effects of somatic mutations in cancer remains a significant challenge for the implementation of precision medicine, especially in the context of variants of unknown significance. Berger and colleagues [26] addressed this challenge by developing a method called expression-based variant-impact phenotyping that uses gene expression changes to distinguish impactful from neutral somatic mutations. Leveraging the L1000 profiling technology, they successfully classified the function of 194 genetic variants in lung adenocarcinoma into 4 categories: gain-of-function, loss-of-function, change-of-function, and neutral; 69% as impactful and 31% as functionally neutral. Some of the variants classified as impactful are rare somatic mutations, including *EGFR* S645C, *ARAF* S214C and S214F, and *ERBB2* S418T, demonstrating that rare mutations can be functionally relevant in cancer. Notably, some of these impactful variants, such as *EGFR* S645C and *ERBB2* S418T, were found to promote tumor formation in vivo.

Busby and colleagues [27] investigated the combination of connectivity mapping and pharmacoepidemiology as a way to identify medications that altered breast cancer risk. However, this novel approach did not identify any additional medications that were substantially associated with breast cancer risk. They suggested that this failure to identify novel factors was possibly due to the use of cell line models for the connectivity mapping process because they might not accurately translate to the human body. Alternatively, the heterogeneous nature of breast cancers that are made up of different subtypes could potentially mask the crucial signals for specific breast cancer subtypes.

EXPANDING THE CONNECTIVITY MAP CONCEPT TO DIFFERENT "OMICS" DATA SOURCES

The ultimate goal of the CMap concept is to develop a functional look-up table for systems biology, which is analogous to the periodic table in chemistry (see Fig. 1). To accomplish this, several recent efforts focus on expanding the CMap concept to different "omics" data sources. Table 2 summarizes the technologies and computational tools that have implemented the CMap concept in different "omics" data sources.

Proteomics Data

Proteomic changes represent an additional dimension to transcriptional changes in cellular responses to perturbations. The accurate profiling of proteomic changes is particularly important in capturing the cellular changes on genetic and/or pharmacologic perturbations. To profile these protein-level changes, Abelin and colleagues [28] have developed a high-throughput and reproducible proteomic platform known as P100 to profile the phosphosignaling changes across thousands of samples. This technological platform used targeted liquid chromatography-mass spectrometry assays to measure the levels of ~100 diverse phosphosites in a single experiment. By using this assay, Litichevskiy and colleagues [29] profiled phosphosignaling induced by 90 drugs in 6 cell lines to generate their proteomic signatures.

TABLE 2
Connectivity Map and Related Web Applications

Method	Descriptions	URL Link
Transcriptomics data		
CMap	• Collects microarray-based gene expression profiles from cultured human cancer cells treated using a wide range of experimentally and clinically used small molecules • Contains 6100 instances of unique treatment-control pairs of 1309 drugs	https://portals.broadinstitute.org/cmap/
L1000	• Catalogs how human cells globally respond to chemical, genetic, and disease perturbations • Collects the gene-expression profiles of small-molecule treatments, genetic manipulation for knocking-down genes by shRNA or overexpressing genes by cDNA	https://clue.io
Ujishima datasets	• Provides cancer researchers gene expression database and related analysis tools to evaluate potential mode of action of chemical compounds in comparison with clinically used anticancer agents	http://scads.jfcr.or.jp/db/cs/
Proteomics data		
P100	• Contains the levels of ~100 diverse phosphosites for CMap approach	https://clue.io/proteomics
Epigenomics data		
GCP	• Measures global modifications to histones for CMap approach	https://clue.io/proteomics
Kinase selectivity data		
K-Map	• Connects a set of query kinases to kinase inhibitors based on the quantitative profiles of the kinase inhibitor selectivity assay	http://tanlab.ucdenver.edu/kMap
Drug sensitivity data		
GDSC	• Collects and annotates large datasets on drug sensitivity in cancer cells • Links these data to detailed genomic information to facilitate the discovery of molecular biomarkers of drug response	https://www.cancerrxgene.org/
Cancer Cell Line Encyclopedia		
CCLE	• Compilation of gene expression, chromosomal copy number, and massively parallel sequencing data of human cancer cell lines • Provides identification of genetic, lineage, and gene expression–based predictors of drug sensitivity when coupled with pharmacologic profiles for 24 anticancer drugs	https://portals.broadinstitute.org/ccle
Cancer Therapeutics Response Portal		
CTRP	• Links genetic, lineage, and other cellular features of cancer cell lines to small-molecule sensitivity	https://portals.broadinstitute.org/ctrp/

(continued on next page)

TABLE 2
(*continued*)

Method	Descriptions	URL Link
DeSigN	• Correlates phenotype-specific gene expression signatures derived from differentially expressed genes with predefined gene expression profiles associated with drug response data (IC_{50}) from 140 small molecules inhibitors available in GDSC	http://design-v2.cancerresearch.my/query
Cell morphology data		
Cell Painting assay	• Detects subtle phenotypic changes or biological similarities among samples on genetic or pharmacologic perturbations for CMap approach	https://clue.io/morphology

Epigenomics Data

Epigenetics plays a crucial role in regulating the function of a genome in diverse cellular processes, such as cell lineage commitment and responses to environmental cues. In addition, dysregulation of epigenetic regulations has been implicated in various disease causes. Creech and colleagues [30] developed a robust, high-throughput platform, known as the global chromatin profiling (GCP) assay, to rapidly profile the core histone modifications of chromatin. The GCP assay used a targeted quantitative mass spectrometry method to interrogate the epigenetic landscape of a cell. The GCP assay allows comparisons among cells with different genetic backgrounds under pharmacologic and/or genetic perturbations. Litichevskiy and colleagues [29], in parallel with their proteomic study, also performed the GCP assay across 6 cell lines treated with 90 drugs to generate the first-ever epigenetic signatures similar to the gene expression signatures.

Kinome Selectivity Data

Protein kinases play essential roles in regulating signal transduction in eukaryotic cells and represent one of the largest "druggable" and well-studied families in the human genome [31]. Kim and colleagues [32] explored these protein kinase avenues by incorporating 2 large-scale kinase inhibitor selectivity studies [33,34] in their tool called K-Map, which can systematically connect a set of query kinases to kinase inhibitors based on the quantitative profiles of the kinase inhibitor activities. Kim and colleagues [35] performed an essential kinome RNA interference screen to identify kinases mediating resistance to the *EGFR* inhibitor gefitinib in an *EGFR* mutant non–small cell lung cancer (NSCLC) cell line. By using essential kinases for querying, K-Map predicted bosutinib to be a more effective drug than gefitinib in killing *EGFR* mutant NSCLC cells. The prediction of K-Map was subsequently validated by in vitro experiments, whereby bosutinib alone was a more effective agent than gefitinib, and the combination of bosutinib and gefitinib showed a synergistic effect in *EGFR* mutant NSCLC cells.

Cell Morphology Data

Cells will undergo morphologic changes when perturbed by external cues. Method that could measure the morphologic changes of cells is particularly useful in drug discovery and the drug development pipeline known as the phenotypic screening assay [36]. Carpenter and colleagues developed a tool called CellProfiler [37,38], an image analysis software for identifying and quantifying cell phenotypes from microscopy images. This Cell Painting assay can measure approximately 1700 morphologic features (such as size, shape, texture, and intensity) to produce a rich morphologic profile. By generating these profiles, the user can detect subtle phenotypic changes or biological similarities among samples on genetic or pharmacologic perturbations [39]. Bray and colleagues [40] recently used the Cell Painting assay to generate the morphologic profiles of 30,616 compounds in U2OS cells, which is the most extensive collection of cell images and morphologic patterns generated to date. As an example, Gustafsdottir and colleagues [41] applied hierarchical clustering to the morphologic profiles and demonstrated that this approach could reveal MoAs for related compounds. This assay provides a complementary approach for developing probes and therapeutics based on morphologic changes related to disease- or gene-related phenotypes.

Drug Sensitivity Signatures Data

To date, large publicly funded projects have generated extensive and freely available data sources and bioinformatics, and statistical tools explicitly designed for such kinds of analyses are evolving. Single-agent drug sensitivity databases, such as Genomics of Drug Sensitivity in Cancer (GDSC) [42], Cancer Cell Line Encyclopedia (CCLE) [43], and Cancer Therapeutics Response Portal (CTRP) [44], are examples of public databases containing responses to hundreds of small molecules by more than a thousand human cell lines. These resources will make the rapid development of new biomarkers of drug responses a real possibility. Drug sensitivity patterns of these cancer cell lines can be mined and correlated with the gene expression data to identify genetic features that are predictive of sensitivity. Lee and colleagues [45], for example, developed the drug repurposing tool called DeSigN that correlates phenotype-specific gene expression signatures derived from differentially expressed genes with predefined gene expression profiles associated with drug response data (50% inhibitory concentration [IC_{50}]) from 140 small molecule inhibitors available in GDSC. From this study, a *Src/Abl* kinase inhibitor, bosutinib, was predicted by DeSigN to be a sensitive inhibitor of oral squamous cell carcinoma, and its drug sensitivity efficacy in vitro was validated. Similar to single-agent drug sensitivity databases, combinations of multiple drugs are gaining more and more interest, motivated by factors such as higher efficacy [46], fewer side effects [47], and less toxicity [48] in comparison with single-drug treatments. Recently, several large-scale drug combination databases were published, namely NCI-ALMANAC [49], Merck Research Laboratories [50], and the AstraZeneca-Sanger Drug Combination Prediction DREAM Challenge [51], which undoubtedly will accelerate the discovery of more favorable drug combinations to be used for treating human diseases.

SUMMARY

In this article, the authors reviewed the CMap concept as a functional look-up table for systems biology, by which large-scale public databases such as CMap and LINCS have been used to repurpose drugs for diseases that would otherwise have limited therapeutic options. Some of the analytical pattern-matching software tools that facilitate this type of functional mapping are described. The authors also reviewed recent developments in implementing the CMap concept in other "omics" data sources. The CMap as a means of drug discovery has other utilities that have yet to be explored. For instance, a patient-centric clinical outcome CMap would enable researchers to mine patient drug response data instead of cell line data, which could accelerate the personalized medicine in treating individual patients based on their underlying gene signatures.

ACKNOWLEDGMENTS

The authors thank the editor and reviewers for their constructive comments for improving the presentations of this article.

REFERENCES

[1] Lamb J, Crawford ED, Peck D, et al. The connectivity map: using gene-expression signatures to connect small molecules, genes, and disease. Science 2006;313(5795):1929–35.
[2] Subramanian A, Narayan R, Corsello SM, et al. A next generation connectivity map: L1000 platform and the first 1,000,000 profiles. Cell 2017;171(6):1437–52.e17.
[3] Duan Q, Flynn C, Niepel M, et al. LINCS Canvas browser: interactive web app to query, browse and interrogate LINCS L1000 gene expression signatures. Nucleic Acids Res 2014;42(Web Server issue):W449–60.
[4] Vidović D, Koleti A, Schurer SC. Large-scale integration of small molecule-induced genome-wide transcriptional responses, kinome-wide binding affinities and cell-growth inhibition profiles reveal global trends characterizing systems-level drug action. Front Genet 2014;5:342.
[5] Peck D, Crawford ED, Ross KN, et al. A method for high-throughput gene expression signature analysis. Genome Biol 2006;7(7):R61.
[6] Ushijima M, Mashima T, Tomida A, et al. Development of a gene expression database and related analysis programs for evaluation of anticancer compounds. Cancer Sci 2013;104(3):360–8.
[7] Zhang SD, Gant TW. A simple and robust method for connecting small-molecule drugs using gene-expression signatures. BMC Bioinformatics 2008;9:258.
[8] Cheng J, Yang L, Kumar V, et al. Systematic evaluation of connectivity map for disease indications. Genome Med 2014;6(12):540.
[9] Cheng J, Xie Q, Kumar V, et al. Evaluation of analytical methods for connectivity map data. In: Altman RB, Dunker AK, Hunter L, editors. Pacific Symposium on Biocomputing. Kohala Coast (HI): 2013. p. 5–16.
[10] Chen B, Ma L, Paik H, et al. Reversal of cancer gene expression correlates with drug efficacy and reveals therapeutic targets. Nat Commun 2017;8:16022.
[11] Musa A, Ghoraie LS, Zhang SD, et al. A review of connectivity map and computational approaches in pharmacogenomics. Brief Bioinform 2017;18(5):903.
[12] Subramanian A, Tamayo P, Mootha VK, et al. Gene set enrichment analysis: a knowledge-based approach for interpreting genome-wide expression profiles. Proc Natl Acad Sci U S A 2005;102(43):15545–50.

[13] Jahchan NS, Dudley JT, Mazur PK, et al. A drug repositioning approach identifies tricyclic antidepressants as inhibitors of small cell lung cancer and other neuroendocrine tumors. Cancer Discov 2013;3(12):1364–77.
[14] Sirota M, Dudley JT, Kim J, et al. Discovery and preclinical validation of drug indications using compendia of public gene expression data. Sci Transl Med 2011; 3(96):96ra77.
[15] Raghavan R, Hyter S, Pathak HB, et al. Drug discovery using clinical outcome-based connectivity mapping: application to ovarian cancer. BMC Genomics 2016;17(1): 811.
[16] Liu Z, Fang H, Slikker W, et al. Potential reuse of oncology drugs in the treatment of rare diseases. Trends Pharmacol Sci 2016;37(10):843–57.
[17] Xiao SJ, Zhu XC, Deng H, et al. Gene expression profiling coupled with connectivity map database mining reveals potential therapeutic drugs for Hirschsprung disease. J Pediatr Surg 2018;53(9):1716–21.
[18] Dudley JT, Sirota M, Shenoy M, et al. Computational repositioning of the anticonvulsant topiramate for inflammatory bowel disease. Sci Transl Med 2011;3(96): 96ra76.
[19] Brum AM, van de Peppel J, Nguyen L, et al. Using the connectivity map to discover compounds influencing human osteoblast differentiation. J Cell Physiol 2018; 233(6):4895–906.
[20] Malcomson B, Wilson H, Veglia E, et al. Connectivity mapping (ssCMap) to predict A20-inducing drugs and their antiinflammatory action in cystic fibrosis. Proc Natl Acad Sci U S A 2016;113(26):E3725–34.
[21] Kim BY, Song KH, Lim CY, et al. Therapeutic properties of Scutellaria baicalensis in db/db mice evaluated using connectivity map and network pharmacology. Sci Rep 2017;7:41711.
[22] Yoo M, Shin J, c Kim H, et al. Exploring the molecular mechanisms of traditional Chinese medicine components using gene expression signatures and connectivity map. Comput Methods Programs Biomed 2018;174: 33–40.
[23] Lv C, Wu X, Wang X, et al. The gene expression profiles in response to 102 traditional Chinese medicine (TCM) components: a general template for research on TCMs. Sci Rep 2017;7(1):352.
[24] De Bastiani MA, Pfaffenseller B, Klamt F. Master regulators connectivity map: a transcription factors-centered approach to drug repositioning. Front Pharmacol 2018; 9:697.
[25] De Wolf H, Cougnaud L, Van Hoorde K, et al. High-throughput gene expression profiles to define drug similarity and predict compound activity. Assay Drug Dev Technol 2018;16(3):162–76.
[26] Berger AH, Brooks AN, Wu X, et al. High-throughput phenotyping of lung cancer somatic mutations. Cancer Cell 2016;30(2):214–28.
[27] Busby J, Murray L, Mills K, et al. A combined connectivity mapping and pharmacoepidemiology approach to identify existing medications with breast cancer causing or preventing properties. Pharmacoepidemiol Drug Saf 2018;27(1):78–86.
[28] Abelin JG, Patel J, Lu X, et al. Reduced-representation phosphosignatures measured by quantitative targeted MS capture cellular states and enable large-scale comparison of drug-induced phenotypes. Mol Cell Proteomics 2016;15(5):1622–41.
[29] Litichevskiy L, Peckner R, Abelin JG, et al. A library of phosphoproteomic and chromatin signatures for characterizing cellular responses to drug perturbations. Cell Syst 2018;6(4):424–43.e7.
[30] Creech AL, Taylor JE, Maier VK, et al. Building the connectivity map of epigenetics: chromatin profiling by quantitative targeted mass spectrometry. Methods 2015; 72:57–64.
[31] Cohen P. Protein kinases–the major drug targets of the twenty-first century? Nat Rev Drug Discov 2002;1(4): 309–15.
[32] Kim J, Yoo M, Kang J, et al. K-Map: connecting kinases with therapeutics for drug repurposing and development. Hum Genomics 2013;7:20.
[33] Anastassiadis T, Deacon SW, Devarajan K, et al. Comprehensive assay of kinase catalytic activity reveals features of kinase inhibitor selectivity. Nat Biotechnol 2011; 29(11):1039–45.
[34] Davis MI, Hunt JP, Herrgard S, et al. Comprehensive analysis of kinase inhibitor selectivity. Nat Biotechnol 2011;29(11):1046–51.
[35] Kim J, Vasu VT, Mishra R, et al. Bioinformatics-driven discovery of rational combination for overcoming EGFR-mutant lung cancer resistance to EGFR therapy. Bioinformatics 2014;30(17):2393–8.
[36] Moffat JG, Rudolph J, Bailey D. Phenotypic screening in cancer drug discovery—past, present and future. Nat Rev Drug Discov 2014;13(8):588–602.
[37] Carpenter AE, Jones TR, Lamprecht MR, et al. CellProfiler: image analysis software for identifying and quantifying cell phenotypes. Genome Biol 2006;7(10):R100.
[38] Kamentsky L, Jones TR, Fraser A, et al. Improved structure, function and compatibility for CellProfiler: modular high-throughput image analysis software. Bioinformatics 2011;27(8):1179–80.
[39] Bray MA, Singh S, Han H, et al. Cell painting, a high-content image-based assay for morphological profiling using multiplexed fluorescent dyes. Nat Protoc 2016; 11(9):1757–74.
[40] Bray MA, Gustafsdottir SM, Rohban MH, et al. A dataset of images and morphological profiles of 30 000 small-molecule treatments using the Cell Painting assay. Gigascience 2017;6(12):1–5.
[41] Gustafsdottir SM, Ljosa V, Sokolnicki KL, et al. Multiplex cytological profiling assay to measure diverse cellular states. PLoS One 2013;8(12):e80999.
[42] Garnett MJ, Edelman EJ, Heidorn SJ, et al. Systematic identification of genomic markers of drug sensitivity in cancer cells. Nature 2012;483(7391):570–5.

[43] Barretina J, Caponigro G, Stransky N, et al. The cancer cell line encyclopedia enables predictive modelling of anticancer drug sensitivity. Nature 2012;483(7391):603–7.
[44] Basu A, Bodycombe NE, Cheah JH, et al. An interactive resource to identify cancer genetic and lineage dependencies targeted by small molecules. Cell 2013;154(5):1151–61.
[45] Lee BKB, Tiong KH, Chang JK, et al. DeSigN: connecting gene expression with therapeutics for drug repurposing and development. BMC Genomics 2017;18(Suppl 1):934.
[46] Wang G, Ye Y, Yang X, et al. Expression-based in silico screening of candidate therapeutic compounds for lung adenocarcinoma. PLoS One 2011;6(1):e14573.
[47] Gupta EK, Ito MK. Lovastatin and extended-release niacin combination product: the first drug combination for the management of hyperlipidemia. Heart Dis 2002;4(2):124–37.
[48] Sun X, Vilar S, Tatonetti NP. High-throughput methods for combinatorial drug discovery. Sci Transl Med 2013;5(205):205rv1.
[49] Holbeck SL, Camalier R, Crowell JA, et al. The National Cancer Institute ALMANAC: a comprehensive screening resource for the detection of anticancer drug pairs with enhanced therapeutic activity. Cancer Res 2017;77(13):3564–76.
[50] O'Neil J, Benita Y, Feldman I, et al. An unbiased oncology compound screen to identify novel combination strategies. Mol Cancer Ther 2016;15(6):1155–62.
[51] Menden MP, Wang D, Guan Y, et al. Community assessment to advance computational prediction of cancer drug combinations in a pharmacogenomic screen. Nat Commun 2019;10(1):2674.

Kolibri 360 GmbH
Ferdinand-Jühlke-Straße 7
99095 Erfurt, Deutschland
produktsicherheit@kolibri360.de